Endocrine Surgery
Third Edition

Take a look at the other great titles in the Companion Series...

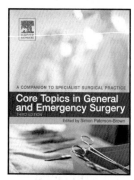

**Paterson-Brown
Core Topics in
General and
Emergency Surgery**
3rd Edition
0702027332

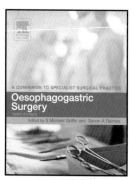

**Griffin & Raimes
Oesophagogastric
Surgery**
3rd Edition
0702027359

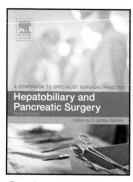

**Garden
Hepatobiliary and
Pancreatic Surgery**
3rd Edition
0702027367

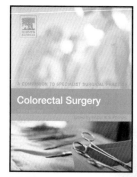

**Phillips
Colorectal Surgery**
3rd Edition
0702027324

**Dixon
Breast Surgery**
3rd Edition
0702027383

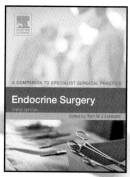

**Lennard
Endocrine Surgery**
3rd Edition
0702027391

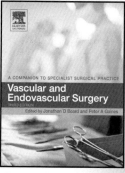

**Beard & Gaines
Vascular and
Endovascular
Surgery**
3rd Edition
0702027340

**Forsythe
Transplantation**
3rd Edition
0702027375

ELSEVIER
SAUNDERS

Order either through your local bookshop, direct from Elsevier
(call customer services on +44 (0)1865 474000) or log on to
http://www.elsevierhealth.com/surgery

A Companion to Specialist Surgical Practice
Third Edition

Series Editors
O. James Garden
Simon Paterson-Brown

Endocrine Surgery
Third Edition

Edited by
Tom W.J. Lennard
Professor of Breast and Endocrine Surgery and
Head of School of Surgical and Reproductive Sciences
University of Newcastle upon Tyne

ELSEVIER
SAUNDERS

ELSEVIER
SAUNDERS

An imprint of Elsevier Limited

© 2006, Elsevier Limited. All rights reserved.

First edition 1997
Second edition 2001
Third edition 2006
Reprinted 2006, 2007

The right of T.W.J. Lennard to be identified as editor of this work has been asserted by him in accordance with the Copyright, Designs and Patents Act 1988.

EAN 9780702027390
ISBN 0 7020 2739 1

British Library Cataloguing in Publication Data
A catalogue record for this book is available from the British Library

Library of Congress Cataloging in Publication Data
A catalog record for this book is available from the Library of Congress

Notice
Medical knowledge is constantly changing. Standard safety precautions must be followed, but as new research and clinical experience broaden our knowledge, changes in treatment and drug therapy may become necessary or appropriate. Readers are advised to check the most current product information provided by the manufacturer of each drug to be administered to verify the recommended dose, the method and duration of administration, and contraindications. It is the responsibility of the practitioner, relying on experience and knowledge of the patient, to determine dosages and the best treatment for each individual patient. Neither the Publisher nor the editor assumes any liability for any injury and/or damage to persons or property arising from this publication.
The Publisher

Printed in The Netherlands
Last digit is the print number: 9 8 7 6 5 4 3

Commissioning Editor: Laurence Hunter
Project Development Manager: Sheila Black
Editorial Assistants: Kathryn Mason, Liz Brown
Project Manager: Cheryl Brant
Design Manager: Jayne Jones
Illustration Manager: Mick Ruddy
Illustrator: Martin Woodward
Marketing Managers: Gaynor Jones (UK), Ethel Cathers (USA)

Contents

Colour plate section follows p. 212

Contributors

Göran Åkerström MD PhD
Professor and Head of Endocrine
Surgery
University Hospital
Uppsala, Sweden

**Stephen G. Ball BSc PhD MB BS
FRCP**
Senior Lecturer
University of Newcastle;
Honorary Consultant
Endocrine Unit
Newcastle Hospitals NHS Trust
Newcastle upon Tyne, UK

Richard D. Bliss MB FRCS
Consultant Surgeon
Royal Victoria Infirmary
Newcastle upon Tyne, UK

**Fiona S. Douglas MB BS MRCP
FRCP**
Consultant in Clinical Genetics
Institute of Human Genetics
International Centre for Life
Newcastle upon Tyne, UK

**Barnard J. Harrison MB BS MS
FRCS FRCS(Ed)**
Consultant Endocrine Surgeon
Royal Hallamshire Hospital
Sheffield, UK

Per Hellman MD PhD
Associate Professor and
Consultant Surgeon
University Hospital
Uppsala, Sweden

Jean-François Henry MD
Professor of Surgery and Chairman
Department of Endocrine Surgery
University Hospital La Timone
Marseilles, France

Ola Hessman MD PhD
Consultant Surgeon
University Hospital
Uppsala, Sweden

William B. Inabnet MD FACS
Chief, Section of Endocrine
Surgery
Columbia University
College of Physicians and
Surgeons
New York, NY, USA

James A. Lee MD
Endocrine Surgery Fellow
Columbia University Medical
Center
New York, NY, USA

**Tom W.J. Lennard MD LRCP
MRCS FRCS(Ed) FRCS**
Professor of Breast and Endocrine
Surgery
Head of School of Surgical and
Reproductive Sciences
University of Newcastle upon Tyne
Newcastle upon Tyne, UK

Jeffrey A. Norton MD
Professor of Surgery
Chief of Surgical Oncology
Stanford University Medical Center
Stanford, CA, USA

Zenon Rayter MS FRCS
Consultant Surgeon
Bristol Royal Infirmary
Bristol, UK

**Gregory P. Sadler MD FRCS(Ed)
FRCS(Gen Surg)**
Consultant Endocrine Surgeon
John Radcliffe Hospital
Headington
Oxford, UK

Frédéric Sebag MD
Assistant Surgeon
Department of Endocrine Surgery
University Hospital La Timone
Marseilles, France

**Anthony E. Young MA MChir
FRCS**
Consultant Surgeon
St Thomas' Hospital
London, UK

Preface

The *Companion to Specialist Surgical Practice* series was designed to meet the needs of surgeons in higher training and practising consultants who wish up-to-date and evidence-based information on the subspecialist areas relevant to their surgical practice. In trying to meet this aim, we have recognised that the series will never be as all-encompassing as many of the larger reference surgical textbooks. However, by their very size, it is rare that the latter are completely up to date at the time of publication. The first edition of this series was published in 1997, with the second following in 2001. In this third edition, we have been able to bring up to date the relevant specialist information that we and the individual volume editors consider important for the practising subspecialist surgeon. Where possible, all contributors have attempted to identify evidence-based references to support key recommendations within each chapter. These should all be interpreted with the help of the guidance summary 'Evidence-based practice in surgery', which follows this preface.

We are extremely grateful to all volume editors and to their contributors to this third edition. It is thanks to their enthusiasm and hard work that the relatively short time frame between each of the editions has been maintained, thereby providing to the reader the most accurate and up-to-date infor-

mation possible. We were all immensely saddened by the sudden and tragic death of Professor John Farndon, who edited the first and second editions of the volumes *Breast Surgery* and *Endocrine Surgery*. While recognising that he was a unique and talented individual, we are pleased to welcome the additional editorial skills of Mike Dixon and Tom Lennard for this third edition.

We are also grateful for the support and encouragement of Elsevier Ltd and hope that our aim – of providing up-to-date and affordable surgical texts – has been met and that all readers, whether in training or in consultant practice, will find this third edition a valuable resource.

O. James Garden BSc, MB, ChB, MD, FRCS(Glasg), FRCS(Ed), FRCP(Ed)
Regius Professor of Clinical Surgery, Clinical and Surgical Sciences (Surgery), University of Edinburgh, and Honorary Consultant Surgeon, Royal Infirmary of Edinburgh

Simon Paterson-Brown MB, BS, MPhil, MS, FRCS(Ed), FRCS
Honorary Senior Lecturer, Clinical and Surgical Sciences (Surgery), University of Edinburgh, and Consultant General and Upper Gastrointestinal Surgeon, Royal Infirmary of Edinburgh

EVIDENCE-BASED PRACTICE IN SURGERY

The third edition of the *Companion to Specialist Surgical Practice* series has attempted to incorporate, where appropriate, **evidence-based practice in surgery**, which has been highlighted in the text and relevant references. A detailed chapter on evidence-based practice in surgery, written by Kathryn Rigby and Jonathan Michaels, has been included in the volume *Core Topics in General and Emergency Surgery*, to which the reader is referred for further information on assessing levels of evidence. We are grateful to them for providing this summary for each volume.

Critical appraisal for developing evidence-based practice can be obtained from a number of sources, the most reliable being randomised controlled clinical trials, systematic literature reviews, meta-analyses and observational studies. For practical purposes three grades of evidence can be used, analogous to the levels of 'proof' required in a court of law:

1. **Beyond reasonable doubt** – such evidence is likely to have arisen from high-quality randomised controlled trials, systematic reviews, or high-quality synthesised evidence such as decision analysis, cost-effectiveness analysis or large observational data sets. The studies need to be directly applicable to the population of concern and have clear results. The grade is analogous to burden of proof within a crimimal court and may be thought of as corresponding to the usual standard of 'proof' within the medical literature (i.e. $P<0.05$).

2. **On the balance of probabilities** – in many cases a high-quality review of literature may fail to reach firm conclusions owing to conflicting or inconclusive results, trials of poor methodological quality or the lack of evidence in the population to which the guidelines apply. In such cases it may still be possible to make a statement as to the best treatment on the 'balance of probabilities'. This is analogous to the decision in a civil court where all the available evidence will be weighed up and the verdict will depend upon the balance of probabilities.

3. **Not proven** – insufficient evidence upon which to base a decision or contradictory evidence.

Depending on the information available three grades of recommendation can be used:

a. strong recommendation, which should be followed unless there are compelling reasons to act otherwise;

b. a recommendaton based on evidence of effectiveness but where there may be other factors to take into account in decision-making, for example the user of the guidelines may be expected to take into account patient preferences, local facilities, local audit results or available resources;

c. a recommendation made where there is no adequate evidence as to the most effective practice, although there may be reasons for making a recommendation in order to minimise cost or reduce the chance of error through a locally agreed protocol.

The text and references that are considered to be associated with reasonable evidence are highlighted in this volume with a 'scalpel code', leaving the reader to reach his or her own conclusion.

Editor's note

I have made significant changes to the contributors to this third edition and am most grateful to my friends and colleagues who took on the task of updating, and in some cases completely rewriting, the chapters for this book. The contributors represent leading experts in their field from around the world, who are all busy practising surgeons or clinicians, and their keeping to the tight timelines for the production of this book has been much appreciated. Beyond that, they have also contributed excellent content and illustrations, which update and advance our knowledge on the subject of endo-crine surgery up to the present day. I hope that those who read these chapters will find them informative and enjoyable and that the information transmitted within them will assist us all in the better management of our patients with endocrine disease.

Tom W.J. Lennard MD, LRCP, MRCS, FRCS(Ed), FRCS
Professor of Breast and Endocrine Surgery and Head of School of Surgical and Reproductive Sciences, University of Newcastle upon Tyne

Dedication

To the memory of John Farndon, a close friend, a mentor for me and for many, and a huge contributor to the clinical and academic subject of endocrine surgery.

TWJL

One

Parathyroid disease

William B. Inabnet,
James A. Lee,
Jean-François Henry and
Frédéric Sebag

● **Part 1** ●

Parathyroid disease, syndromes and pathophysiology

William B. Inabnet and James A. Lee

INTRODUCTION

Hyperparathyroidism is a disease characterised by elevated serum calcium and inappropriately elevated parathyroid hormone (PTH) levels, that occurs with a prevalence of 3/1000 in the general population.[1] The modern era of treating parathyroid disease began in 1925 when Mandl performed the first parathyroidectomy in a patient with severe bone disease.[2] Early in the history of hyperparathyroidism, patients presented with advanced clinical disease, including fractures, skeletal deformities, kidney stones and kidney failure. The discovery of the peptide PTH in the early 1970s coupled with the development of a chemical analyser to measure calcium permitted the biochemical diagnosis of hyperparathyroidism much earlier in the disease course.[3,4] During this era, bilateral neck exploration was the standard approach resulting in a cure rate ranging from 92 to 96% when performed by a skilled surgical team.[5,6] Over the last 20 years, the treatment of hyperparathyroidism has experienced a dramatic change with the development of new technology to permit accurate preoperative localisation of abnormal glands, and intraoperative confirmation of the completeness of parathyroid resection.

EMBRYOLOGY AND ANATOMY

In order to successfully diagnose and treat disorders of the parathyroid glands, a keen understanding of parathyroid embryology and anatomy is essential. The parathyroid glands are small, brownish-tan glands located in the space around the thyroid gland. During the fifth week of fetal development, the inferior parathyroid glands arise from the dorsal aspect of the third pharyngeal pouch.[7] Following development of the thymus from the ventral aspect of the third pharyngeal pouch, the inferior parathyroid glands and thymus descend in a caudal and medial direction to rest in the inferior neck and thorax respectively. The superior parathyroid glands arise from the dorsal wing of the fourth pharyngeal pouch and descend in a caudal direction with the thyroid gland.[7]

Because of the longer pathway of descent, the inferior parathyroid glands have a higher variability of location compared with the superior parathyroid glands, an observation that is important during parathyroid surgery.

In an autopsy series of 503 human subjects, Akerstrom et al. showed that four parathyroid glands were present in 84% of cases, whereas 3% of patients had only three glands and 13% had supernumerary glands.[8] The presence of missed hyperfunctioning supernumerary glands is an important but infrequent cause of persistent hyperparathyroidism and should be considered in all cases of persistent disease.[9] In 80% of cases, the location of the inferior and superior glands is symmetrical when compared with the glands on the contralateral side of the neck.[8] The superior parathyroid glands are most commonly found immediately superior to the junction of the recurrent laryngeal nerve and the inferior thyroid artery and can be located inside the thyroid gland in 0.2% of cases.[8] Approximately 50% of inferior parathyroid glands are located in the vicinity of the inferior pole of the thyroid gland and about 30% are found in the thyrothymic ligament.

CALCIUM AND PARATHYROID HORMONE (PTH) REGULATION

The parathyroid glands play a central role in regulating serum levels of calcium through a complex feedback loop involving PTH, serum ionised calcium levels and vitamin D. The key organ systems involved in this process include the parathyroid glands, gastrointestinal tract, kidneys and skin. Although multiple factors influence parathyroid function, it is now clear that calcium is the single most potent stimulator of PTH release. Calcium-sensing receptors (CSRs), which are located on the surface of the parathyroid chief cells and are coupled with a G-protein receptor, are able to detect minuscule changes in serum levels of extracellular ionised calcium.[10,11] When serum levels of calcium decrease, the CSRs are activated thereby stimulating the synthesis and release of PTH.[12] In primary hyperparathyroidism (PHP), the set point of the CSRs is adjusted upwards, probably through a mutation of unknown aetiology, causing the parathyroid chief cell to 'believe' that serum calcium levels are low when in fact they are not. As a result

of this alteration in the CSR set point, the parathyroid chief cell increases production of PTH, ultimately leading to hypercalcaemia. Calcium-sensing receptors are also present on other tissues such as the kidneys and gastrointestinal tract, where calcium homeostasis is influenced.[11,13,14] In the kidney, the CSRs regulate renal calcium excretion and influence the transepithelial movement of water and other electrolytes.[11] In the gastrointestinal tract, CSRs are present in the gastrin-secreting G-cells and acid-secreting parietal cells, thereby providing a molecular link between hypercalcaemia and acid hypersecretion.[13] These facts also underscore the complexity of calcium homeostasis in influencing cellular function throughout the body.

PTH is an intact 84-amino-acid peptide with amino and carboxy terminals.[15] Production of PTH begins in the endoplasmic reticulum of the parathyroid chief cells as a 115-amino-acid molecule, which undergoes a series of cleavages before being released from the cytoplasm as the biologically active (1–84) PTH molecule. The circulating (1–84) PTH molecule, which has a half-life of 3–5 minutes in patients with normal renal function, is initially cleaved in the liver, yielding an inactive C-terminal fragment, which is ultimately cleared by the kidneys.[15,16] The N-terminal fragment is the part of the peptide that is responsible for the biological activity of PTH on peripheral tissues.

PTH acts directly on the kidneys, bone and gastrointestinal tract to activate several intracellular second messengers including cyclic AMP and calcium.[17–19] In the kidneys, PTH increases serum calcium levels by acting on the renal tubule to increase resorption of calcium and to increase the hydroxylation of 25-hydroxyvitamin D to the biologically active 1,25-dihydroxyvitamin D.[19,20] PTH also stimulates the renal tubular secretion of phosphate and bicarbonate. In the bone, PTH acts on osteoblasts and osteoclasts to increase bone turnover, thereby providing a large source of calcium for the extracellular space.[21]

Vitamin D is a fat-soluble vitamin that is prevalent in dairy products. After being absorbed by the gastrointestinal tract, it is hydroxylated in the liver to become 25-hydroxyvitamim D, which in turn is hydroxylated in the kidneys to become 1,25-dihydroxyvitamin D. The latter plays an important role in calcium homeostasis by increasing the resorption of phosphorus in the kidneys and increasing the absorption of calcium from the gastrointestinal tract.[20] Calcitonin, which is synthesised by the parafollicular C cells of the thyroid gland, acts as the physiological antagonist to PTH. Calcitonin decreases serum levels of calcium by decreasing bone turnover and in fact can be used to treat patients in hypercalcaemic crisis.[22]

PRIMARY HYPERPARATHYROIDISM

Incidence

Early in the history of PHP, patients presented with manifestations of severe hypercalcaemia and advanced disease, but the true incidence of hyperparathyroidism was not known due to the inability to routinely measure serum calcium levels. The development of the automated serum chemical analyser and the practice of widespread biochemical screening permitted the detection of mild increases in serum calcium levels, thereby allowing earlier recognition of abnormalities in calcium homeostasis.

Multiple factors influence the incidence of PHP, including the region of the world under evaluation, the nutritional status of the studied population, iatrogenic factors, and the availability of routine biochemical screening. In the 1970s, there was a dramatic fivefold increase in the incidence of PHP largely due to the 'catch-up' effect of identifying patients who had PHP prior to the development of the automated calcium analyser.[1] During the 1980s, the incidence of PHP in North America actually decreased as the impact of the 'catch-up' effect levelled off.[23] The number of patients with a history of irradiation to the head and neck region for benign disorders decreased in the 1980s, which may also have contributed to the decreased incidence of PHP, as head and neck irradiation is a known risk factor for parathyroid hypersecretion.

PHP occurs more frequently in women than men, but the overall incidence increases with age in both sexes. In North America, the incidence of PHP in the general population is 4.3/1000, whereas in Europe the incidence is 3/1000.[1,23] In women aged between 55 and 75 years, the incidence of PHP is 21/1000.[1] Possible explanations for the increased incidence

with age include the lower rate of biochemical screening in patients less than 50 years of age and the increased use of bone density measurements in postmenopausal women as a routine part of healthcare screening. The detection of osteopenia and/or osteoporosis that is out of proportion to age-matched controls often leads the clinician to measure serum calcium and PTH levels, thereby identifying hyperparathyroidism as the cause of increased bone loss. Vitamin D deficiency also influences the true detected incidence of PHP as this condition may cause serum calcium levels to be normal in patients with hyperparathyroidism. For example, the incidence of vitamin D deficiency in southern Europe is high, leading to an underestimation of the true incidence of hyperparathyroidism in this region of the world.[1]

Clinical manifestations

The clinical presentation of patients with PHP is highly variable, ranging from none to profound symptoms of hypercalcaemia, such as excessive thirst, dehydration, kidney stones, muscle weakness, and pathological fracture. Generally speaking, the clinical manifestations of PHP can be broadly classified by organ system (**Box 1.1**). Since many of these symptoms overlap with other clinical conditions, particularly in the elderly, the diagnosis of hyperparathyroidism is often delayed until hypercalcaemia is recognised on biochemical screening. Often the presence of a classic symptom, such as nephrolithiasis, will lead the astute clinician to assess the patient for PHP. By far, fatigue is one of the most common symptoms of hyperparathyroidism, being present in >80% of patients.[23] Numerous studies have shown that a high percentage of patients that are thought to be asymptomatic actually have occult symptoms attributable to PHP.[23]

There are numerous medical conditions that are associated with and/or exacerbated by PHP, including hypertension, diabetes, pancreatitis, nephrolithiasis, gout and peptic ulcer disease.

Diagnosis

Prior to the 1970s and the advent of routine serum calcium measurements as part of the basic metabolic profile, the diagnosis of PHP was made primarily

Box 1.1 • Symptoms of primary hyperparathyroidism classified by organ system

Gastrointestinal

- Nausea/vomiting
- Epigastric pain
- Pancreatitis
- Peptic ulcer disease
- Anorexia
- Weight loss
- Constipation

Cardiovascular

- Hypertension
- Shortened Q–T interval, wide T wave
- Bradycardia
- Heart block
- Lethal arrhythmias

Renal

- Renal colic
- Polyuria/oliguria/anuria
- Thirst/dehydration
- Renal failure

Neuropsychiatric

- Anxiety
- Headaches
- Dementia/paranoia
- Confusion
- Depression
- Muscle weakness
- Hyporeflexia
- Ataxia
- Coma

Miscellaneous

- Visual changes
- Band keratopathy
- Conjunctivitis
- Myalgia
- Pruritus

on clinical findings. Walter St Goar immortalised this constellation of findings in the mnemonic 'bones, stones and groans'. However, with routine serum calcium measurements, an elevated serum calcium level has become the most common presentation. PHP is confirmed by elevated serum calcium and serum PTH levels and can be suggested by other laboratory values (see below).

- **Elevated serum calcium:** While a useful screening tool, many conditions can lead to inaccuracies in the measured total serum calcium levels. For example, hypoalbuminaemia and acidosis can create 'normal' serum calcium levels. Given these variables, many groups favour measuring the ionised serum calcium level instead. Monchik found in a number of series that an elevated serum ionised calcium correlated better with the presence of PHP as confirmed by surgery.[24]
- **Elevated serum PTH:** Current antibody-driven assays for serum intact parathyroid hormone (iPTH) levels are highly accurate.
- **Chloride:phosphate ratio:** A recent retrospective study suggests that a chloride:phosphate ratio ≥33 is indicative of PHP in both hypercalcaemic as well as normocalcaemic patients.[25]
- **Hypercalciuria:** The presence of hypercalciuria rules out benign familial hypercalcaemic hypocalciuria, which can mimic PHP.
- **Hypophosphataemia:** Due to the decreased resorption of phosphate by the renal tubule, phosphate levels decrease in approximately 50% of patients with PHP.

Normocalcaemic hyperparathyroidism

There is a small subset of patients with PHP who present with normal or only intermittently elevated calcium levels. Mather first described normocalcaemic hyperparathyroidism in 1953 in a woman who presented with osteitis fibrosa cystica.[26] Since that time, this variation of PHP has been an infrequent but recognised entity. While still uncommon when compared with hypercalcaemic PHP, recent population studies have shown that this variant of the disease may be more prevalent than previously believed and that improved screening may help identify mildly symptomatic or asymptomatic patients.[27]

The exact biochemical mechanisms of normocalcaemic PHP remain elusive. Some investigators postulate that the normocalcaemic variant of PHP represents an early or preclinical phase that progresses to typical hypercalcaemic PHP.[28,29] Others have found distinct differences in the biological response to PTH in patients with normocalcaemic vs. hypercalcaemic hyperparathyroidism.[30] For example, Maruani et al. found that patients with normocalcaemic hyperparathyroidism displayed a resistance to the renal and bony effects of PTH as measured by a lower fasting urine calcium excretion and renal tubular calcium resorption as well as lower values of markers of bone turnover.[30,31] While most patients with normocalcaemic PHP present with nephrolithiasis, recent data show that other classic constitutional symptoms are just as prevalent in normocalcaemic patients as in hypercalcaemic PHP patients, suggesting that there is a larger unidentified population with PHP.[32,33]

The majority of patients with normocalcaemic PHP present with renal calculi and hypercalciuria. However, the most common cause of renal calculi and hypercalciuria is idiopathic hypercalciuria (IH). To further confound the matter, some variants of IH have elevated PTH levels. It is vitally important to distinguish between these two entities since surgical parathyroidectomy effectively cures normocalcaemic PHP whereas postsurgical IH patients continue to form stones.[32,34]

Many tests are helpful in differentiating between the two diseases, but none has been shown to be conclusive enough to be used in isolation. The best diagnostic yield is to use two or more tests in combination.

- **Thiazide administration:** Administration of thiazide diuretics leads to a decrease in urinary calcium excretion. Patients with normocalcaemic PHP will have persistently elevated PTH levels, whereas those with idiopathic hypercalciuria will have a normalisation of PTH.[35,36]
- **Phosphate deprivation:** After restricting phosphate to 350 mg/day and administering 650 mg of aluminium hydroxide four times/day (while on a normal calorie and normal calcium diet), serum calcium and phosphorus levels are checked every day for 4 days. Patients with subsequent hypercalcaemia or persistent hypercalciuria usually have normocalcaemic PHP.[37] This test is not used routinely anymore.
- **Calcium loading test:** After administration of either 350 or 1000 mg of oral calcium, serum calcium and urine calcium are measured. Patients with normocalcaemic PHP have a significant increase in serum calcium (due to increased intestinal absorption) and an increase in urine calcium excretion whereas intestinal absorption of calcium varies widely in patients with IH.[38,39] In a recent study, after administration of 1 g of oral calcium, the combined parameters of (i) circulating PTH nadir (pg/mL) × peak calcium concentration (mg/dL) and (ii) relative PTH decline/relative calcium increment, diagnosed normocalcaemic PHP with 100% sensitivity and 87% specificity.[40] Furthermore, calcium loading suppressed urinary cAMP[39] but did not suppress PTH levels below 70% of baseline.[24]
- **Serum ionised calcium:** An elevated ionised calcium, in conjunction with an elevated PTH, is increasingly gaining acceptance as an excellent means of distinguishing normocalcaemic PHP from IH.[24,30,34,41]

As mentioned previously, the mainstay of treatment for normocalcaemic PHP is operative parathyroidectomy.

Hypercalcaemic crisis

Hypercalcaemia is seen in approximately 0.5% of the general population and up to 5% of the hospital population.[42,43] The majority of cases of hypercalcaemia are classified as mild to moderate (<12 mg/dL or 12–14 mg/dL respectively), and the patient is asymptomatic. This group responds to dietary measures and treatment of the underlying aetiology. However, a subset of patients will present in hypercalcaemic crisis, with serum calcium >14 mg/dL, and are severely symptomatic. These patients require hospitalisation and aggressive reduction of serum calcium. Fortunately, except in cases of malignancy, treatment for hypercalcaemia is typically successful.

Since the calcium ion plays a crucial role in membrane potentials throughout the body, the symptoms of hypercalcaemia are varied and potentially life-threatening. The classic presentation of severe hypercalcaemia includes acute confusion, abdominal pain, vomiting, dehydration and anuria. In addition, patients may develop lethal arrhythmias due to decreased conduction velocities and shortened refractory periods, which manifest on an electrocardiogram as a prolonged P–R interval, a shortened Q–T interval, and arrhythmia. Hypercalcaemic crisis is the most extreme form of hypercalcaemia and is defined as severe hypercalcaemia in association with profound dehydration and obtundation.[44] At serum calcium levels of 15–18 mg/dL, coma and cardiac arrest may occur.

The most common aetiology of hypercalcaemia in non-hospitalised patients is PHP, while malignancy accounts for almost two-thirds of the hypercalcaemic in-patient population.[45] It is crucial to identify the underlying cause of hypercalcaemia in order to effectively and definitively address the acute event. **Box 1.2** lists the differential diagnoses for hypercalcaemia. The treatment of severe hypercalcaemia revolves around aggressive rehydration, increasing renal excretion of calcium, blunting of calcium release from skeletal stores, and treating the underlying cause of the hypercalcaemia.[46]

The primary goal of treatment is to achieve adequate volume resuscitation, which in turn increases calcium excretion in the kidneys.[46,47] Patients are invariably dehydrated due to poor oral intake and vomiting. The resultant decrement in glomerular filtration rate leads to a decrease in renal excretion of calcium. Typically, 200–500 mL/h of normal saline is given to maintain urine output above 100 mL/h with the caveat that comorbidities may limit the rate of resuscitation. Using normal saline lends substrate for the resultant natriuresis. Once the intravascular volume is restored, loop diuretics such as furosemide may be given to enhance calciuresis by inhibiting calcium resorption in the thick ascending limb of the loop of Henle. During the resuscitative phase, the patient must be monitored closely for signs of fluid overload, hypokalaemia and hypomagnesaemia. Serum calcium levels can be reduced by 1.6–2.5 mg/dL within 24 hours by volume repletion and loop diuretic administration alone.[44] However, when serum

Box 1.2 • Differential diagnosis of hypercalcaemia

Malignancy

- Solid tumour (parathyroid hormone-related peptide mediated): lung, kidney, squamous cell carcinoma of head/neck/oesophagus/female genital tract
- Metastases (osteoclastic lesions): breast, prostate
- Haematological: multiple myeloma, lymphoma, leukaemia

Hyperparathyroidism

- Primary hyperparathyroidism
- Familial: multiple endocrine neoplasia (MEN) types I and II, benign familial hypocalciuric hypercalcaemia, idiopathic hypercalcaemia of infancy
- Lithium

Increased bone turnover

- Vitamin A intoxication
- Thiazide diuretics
- Hyperthyroidism
- Immobilisation
- Paget's disease

Excess vitamin D

- Vitamin D intoxication
- Increased 1,25-dihydroxylated vitamin D: granulomatous disease

Renal failure

- Milk alkali syndrome
- Secondary hyperparathyroidism
- Aluminium intoxication

Miscellaneous

- Addisonian crisis
- Laboratory error: haemoconcentration, hypoproteinaemia

calcium exceeds 12 mg/dL or hypercalcaemia is caused by malignancy, intravenous fluids and diuretics alone are usually insufficient to normalise calcium levels.

Numerous agents are available to blunt the release of calcium from bone resorption and treat the underlying disease.[44,46,47] **Table 1.1** provides an

Table 1.1 • Treatment of hypercalcaemia

Treatment	Onset	Duration	Effectiveness (% normalised)	Advantages	Disadvantages
First-line therapy					
Normal saline	Hours	During use	0–10	Almost always dehydrated	Congestive heart failure Hypokalaemia/ hypomagnesaemia
Loop diuretic	Hours	2–6 hours	0–10	Fast onset	Electrolyte abnormalities Dehydration
Bisphosphonates: Etidronate (first-generation)	1–2 days	5–7 days	30–80	Intermediate onset	Hyperphosphataemia 3-day infusion Fever (20%)
Pamidronate (second-generation)	1–2 days	10–14 days	70–100	High potency Prolonged duration Intermediate onset	Hypophosphataemia/ hypocalcaemia Hypomagnesaemia
Calcitonin (salmon)	Hours	2–3 days	10–20	Fast onset Bridge until intermediate-action drugs take effect	Tachyphylaxis Flushing Nausea/vomiting
Second-line therapy					
Plicamycin	1–2 days	Days	75–85	High potency	Hepatocellular necrosis Bleeding (decreased clotting factors) Thrombocytopenia Renal failure Electrolyte abnormalities Hypocalcaemia
Gallium nitrate	Day 6	7–10 days	75–82	High potency	5-day infusion Contraindicated in renal failure Hypophosphataemia Anaemia Nausea/vomiting Rare hypotension
Glucocorticoids	5–7 days	Days–weeks	Variable	Oral therapy Cidal effect on haematological and breast cancers	Only effective in vitamin D excess or granulomatous disease Immunosuppression Cushing's syndrome
Phosphates: Oral	24 hours	During use	Variable	Low toxicity	Only effective in hyperphosphataemia
Intravenous	Hours	1–2 days	Variable	High potency Rapid action	Severe hypocalcaemia Organ damage Potentially lethal

overview of agents available to combat hyper-calcaemia and their relative strengths and weaknesses.

Bisphosphonates: pamidronate 60–90 mg i.v. Bisphosphonates are pyrophosphate analogues that are concentrated in areas of high bone turnover and inhibit osteoclast activity. Endogenous phosphatases cannot hydrolyse the central carbon-phosphorus-carbon bond making this drug stable in vivo. Bisphosphonates should be given intravenously due to their poor absorption by the gastrointestinal tract. In the USA, only etidronate (first generation) and pamidronate (second generation) are approved for use in treating hypercalcaemia. Pamidronate has widely supplanted etidronate as the bisphosphonate of choice due to its faster onset, increased duration of action, increased efficacy, and minimal adverse effect on mineralisation. One dose of intravenous pamidronate normalises serum calcium for 10–14 days in 80 to 100% of patients with hypercalcaemia of malignancy. Newer, more potent generations of bisphosphonates may replace pamidronate as the standard as more clinical data become available.[48]

Calcitonin: salmon calcitonin 4–8 U/kg s.c./i.v. Calcitonin diminishes osteoclast activity and increases calciuresis within minutes of adminis-tration. However, the duration of action is limited to only a few days. Calcitonin therapy only rarely results in normocalcaemia. Tachyphylaxis limits the long-term use of calcitonin. Currently, calcitonin is used primarily as an immediate hypocalcaemic agent that temporises until the more sustained effects of other agents begin.

Gallium nitrate: 200 mg/m² i.v. q.d. for 5 days Gallium nitrate inhibits bone resorption by reducing the solubility of hydroxyapatite crystals. This drug induces a normocalcaemia within 2–3 days that lasts for 5–6 days in approximately 75% of patients. The use of gallium nitrate has been limited by its nephrotoxicity, the need for continuous infusion, and lack of clinical data.

Plicamycin: 25 μg/kg Plicamycin is an osteoclast cytotoxin originally used in chemotherapy. Due to its serious side effects (hepatic, renal and bone marrow toxicity), plicamycin is reserved for patients

who fail bisphosphonate therapy. Since toxicities are related to the frequency and total dosage, administration is limited to one dose with additional dosing only if hypercalcaemia recurs.

Glucocorticoids: prednisone 40–100 mg p.o. q.d. or hydrocortisone 200–300 mg i.v. for 3–5 days Glucocorticoids are used primarily to augment the effect of calcitonin or in diseases associated with vitamin D excess (i.e. granulomatous diseases, vitamin D toxicity, and multiple myeloma). Gluco-corticoids increase calciuresis, decrease intestinal absorption of calcium, and have a direct tumoricidal effect on certain haematological malignancies as well as breast cancer.

Oral inorganic phosphate: phosphate 1–1.5 g p.o. q.d. Oral inorganic phosphate has a limited effect in normalising serum calcium in patients who are hypophosphataemic by increasing calcium uptake by bone and intestinal absorption of calcium. Intravenous phosphate is one of the swiftest means to reduce serum calcium levels. However, it can cause fatal hypocalcaemia and severe organ failure by calcium-phosphate precipitation. As such, intra-venous phosphate is reserved for life-threatening hypercalcaemia, and even then, must be used with extreme caution.

Dialysis Dialysis is the treatment of choice for patients with hypercalcaemia and renal or heart failure. Dialysis may also be considered in hyper-calcaemic patients who fail standard therapies. Haemodialysis and peritoneal dialysis can remove up to 250 mg of calcium/hour. Care must be taken to avoid the hypophosphataemia that often accompanies dialysis.

The underlying cause of hypercalcaemic crisis must always be addressed as part of the definitive management.[46] In patients with an elevated PTH level and clinical factors suggestive of PHP, parathyroidectomy is the fastest way to decrease PTH levels and consequently serum calcium levels. Therefore, expedient operative intervention should always be considered in this subgroup of patients.[49] In contrast, patients with malignancy-associated hypercalcaemic crisis typically present at advanced or terminal stages of their disease with a mean survival of only months. In this setting, discussion with the patient and family regarding end-of-life decisions will be appropriate.

Imaging and localisation

In the hands of experienced surgeons, bilateral neck exploration for PHP cures 95% of cases.[50–52] Furthermore, prior to recent advances in imaging technology, the sensitivity of localisation studies was approximately 60–70%. Given these facts, the National Institute of Health released guidelines in 1990 for the treatment of PHP that included the recommendation that preoperative localisation was not indicated.[53] Localisation studies were to be limited to re-operative cases. However, the advent of rapid intraoperative PTH assays and the highly sensitive and specific sestamibi scan (see below) have rekindled interest in preoperative localisation for directed unilateral exploration – the so-called focused approach.

Most patients with PHP have a single adenoma, while entities such as multiple adenoma and four-gland hyperplasia are considerably less frequent. In a meta-analysis comprising 6331 patients (excluding familial hyperparathyroid cases) with PHP, Denham and Norman found that 87% had single adenomas, 9% had four-gland hyperplasia, 3% had multiple adenomas, and fewer than 1% had cancer.[54] These statistics are consistent across the literature.[55–57] The fact that the overwhelming majority of patients have unilateral disease or bilateral disease that can be identified by unilateral exploration raises the issue of whether bilateral exploration is mandated in every case. Is it reasonable to expose the patient to the increased morbidity of bilateral exploration to identify the less than 3% of people who will have a second adenoma on the contralateral side? These issues have led many endocrine surgeons to investigate the feasibility of preoperative local-isation and directed unilateral exploration. This trend, along with the need to localise pathology in re-operative situations, has spurred the refinement of imaging techniques for parathyroid disease. **Table 1.2** provides a summary of the current imaging modalities.

ULTRASOUND (US)

Ultrasound was one of the first localisation techniques to be widely used. Typically this test is performed with the 7.5- or 10-MHz probes to optimise penetration and resolution. It is fast, non-invasive, non-irradiating and inexpensive. Furthermore, it allows visualisation of the thyroid, carotid, jugular and cervical areas. However, ultrasound is dependent on operator experience and size of pathology (limit is approximately 5 mm). This tech-nique also has difficulty locating abnormalities in the retro-oesophageal, retrosternal, retrotracheal and deep cervical areas. False-positive results (15–20%) are due to muscles, vessels, thyroid nodules, lymph-adenopathy and oesophageal pathology.[58,59] Image quality may be limited by patient motion or metallic clips from previous operations. The reported sensitivity of ultrasound is between 71 and 80%, but falls to 40% for re-operative localisation.[60]

Endoscopic US has also been used to evaluate posterior, deep cervical and perioesophageal glands. Endoscopic US correctly identified 12 of 23 adenomas (the remaining 11 were in either the anterior or lateral neck) in one series and had a sensitivity of 71% in another.[61,62] Endoscopic US appears to have a role in localising certain parathyroid lesions for recurrent or persistent hyperparathyroidism.

Given these limitations, US is perhaps most useful when used in conjunction with other modalities. US combined with thyroid scintigraphy has the specific benefits of identifying intrathyroidal adenomas and distinguishing adenomas from thyroid nodules.[63–65] Performing US-guided fine-needle aspiration (FNA) increases the sensitivity of US localisation by confirming the presence of PTH in the mass. Cytological studies of the aspirate are not useful and often cannot even distinguish between thyroid and parathyroid tissue. In one small series, PTH analysis of the aspirate made the diagnosis in 100% of cases.[66] Finally, US provides a useful means to define the depth and singularity of adenomas found by scintigraphy.

COMPUTED TOMOGRAPHY (CT)

With the new-generation CT scanners, the accuracy of CT has improved greatly. Now the limitations of CT are based primarily on the size of the adenoma. CT scan is able to visualise the retro-oesophageal, retrotracheal and mediastinal areas. However, CT scan has difficulty in localising adenomas in the lower neck (at the level of the shoulders), and close

Table 1.2 • Imaging methods for localisation in primary hyperparathyroidism

Study	Sensitivity (%)	Specificity (%)	Re-operative sensitivity (%)	False positives (%)	Advantages	Disadvantages
Ultrasound guidance	71–80	80	40	15–20	Inexpensive Fast Morphology No radiation/no i.v. contrast Confirms findings Can combine with fine-needle aspiration (FNA)	Difficulty with posterior areas and mediastinum Operator dependent Cannot detect lesions below 5 mm
Endoscopic ultrasound	71	–	–	–	Posterior/perioesophageal areas	Difficulty with anterior/lateral areas
CT scan with i.v. contrast	46–80	80	–	50	Mediastinum Retro-oesophageal/retrotracheal areas Can combine with FNA	Difficulty with lower neck around shoulders/thyroid area Previous surgery yields artefact Radiation Needs i.v. contrast
Magnetic resonance imaging	64–88	88–95	50–88	18	Localising ectopic glands Used if scintigraphy fails to localise lesion No i.v. contrast	Expensive Cannot be combined with FNA Compliance sometimes limited by claustrophobia Cannot detect lesions below 5 mm
Thallium-technetium scan	75	73–82	50	25	Wide availability Minimal radiation	Poor anatomical detail Average sensitivity
Technetium-sestamibi scan	90.7	98.8	–	Low	Best localisation modality Minimal radiation Widely available SPECT offers excellent anatomical localisation Not operator dependent	May not identify four-gland hyperplasia or multiple adenomas
Angiography	–	–	60	–	Precise anatomical localisation Re-operative localisation Identifies multiple adenoma and four-gland hyperplasia	Neurological complications Embolisation Dye-induced renal failure
Angiography and venous sampling	–	96–98	91–95	Low		
Venous sampling	–	–	80	6–18		

to or within the thyroid. Furthermore, CT scan is inaccurate in differentiating between upper and lower pole glands.[67,68] CT scans with intravenous contrast have sensitivities in the 80% range, but prior operations in the neck can produce artefacts, such as the 'sparkler effect' (seen with surgical clips), which reduce this number.[69,70] The false-positive rate, at 50%, is higher than in other imaging modalities.[71,72]

While CT scan alone has many limitations, it can be a useful adjunct in combination with other localisation studies for recurrent disease. CT is especially useful for identifying mediastinal adenomas. As with US, CT may be used in conjunction with FNA to increase diagnostic yield.[73]

MAGNETIC RESONANCE IMAGING (MRI)

MRI is superior to CT scanning in that it does not require intravenous contrast nor is it subject to the 'sparkler effect' or shoulder artefact. On T2-weighted imaging, enlarged parathyroid glands have significantly increased intensity. T2-weighted MRI is an excellent means of localising ectopic glands in patients undergoing re-operation for PHP, though it was less useful for identifying lesions in normal positions. Aufferman et al. found that MRI located 79% of ectopic adenomas while localising only 59% of those in the normal anatomical position.[74] Overall sensitivities are in the 50–88% range for re-operative localisation.[70,75] Despite better sensitivities (64–88%) than CT scanning, MRI has significant drawbacks.[70–72,76,77] This modality cannot image normal glands or adenomas less than 5 mm in size. Furthermore, it has difficulty localising superior parathyroid glands since they lie posterior to the thyroid. False positives can result from thyroid nodules and lymphadenopathy.[78] Finally, MRI is expensive, cannot be combined with FNA, and patient compliance is sometimes limited by claustrophobia. Given all these factors, MRI is best reserved for localisation in re-operation for PHP or when parathyroid scintigraphy is negative or equivocal.[79,80]

THALLIUM-201–TECHNETIUM-99M PERTECHNETATE SCAN (TL-99MTC SCAN)

Tl-Tc scanning is an image subtraction technique that is rapidly being replaced by sestamibi scanning (see below). Tl-Tc scanning relies on the fact that the thyroid and parathyroid tissues (especially hyperfunctioning glands) take up thallium while the thyroid alone takes up technetium. By subtracting the two images, one can localise the parathyroid tumour. The sensitivity of Tl-Tc scanning is 75% for first-time operations and only 50% for re-operations.[70,81] The false-positive rate is approximately 25% and occurs with metastatic nodal disease and thyroid pathology.[70,81] Given the average sensitivity and poor anatomical detail of Tl-Tc scanning, this mode has been relegated to second-line imaging status.

TECHNETIUM-99M SESTAMIBI SCAN (SESTAMIBI SCAN)

Ever since Coakley et al. fortuitously discovered that technetium-99m sestamibi concentrated in abnormal parathyroid glands, sestamibi scanning has revolutionised the practice of parathyroid surgery making directed unilateral exploration a reasonable alternative to routine bilateral exploration.[82] Sestamibi is a derivative of technetium that avidly incorporates itself into mitochondria. The large amount of mitochondria in hyperactive parathyroid glands allows more intense labelling of parathyroid tumours relative to the thyroid and surrounding tissue.[83] The radiotracer also washes out much more slowly from the parathyroid than the thyroid. This differential uptake can be accentuated by pretest medical thyroid suppression. Sestamibi exploits these differences in uptake and retention to localise parathyroid adenomas. This radioisotope has a short half-life and produces high-energy photon emission that allows for low doses of radiation and high-definition imaging. Also, sestamibi scanning images both in the antero-posterior and lateral views, which allows for more precise localisation of the pathology.

There are three basic protocols for sestamibi scanning in current use:

- **Single-isotope dual-phase scan:** After intravenous administration of 15–25 mCi of sestamibi, images are taken at 10, 15, 120, and 180 minutes post-injection. A positive scan demonstrates increased uptake of tracer in the thyroid gland and parathyroid adenoma in early phases with washout of tracer from the thyroid gland but not the parathyroid adenoma in the late-phase images. This is the simplest and most widely used protocol. However, two potential pitfalls of this technique are: (i) sestamibi can accumulate and remain in thyroid nodules; and (ii) rapid washout of sestamibi can lead to false-negative results. To counter the first problem, many investigators are experimenting with dual isotope subtraction scanning. **Figure 1.1** illustrates a typical parathyroid adenoma in the early-phase scan.

- **Dual-isotope subtraction scanning:** Sestamibi and another radioisotope that amasses in the thyroid (such as ^{123}I or thallium chloride) are administered and the two views are subtracted to reveal the parathyroid pathology. Images are taken in both early and late phases. Late-phase imaging helps to exclude false-positive results by allowing more time for thyroid nodules to wash out. Numerous protocols and isotopes are currently being investigated but none has yet proven superior to the rest. **Figure 1.2** demonstrates a dual-isotope subtraction scan. Panel A demonstrates ^{123}I tracer uptake in only the thyroid gland. Panel B demonstrates an early-phase image with uptake of sestamibi tracer in the right lower parathyroid adenoma (arrow) and parts of the thyroid gland. Panel C demonstrates persistent tracer in the parathyroid adenoma (arrow) and washout of tracer from the thyroid gland.

- **SPECT (single-photon emission computed tomography) analysis:** This protocol allows for three-dimensional images to be created, which allows for better anatomical localisation, especially within the mediastinum, without any significant increase in sensitivity.[84,85] While this enhanced anatomical delineation may be useful in re-operative PHP, the significantly increased cost of this modality does not justify its routine use in preoperative localisation. **Figure 1.3** (see also Plate 1, facing p. 212) demonstrates a CT-enhanced SPECT scan (CT-SPECT). The top two rows of images mark the parathyroid adenoma on a CT scan (crosshair). The bottom row of images marks the parathyroid adenoma on SPECT scan (crosshair).

Irrespective of the protocol, depending on the series quoted, sestamibi scanning localises parathyroid adenomas in 80–100% of cases and has a

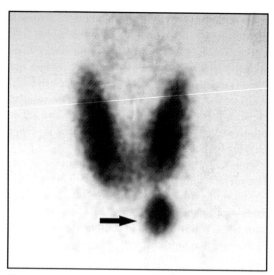

Figure 1.1 • Single-isotope dual-phase sestamibi scan. Sestamibi tracer can be seen concentrating in both the thyroid gland and a left lower pole parathyroid adenoma (arrow) in this early-phase image. Delayed-phase images would demonstrate washout of tracer from the thyroid gland but not the parathyroid adenoma.

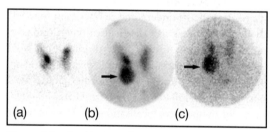

(a)   (b)   (c)

Figure 1.2 • Dual-isotope dual-phase sestamibi scan using both sestamibi and iodine-123. Panel A demonstrates the ^{123}I-only scan that delineates the thyroid gland only. Panel B demonstrates a right lower lobe parathyroid adenoma (arrow) in the early phase image with concomitant thyroid uptake of [123]I. Panel C demonstrates the same right lower lobe parathyroid adenoma (arrow) with thyroid 'washout' seen in this late-phase image.

specificity of around 90%.[54,86–91] The false-positive rate is low and is usually due to thyroid adenomas. The false-negative rate is relatively low, but perhaps the major drawback of sestamibi scanning is that it does not always identify patients with multiple adenomas or four-gland hyperplasia.[85,91,92] The false-negative rate is low and is usually related to small-sized glands or failure to recognise hyperplasia. In a meta-analysis of the English-language

Figure 1.3 • Computed tomography (CT)-enhanced SPECT scan. This image shows a mediastinal parathyroid adenoma identified precisely by SPECT enhancement and CT. The top two rows of images mark the parathyroid adenoma on CT scan (crosshair). The bottom row of images mark the parathyroid adenoma on SPECT scan.

literature over the last ten years, comprising 6331 patients, Denham and Norman found that 87% of patients had a single adenoma that sestamibi scan localised with an average sensitivity and specificity of 90.7% and 98.8% respectively.[54] Sestamibi-guided unilateral exploration led to an average cost saving of US$650 per operation. This study demonstrated that preoperative localisation with sestamibi scan was specific enough to make unilateral exploration both safe and cost-effective. If a single focus of uptake is noted, then unilateral exploration is likely to be successful. If no uptake or multiple areas of uptake are seen then bilateral exploration should be planned. Other radioisotopes, such as ^{99m}Tc-Tetrofosmin and $2[^{18}F]$-fluoro-2-deoxyglucose, are currently being evaluated. For the time, sestamibi scanning remains the standard for non-invasive localisation modalities.

PARATHYROID ANGIOGRAPHY AND VENOUS SAMPLING FOR PTH

Parathyroid angiography involves examination of both thyrocervical trunks, both internal mammary arteries, and both carotids with occasional selective superior thyroid artery catheterisation. The highly vascular parathyroid adenomas appear as a persistent oval or round 'stain' on angiography. Glands 4 mm in size or greater may be readily visualised. False positives are typically due to thyroid nodules or inflamed lymph nodes. Due to potentially serious complications like dye-induced renal failure, embolisation and neurological damage, angiography is usually reserved for re-operative localisation. The sensitivity of parathyroid angiography in this situation approaches 60%.[60,93,94]

Selective venous sampling for PTH allows for precise localisation of adenomas in the hands of an experienced interventionalist. The venous drainage of the lesion is established when there is a twofold drop in PTH between the sampled blood and the serum PTH. The technique has a sensitivity of 80% and is equally effective in localising mediastinal and cervical adenomas.[59,60,95,96] Venous sampling also allows for the identification of pathology in multiple glands. Venous sampling without concomitant angiography has a false-positive rate of 6–18%.[96]

When combined, the sensitivity for parathyroid angiography and selective venous sampling for PTH have a sensitivity of 91–95%, with a low false-positive rate.[93] Furthermore, the combination of the two modalities allows for precise localisation of single or multiple adenomas, even in ectopic locations and hyperplasia. However, the significant potential complications limit this study to use in localisation for re-operative PHP.

Pathology

PHP can be caused by single adenomas (87–90%), multiple adenomas (3%), four-gland hyperplasia (9%) or carcinoma (1%). Pathological criteria for differentiation of these entities are not universally accepted. In fact, in a small series of patients with single adenomas reported by Wang et al., none of the patients with histological evidence of hyperplasia in the remaining glands had recurrent or persistent PHP, suggesting that microscopic criteria for identifying pathological lesions are not very accurate.[97] Due to the imprecise nature of histological diagnosis for PHP, frozen section often does not help intraoperative distinction between different lesions. The best indicators that a gland is abnormal are its size and weight. While normal parathyroid glands weigh 40 mg on average, diseased glands weigh anywhere from 70 mg to 20 g. Indeed, some authors suggest that the only role for frozen section is to determine the weight of the specimen.[98] Numerous markers and special stains have been proposed to aid in differentiation, but none has gained wide acceptance.

ADENOMA

The gross appearance of an adenoma is typically large and tan or beefy red. Some authors have described the classic adenoma as a 'little kidney in the neck or mediastinum'.[99] The other glands appear atrophic or normal in size. While normal para-

Figure 1.4 • Parathyroid adenoma. This photomicrograph demonstrates the characteristic hypercellularity, loss of fat, loss of lobulation, and oxyphilic change of adenomatous degeneration (×40).

thyroids contain predominantly chief cells with scattered oxyphil cells, adenomas contain solid sheets of chief cells, oxyphil cells, or a combination of both surrounded by a fibrous capsule. Classically, there is a rim of compressed normal parathyroid surrounding the adenoma, which can be found in 20–30% of patients. **Figure 1.4** (see also Plate 2, facing p. 212) demonstrates the characteristic hypercellularity, loss of fat, loss of lobulation, and oxyphilic change of adenomatous degeneration. Pleomorphism and multinucleation may be present, but mitotic figures are rare and more strongly associated with carcinoma. There is less stromal fat in adenomas compared with normal parathyroids. Research demonstrates that parathyroid adenomas are typically monoclonal and may have very specific mutations in certain genes such as the *MEN1* tumour suppressor gene and the *PRAD1* oncogene.[100]

DOUBLE ADENOMA

Although uncommon, this form of PHP may lead to recurrent or persistent PHP if diseased glands are located on the contralateral side of a unilateral exploration. Finding two abnormal glands on one side mandates bilateral exploration.

HYPERPLASIA

A polyclonal expansion of parathyroid cells is called hyperplasia. This is more typical of familial hyperparathyroidism but may be found in sporadic

Figure 1.5 • Parathyroid hyperplasia. This photomicrograph demonstrates the characteristic hypercellularity, loss of fat and retained lobulation of parathyroid hyperplasia (×40).

Figure 1.6 • Parathyroid carcinoma. This photomicrograph demonstrates the characteristic thickened fibrous septa, nuclear atypia and capsular invasion of parathyroid carcinoma (×40).

cases. Grossly, the hyperplasia is typically not uniform. One gland may appear much larger than the rest giving the false impression of adenomatous disease, but on histological examination, each gland is hyperplastic. Microscopically, the chief cells are mainly affected. Moreso than with adenomas, the absence of parathyroid fat supports the diagnosis of hyperplasia. **Figure 1.5** (see also Plate 3, facing p. 212) demonstrates the characteristic hypercellularity, loss of fat, and retained lobulation of parathyroid hyperplasia. Diffuse hyperplasia warrants four-gland exploration with three-and-a-half gland parathyroidectomy or four-gland excision with autotransplantation.

CARCINOMA

A rare finding, parathyroid carcinoma is a difficult diagnosis to make preoperatively and often is a retrospective diagnosis made only after metastatic disease develops. Patients tend to be younger (50s cf. 60s) than in benign disease and there is an equal distribution among men and women. On preoperative evaluation, carcinoma produces a palpable mass in 30–75% of patients (far more frequently than in benign disease) and serum calcium tends to be higher than for adenomatous disease. Furthermore, recurrent laryngeal nerve involvement is suggestive of malignancy. Classic operative findings for parathyroid carcinoma include adherence or invasion into surrounding structures and dense scarring. Typical histological findings include bizarre nuclear atypia, mitotic figures, and capsular

or vascular invasion. **Figure 1.6** (see also Plate 4, facing p. 212) demonstrates the characteristic thickened fibrous septa, nuclear atypia and capsular invasion. The only definitive criteria for malignancy are metastatic disease (lung, lymph node, liver) and local invasion. There is a recurrence rate of 66%. The 5-year survival is approximately 69%, with death caused by metabolic sequelae of hypercalcaemia.

SECONDARY HYPERPARATHYROIDISM (SHP)

Secondary hyperparathyroidism arises when factors other than primary parathyroid disease cause overproduction of PTH. For example, hypermagnesaemia, osteoporosis, rickets and osteomalacia can all cause SHP. By far the most common cause of SHP is chronic renal failure. Indeed, there is such a strong correlation between the two conditions that some call SHP 'renal hyperparathyroidism'. In fact, almost every renal failure patient will develop some form of SHP.

Pathogenesis

Every aspect of renal failure from the decreased renal synthetic function to the metabolic abnormalities to even the treatment contributes to the pathogenesis of SHP. These factors lead to hypertrophy and hyperplastic transformation of the parathyroid gland with subsequent elevation of PTH levels in a futile attempt to normalise serum calcium levels.

HYPOCALCAEMIA AND HYPERPHOSPHATAEMIA

As outlined previously, hypocalcaemia stimulates PTH secretion in an attempt to normalise levels. Furthermore, phosphate and calcium concentrations are inversely related. As the kidney's ability to excrete phosphates declines and hyperphosphataemia develops, serum calcium levels fall. Further exacerbation of hypocalcaemia comes from the use of calcium-poor dialysates. The consequent decline in calcium levels stimulates PTH overproduction and inhibits the negative-feedback loop.

DECREASED SYNTHESIS OF CALCITRIOL

Calcitriol increases serum calcium by enhancing osteoclast activity and increasing the intestinal absorption of calcium. Calcitriol also acts as part of the negative-feedback loop on the parathyroids to decrease PTH secretion. Decreased renal synthetic function and chronic hyperphosphataemia lead to a reduction in renal 1α-hydroxylase, which in turn leads to a decrement in the conversion of 25-hydroxylated vitamin D_3 (calcidiol) to calcitriol. This dearth of calcitriol not only lowers serum calcium levels leading to increased PTH production, but also dampens an important means of inhibiting the stimulus to secrete PTH.

BONY RESISTANCE TO PTH

Typically, PTH induces bone resorption with a subsequent rise in serum calcium levels by activating osteoclasts. However, experiments have shown that excessive PTH blunts the mobilisation of calcium from osseous stores.[101]

CHANGES IN PTH SET POINT

The PTH set point is defined as the serum calcium level that decreases PTH levels by 50%.[102] As the set point rises, inhibition of PTH secretion is lost and SHP results. Research suggests that changes in set point may be due to alterations in the expression

or sensitivity of the calcium-sensing receptor, but no genetic links have yet been found.[100]

ALUMINIUM INTOXICATION

High aluminium concentrations in renal dialysate and phosphate binders can lead to accumulation in bone. This buildup can lead to osteomalacia, which in turn exacerbates PTH overproduction.

Presentation

As with PHP, many patients are asymptomatic and only come to attention due to serological tests. Symptomatic patients classically present with osseous lesions, pruritus and metastatic calcifications.

OSSEOUS LESIONS

Bone pain is a common complaint in patients with SHP and is due to increased bone remodelling. Adults tend to develop compression fractures of the axial skeleton, but fractures do occur elsewhere. Children can be afflicted by growth retardation. The classic lesion of hyperparathyroidism is osteitis fibrosa cystica, and this can be seen in up to 30% of patients on dialysis.[103] Caused by increased bone resorption and formation, this lesion leads to a chaotic matrix deposition giving the typical 'woven bone' appearance. This compromised bone is inherently weaker than normal bone and may lead to fractures. Other osseous lesions that may develop include pepperpot skull, osteomalacia, and long bone fractures.

PRURITUS

Pruritus is found in 85% of patients on haemodialysis and may become so severe as to be disabling. Significant symptomatic relief is achieved after parathyroidectomy.[104]

METASTATIC CALCIFICATION

Metastatic calcification can affect almost any organ system in the body and may be a significant cause of morbidity in patients with SHP. Perhaps the most common site for calcification is in the vasculature. Other typical areas of calcification include the heart, mitral valve, kidneys, gastrointestinal tract and penis. Parathyroidectomy may decrease the severity of metastatic calcification in all organ systems except the vasculature.[103]

CALCIPHYLAXIS

This is a rare but severe complication, consisting of soft tissue and vascular calcification that may lead to tissue necrosis. The mottled violaceous lesions can progress to ulcers and gangrene. Calciphylaxis may be present anywhere in the body, but is most common in the extremities. The mortality rate of calciphylaxis is approximately 50%. Patients with a high calcium × phosphorus product are at risk for developing calciphylaxis. The mainstays of therapy include phosphate binders and parathyroidectomy.

Treatment

The initial therapy of SHP is primarily medical and revolves around bringing the serum calcium and phosphate to physiological levels. Normalising these removes the major impetus for PTH overproduction. Non-operative therapy includes calcium supplementation (1500 mg/day), phosphate-poor diets, phosphate binders (<1000 mg/day) and vitamin D supplementation. Other therapies include aluminium-binding agents (desferrioxamine) and haemodialysis with calcium-enriched dialysates. However, hypercalcaemia often complicates these treatment regimens. Newly developed calcimimetics bind to the calcium-sensing receptor and lower parathyroid hormone levels without increasing calcium and phosphate levels. Agents like cinacalcet have been shown to effectively reduce PTH levels in contrast to placebo in randomised double-blind studies.[105] The definitive therapy for SHP is renal transplant, although some patients will develop tertiary hyperparathyroidism postoperatively. Operative parathyroidectomy (four-gland with autotransplantation or three-and-a-half gland) is indicated in the 5–10% of patients who fail medical management. Other indications include: (1) intractable bone pain; (2) intractable pruritus; (3) fractures; and (4) symptomatic ectopic calcifications.

TERTIARY HYPERPARATHYROIDISM

Tertiary hyperparathyroidism is a rare condition seen in certain patients with chronic renal failure who have resolution of their renal disease, usually due to a kidney transplant. Prior to transplant, a portion of these patients have parathyroid glands that autonomously produce PTH due to the constant hypocalcaemia caused by the hyperphosphataemia of renal failure. Once freed from the metabolic disarray of their renal disease by transplant, a subset will have parathyroids that continue to produce PTH without the normal feedback inhibition, thus producing hypercalcaemia. Approximately 60% of cases of tertiary hyperparathyroidism resolve spontaneously. Therefore, surgical parathyroidectomy is only indicated if there is persistent hypercalcaemia after 12 months or more of observation.

Key points

- PHP occurs more frequently in women than men.
- PHP is confirmed by elevated serum calcium and serum PTH levels.
- The majority of cases of hypercalcaemia are classified as mild to moderate (<12 mg/dL or 12–14 mg/dL serum calcium respectively), and the patient is asymptomatic.
- Hypercalcaemic crisis consists of serum calcium >14 mg/dL and severe symptoms.
- Treatment of severe hypercalcaemia involves aggressive rehydration, increasing renal excretion of calcium, blunting of calcium release from skeletal stores, and treating the underlying cause of the hypercalcaemia.
- Bilateral neck exploration for PHP cures 95% of cases.
- Of patients with PHP, 87% have single adenomas, 9% have four-gland hyperplasia, 3% have multiple adenomas, and fewer than 1% have cancer.
- Sestamibi scanning localises parathyroid adenomas in up to 80–100% of cases and has a specificity of around 90%, but results in different series vary considerably.
- The most common cause of SHP is chronic renal failure.

REFERENCES

1. Adami S, Marcocci C, Gatti D. Epidemiology of primary hyperparathyroidism in Europe. J Bone Miner Res 2002; 17(suppl. 2):N18–23.

2. Mandl F. Klinisches und Experimenteles zur Frage der lakalisierten und generalisiereten Osteitis Fibrosa. Arch Klin Chir 1926; 143:1.

3. Berson SA, Yalow RS. Parathyroid hormone in plasma in adenomatous hyperparathyroidism, uremia, and bronchogenic carcinoma. Science 1966; 154(751):907–9.

4. Heath H 3rd, Hodgson SF, Kennedy MA. Primary hyperparathyroidism. Incidence, morbidity, and potential economic impact in a community. N Engl J Med 1980; 302(4):189–93.

5. Russell CF, Edis AJ. Surgery for primary hyperparathyroidism: experience with 500 consecutive cases and evaluation of the role of surgery in the asymptomatic patient. Br J Surg 1982; 69(5):244–7.

6. Thompson NW, Eckhauser FE, Harness JK. The anatomy of primary hyperparathyroidism. Surgery 1982; 92(5):814–21.

    An excellent overall review.

7. Moore MA, Owen JJ. Experimental studies on the development of the thymus. J Exp Med 1967; 126(4):715–26.

8. Akerstrom G, Malmaeus J, Bergstrom R. Surgical anatomy of human parathyroid glands. Surgery 1984; 95(1):14–21.

9. Wang C, Mahaffey JE, Axelrod L et al. Hyperfunctioning supernumerary parathyroid glands. Surg Gynecol Obstet 1979; 148(5):711–14.

10. Brown EM. The pathophysiology of primary hyperparathyroidism. J Bone Miner Res 2002; 17(suppl. 2):N24–9.

11. Goodman WG. Calcium-sensing receptors. Semin Nephrol 2004; 24(1):17–24.

12. Tfelt-Hansen J, Schwarz P, Brown EM et al. The calcium-sensing receptor in human disease. Front Biosci 2003; 8:s377–90.

13. Conigrave AD, Franks AH, Brown EM et al. L-Amino acid sensing by the calcium-sensing receptor: a general mechanism for coupling protein and calcium metabolism? Eur J Clin Nutr 2002; 56(11):1072–80.

14. Hofer AM, Brown EM. Extracellular calcium sensing and signalling. Nat Rev Mol Cell Biol 2003; 4(7):530–8.

15. Hoare SR, Usdin TB. Molecular mechanisms of ligand recognition by parathyroid hormone 1 (PTH1) and PTH2 receptors. Curr Pharm Des 2001; 7(8):689–713.

16. Libutti SK, Alexander HR, Bartlett DL et al. Kinetic analysis of the rapid intraoperative parathyroid hormone assay in patients during operation for hyperparathyroidism. Surgery 1999; 126(6):1145–50; discussion 1150–1.

17. Canterbury JM, Levey GS, Reiss E. Activation of renal cortical adenylate cyclase by circulating immunoreactive parathyroid hormone fragments. J Clin Invest 1973; 52(2):524–7.

18. Fujita T, Meguro T, Fukuyama R et al. New signaling pathway for parathyroid hormone and cyclic AMP action on extracellular-regulated kinase and cell proliferation in bone cells. Checkpoint of modulation by cyclic AMP. J Biol Chem 2002; 277(25):22191–200.

19. Brown EM. Extracellular Ca^{2+} sensing, regulation of parathyroid cell function, and role of Ca^{2+} and other ions as extracellular (first) messengers. Physiol Rev 1991; 71(2):371–411.

20. Pak CY. Calcium metabolism. J Am Coll Nutr 1989; 8(suppl.):46S–53S.

21. Carmeliet G, Van Cromphaut S, Daci E et al. Disorders of calcium homeostasis. Best Pract Res Clin Endocrinol Metab 2003; 17(4):529–46.

22. Austin LA, Heath H 3rd. Calcitonin: physiology and pathophysiology. N Engl J Med 1981; 304(5):269–78.

23. Melton JL. The epidemiology of primary hyperparathyroidism in North America. J Bone Miner Res 2002; 17(suppl. 2):N12–N17.

24. Monchik JM. Normocalcemic hyperparathyroidism. Surgery 1995; 118(6):917–23.

25. Boughey JC, Ewart CJ, Yost MJ et al. Chloride/phosphate ratio in primary hyperparathyroidism. Am Surg 2004; 70(1):25–8.

26. Mather H. Hyperparathyroidism with normal serum calcium. Br Med J 1953; 2:424–5.

27. Lundgren E, Rastad J, Thrufjell E et al. Population-based screening for primary hyperparathyroidism with serum calcium and parathyroid hormone values in menopausal women. Surgery 1997; 121(3):287–94.

28. Silverberg SJ, Bilezikian JP. "Incipient" primary hyperparathyroidism: a "forme fruste" of an old disease. J Clin Endocrinol Metab 2003; 88(11):5348–52.

29. Carnaille BM, Pattou FN, Oudar C et al. Parathyroid incidentalomas in normocalcemic patients during thyroid surgery. World J Surg 1996; 20(7):830–4; discussion 834.

    Overview of normocalcaemic hyperparathyroidism.

30. Luong KV, Nguyen LT. Normocalcemic hyperparathyroidism in Vietnamese immigrants living in southern California. Am J Med Sci 2000; 319(6):380–4.

31. Maruani G, Hertig A, Paillard M et al. Normocalcemic primary hyperparathyroidism: evidence for a generalized target-tissue resistance to parathyroid hormone. J Clin Endocrinol Metab 2003; 88(10):4641–8.

32. Siperstein AE, Shen W, Chan AK et al. Normocalcemic hyperparathyroidism. Biochemical and symptom profiles before and after surgery. Arch Surg 1992; 127(10):1157–6; discussion 1161–3.

33. Wu PH, Wang CJ. Normocalcemic primary hyperparathyroidism with fractures. J Arthroplasty 2002; 17(6):805–9.

34. Monchik JM. Normocalcemic hyperparathyroidism. In: Clark OH, Duh Q (eds) Textbook of endocrine surgery. San Francisco: WB Saunders, 1997; p. 335.

35. Parks J, Coe F, Favus M. Hyperparathyroidism in nephrolithiasis. Arch Intern Med 1980; 140:1479–81.

36. Poole GV Jr, Albertson AD, Myers RT. Normocalcemic hyperparathyroidism revisited. Am Surg 1983; 49:668–71.

37. Nichols G Jr, Flanagan B. Normocalcemic hyperparathyroidism. Trans Assoc Am Physicians 1967; 80:314–22.

38. Peacock M. Renal stone disease and bone disease in primary hyperparathyroidism and their relationship to the action of parathyroid hormone on calcium absorption. New York: Excerpta Medica, 1975.

39. Broadus AE, Dominguez M, Bartter FC. Pathophysiological studies in idiopathic hypercalciuria: use of an oral calcium tolerance test to characterize distinctive hypercalciuric subgroups. J Clin Endocrinol Metab 1978; 47(4):751–60.

40. Hagag P, Revet-Zak I, Hod N et al. Diagnosis of normocalcemic hyperparathyroidism by oral calcium loading test. J Endocrinol Invest 2003; 26(4):327–32.

41. Ishikawa Y, Kurita T. [Normocalcemic primary hyperparathyroidism]. Nippon Rinsho 1995; 53(4):915–19.

42. Greenfield MW. Parathyroid glands. In: Lazar J et al. (eds) Surgery: scientific principles and practice, 3rd edn. Philadelphia: Lippincott Williams & Wilkins, 2001; p. 1290.

43. Carroll MF, Schade DS. A practical approach to hypercalcemia. Am Fam Physician 2003; 67(9): 1959–66.

44. Jan de Beur SM LM. Hypercalcemia. In: CW B (ed.) Current therapy in endocrinology and metabolism, 6th edn. New York: Mosby, 1997; p. 552.

45. Ziegler R. Hyperkalzamie. Ther Umsch 2000; 57(6):391–7.

46. Bilezikian, JP. Management of acute hypercalcemia. N Engl J Med 1992; 326:1196–203.

47. Edelson GW, Kleerekoper M. Hypercalcemic crisis. Med Clin N Am 1995; 79:79–92.

48. Oura S. [Malignancy-associated hypercalcemia]. Nippon Rinsho – Jpn J Clin Med 2003; 61(6): 1006–9.

49. Ziegler R. Hypercalcemic crisis. J Am Soc Nephrol 2001; 12(suppl. 17):S3–9.

50. Van Heerden J. Lessons learned. Surgery 1997; 122(6):978–88.

Overview of surgical approach to primary hyperparathyroidism.

51. Kaplan EL, Yashiro T, Salti G. Primary hyperparathyroidism in the 1990s. Choice of surgical procedures for this disease.[see comment]. Ann Surg 1992; 215(4):300–17.

52. Weber C, Burke GJ, McGarity WC. Persistent and recurrent sporadic primary hyperparathyroidism: Histopathology, complications, and results of reoperation. Surgery 1994; 116:991.

53. Consensus Development Conference Panel. Diagnosis and management of asymptomatic primary hyperparathyroidism: Consensus Development Conference statement. Ann Intern Med 1991; 114:593–7.

54. Denham DW, Norman J. Cost-effectiveness of preoperative sestamibi scan for primary hyperparathyroidism is dependent solely upon the surgeon's choice of operative procedure. J Am Coll Surgeons 1998; 186(3):293–305.

55. Wang C, Rieder SV. A density test for the intraoperative differentiation of parathyroid hyperplasia from neoplasia. Ann Surg 1978; 187:63.

56. Verdonk C, Edis AJ. Parathyroid "double adenomas": fact or fiction? Surgery 1981; 90:523.

57. Attie JN, Bock G, August LJ. Multiple parathyroid adenomas: Report of thirty three cases. Surgery 1990; 108:1014.

58. Grant C, Van Heerden JA, Charboneau EM. Clinical management of persistent and/or recurrent primary hyperparathyroidism. World J Surg 1986; 10:555.

59. Rodriquez JM, Tezelman S, Siperstein AE et al. Localization procedures in patients with persistent or recurrent hyperparathyroidism. Arch Surg 1994; 129(8):870–5.

60. Miller D, Doppman MD, Shawker MD et al. Localization of parathyroid adenomas who have undergone surgery. Radiology 1987; 162:133–7.

61. Henry JF, Audiffret J, Denizot A et al. Endosonography in the localization of parathyroid tumors: a preliminary study. Surgery 1990; 108(6):1021–5.

62. Catargi B, Raymond JM, Lafarge-Gense V et al. Localization of parathyroid tumors using endoscopic ultrasonography in primary hyperparathyroidism. J Endocrinol Invest 1999; 22(9):688–92.

63. Casara D, Rubello D, Pelizzo MR et al. Clinical role of 99mTcO4/MIBI scan, ultrasound, and intra-operative gamma probe in the performance of unilateral and minimally invasive surgery in hyperparathyroidism. Eur J Nucl Med 2001; 28:1351–9.

64. Uden P, Aspelin P, Berglund J et al. Preoperative localization in unilateral parathyroid surgery. A cost-benefit study on ultrasound, computed tomography and scintigraphy. Acta Chir Scand 1990; 156(1):29–35.

65. De Feo ML, Colagrande S, Biagini C et al. Parathyroid glands: combination of (99m)Tc MIBI scintigraphy and US for demonstration of parathyroid glands and nodules [see comment]. Radiology 2000; 214(2):393–402.

66. Tikkakoski T, Stenfors LE, Typpo T et al. Parathyroid adenomas: pre-operative localization with ultrasound combined with fine-needle biopsy. J Laryngol Otol 1993; 107(6):543–5.

67. Dijkstra B, Healy C, Kelly LM et al. Parathyroid localisation – current practice. J R Coll Surg Edinb 2002; 47(4):599–607.

68. Giuliano M, Gulec SA, Rubello D et al. Preoperative localization and radioguided parathyroid surgery. J Nucl Med 2003; 44:1443–58.

69. Weber AL, Randolph G, Aksoy F. The thyroid and parathyroid glands: CT and MR imaging and correlation with pathological and clinical findings. Radiol Clin N Am 2000; 38:1105–28.

70. Levin KE, Clark OH. Localization of parathyroid glands. Ann Rev Med 1988; 39:29–40.

71. Erdman WA, Breslau NA, Weinreb JC et al. Noninvasive localization of parathyroid adenomas: a comparison of X-ray computerized tomography, ultrasound, scintigraphy and MRI. Magn Reson Imaging 1989; 7(2):187–94.

72. Levin KE, Gooding GA, Okerlund M et al. Localizing studies in patients with persistent or recurrent hyperparathyroidism. Surgery 1987; 102(6):917–25.

73. Doppman J, Krudy AG, Marx SJ. Aspiration of enlarged parathyroid glands for parathyroid hormone assay. Radiology 1983; 148:31–5.

74. Aufferman W, Gooding G, Okerlund M. Diagnosis of recurrent hyperparathyroidism: Comparison of MR imaging and the other techniques. Am J Roentgenol 1988; 150:1027.

75. Stark D, Clark OH, Moss A. Magnetic resonance imaging of the thyroid, thymus, and parathyroid glands. Surgery 1984; 96(6):1083–90.

76. Kang Y, Rosen K, Clark OH et al. Localization of abnormal parathyroid glands of the mediastinum with MR imaging. Radiology 1993; 189:137–41.

77. Kurbskack A, Wilson SD, Lawson T. Prospective comparison of radionuclide, computed tomography, sonographic, and magnetic resonance localization of parathyroid tumors. Surgery 1989; 106:639.

78. Higgins CB. Role of magnetic resonance imaging in hyperparathyroidism. Radiol Clin N Am 1993; 31(5):1017–28.

79. Fayet P, Hoeffel C, Fulla Y. Technetium-99m-sestamibi, magnetic resonance imaging, and venous blood sampling in persistent and recurrent hyperparathyroidism. Br J Radiol 1997; 70:459–64.

Overview of current state of localisation studies for primary hyperparathyroidism.

80. Gotway M, Reddy G, Webb W et al. Comparison between MR imaging and 99mTc-MIBI scintigraphy in the evaluation of recurrent or persistent hyperparathyroidism: results and factors affecting parathyroid detection. Am J Roentgenol 2001; 166:705–10.

81. Hewin DF, Brammar TJ, Kabala J et al. Role of preoperative localization in the management of primary hyperparathyroidism. Br J Surg 1997; 84(10):1377–80.

82. Coakley AJ, Kettle AG, Wells CP et al. 99Tcm sestamibi – a new agent for parathyroid imaging. Nucl Med Commun 1989; 10(11):791–4.

83. Sandrock D, Merino MJ, Norton JA. Light and electronmicroscopic analyses of parathyroid tumors explain results of Tl201Tc99m parathyroid scintigraphy. Eur J Med 1989; 15:410.

84. Pattou F, Huglo D, Proye C. Radionuclide scanning in parathyroid diseases. Br J Surg 1998; 85(12):1605–16.

85. McHenry C, Lee K, Saddey J et al. Parathyroid localisation with technetium-99m-MIBI scintigraphy to identify anatomy in secondary hyperparathyroidism. J Nucl Med 1996; 37:565–9.

86. O'Doherty MJ, Kettle AG. Parathyroid imaging: preoperative localization. Nucl Med Commun 2003; 24(2):125–31.

87. Casas AT, Burke GJ, Sathyanarayana et al. Prospective comparison of technetium-99m-sestamibi/iodine-123 radionuclide scan versus high-resolution ultrasonography for the preoperative localization of abnormal parathyroid glands in patients with previously unoperated primary hyperparathyroidism. Am J Surg 1993; 166(4):369–73.

88. Thule P, Thakore K, Vansant J et al. Preoperative localization of parathyroid tissue with technetium-99m sestamibi 123I subtraction scanning. J Clin Endocrinol Metab 1994; 78(1):77–82.

89. Casas AT, Burke GJ, Mansberger AR Jr et al. Impact of technetium-99m-sestamibi localization on operative time and success of operations for primary hyperparathyroidism. Am Surg 1994; 60(1):12–16; discussion 16–17.

90. Caixas A, Berna L, Hernandez A et al. Efficacy of preoperative diagnostic imaging localization of technetium 99m-sestamibi scintigraphy in hyperparathyroidism. Surgery 1997; 121(5):535–41.

91. Malhotra A, Silver CE, Deshpande V et al. Preoperative parathyroid localization with sestamibi. Am J Surg 1996; 172(6):637–40.

92. Wei JP, Burke GJ, Mansberger AR Jr. Preoperative imaging of abnormal parathyroid glands in patients with hyperparathyroid disease using combination Tc-99m-pertechnetate and Tc-99m-sestamibi radionuclide scans. Ann Surg 1994; 219(5):568–72; discussion 572–3.

93. Miller DL. Preoperative localization and interventional treatment of parathyroid tumors: When and how? World J Surg 1991; 15:706.

94. Miller DL, Chang R, Doppman J et al. Superselective DSA versus superselective conventional angiography. Radiology 1989; 170:1003.

95. Sugg SL, Fraker DL, Alexander R et al. Prospective evaluation of selective venous sampling for parathyroid hormone concentration in patients undergoing reoperations for primary hyperparathyroidism. Surgery 1993; 114(6):1004–9; discussion 1009–10.

96. Granberg PO, Hamberger B, Johansson G et al. Selective venous sampling for localization of hyperfunctioning parathyroid glands. Br J Surg 1986; 73(2):118–20.

97. Wang CA, Reitz RE, Pollard JJ et al. Localization of hyperfunctioning parathyroids. The surgeons' riddle. Am J Surg 1970; 119(4):462–4.

98. Wang CA. The anatomic basis of parathyroid surgery. Ann Surg 1976; 183:271.

99. Van Heerden J, Farley D. Parathyroid. In: Schwartz S (ed.) Principles of surgery, 7th edn. New York: McGraw-Hill, 1999.

100. Miedlich S, Krohn K, Paschke R. Update on genetic and clinical aspects of primary hyperparathyroidism. Clin Endocrinol 2003; 59:539–54.

101. Rodriguez M, Martin-Malo A, Martinez M. Calcemic response to parathyroid hormone in renal failure: Role of phosphorus and its effect on calcitriol. Kidney Int 1991; 40:1055.

102. Felsenfeld A, Rodriguez M, Dunlay R et al. A comparison of parathyroid gland function in haemodialysis patients with different forms of renal osteodystrophy. Nephrol Dial Transplant 1991; 6:244.

103. Sancho J, Sitges-Sierra A. Metabolic complications for patients with secondary hyperparathyroidism. In: Clark OH, Duh Q (eds) Textbook of endocrine surgery. San Francisco: W.B. Saunders, 1997.

104. Demeure M, McGee D, Wilkes W et al. Results of surgical treatment for primary hyperparathyroidism associated with renal disease. Am J Surg 1990; 160:337.

An overview of the treatment of secondary hyperparathyroidism.

105. Block G, Martin K, de Francisco A et al. Cinacalcet for secondary hyperparathyroidism in patients receiving hemodialysis. N Engl J Med 2004; 350(15):1516–25.

Part 2

Operative strategy for the management of parathyroid disease

Jean-François Henry and Frédéric Sebag

PRIMARY HYPERPARATHYROIDISM

For many years bilateral cervical exploration has been the preferred surgical approach for primary hyperparathyroidism (PHP). When performed by an experienced endocrine surgeon, this procedure is certainly one of the most gratifying of all operations. The success rate is reported to be 95–98%, the morbidity is minimal, the mortality is close to zero and cosmetic results are excellent.[1]

The standard bilateral neck exploration is today challenged by several new minimally invasive techniques. Three main factors have stimulated and allowed these new surgical approaches:

1. The improvement of imaging techniques such as high-resolution ultrasonography and sestamibi scan.
2. The introduction of the quick parathyroid hormone assay (QPTH).
3. The refinement of instrumentation (gamma probe, endoscopic instruments, miniaturised cameras).

Nevertheless, it is imperative to keep in mind the excellent results of conventional parathyroid surgery, which remains the 'gold standard'.

CONVENTIONAL OPEN PARATHYROIDECTOMY

Basic principles of parathyroid surgery

Localisation studies may help the surgeon to discover the pathological gland(s) but the success of a standard bilateral exploration is above all based on a thorough knowledge of the anatomy and an understanding of the embryological evolution of the glands. As Cope wrote in 1960, the initial operation is the 'golden opportunity' to cure the patient.[2]

Ideally, the exploration should allow exposure of the whole of the parathyroid tissue, i.e. of at least four glands, whatever the lesion responsible for the PHP syndrome and the results of preoperative imaging studies. The contribution of frozen section is limited. It has been shown that foci of microscopic hyperplasia observed in biopsy fragments are without functional significance,[3,4] and such hyperplasia may even lead to the performance of unnecessary excisions causing permanent hypoparathyroidism. Frozen section may help the surgeon to confirm or exclude the presence of parathyroid tissue but, it should not be used as grounds for excision of other parathyroid glands.

The pathological nature of the glands is essentially determined from their gross appearance. If the average weight is taken as 40 mg, a gland can only be certainly considered abnormal if above 75 mg. Surgical excision is therefore based on this macroscopic evaluation, which is the more valuable if all the glands have been identified and exposed. However, one must be aware of the risks of devascularisation incurred by too eager a desire to expose a gland.[5,6]

The excision must be selective. The enlarged gland(s) should be removed in toto and the normal glands preserved. Tumoral biopsy is strictly contraindicated, and may be responsible for local spread (parathormatosis).

Management of surgical procedure

The operation is usually performed under general anaesthesia but regional anaesthesia[7] and hypnosedation[8] can also be used.

The patient is positioned symmetrically in dorsal decubitus, with the arms beside the body, in slight procubitus, the neck in hyperextension. The skin incision is a low transverse cervical incision, one or two fingerbreadths above the heads of the clavicles. The cervical approach is made by separation of the strap muscles in the midline.

THE SEARCH FOR SUPERIOR PARATHYROID (P IV)

Exposure of the posterior aspect of the thyroid lobe is made by displacing the gland inwards and forwards and retracting the jugulocarotid bundle outwards. The inferior thyroid artery should be preserved. The recurrent laryngeal nerve should be identified.

In 85% of cases this simple exposure allows identification of the normal P IV in its orthotopic site. It 'floats' in a loose fatty setting immediately adjacent to the inferior cornu of the thyroid cartilage, very close to the recurrent nerve and the most cranial branch of the inferior thyroid artery. These structures constitute three basic landmarks in the search for P IV (**Fig. 1.7**).

When a P IV is abnormal, it tends to migrate posteriorly and downwards (**Fig. 1.8**). Therefore, if it is not found in immmediate contact with the thyroid capsule, it should be sought beside or behind the oesophagus. Its migration may drag it down very low, well below the inferior thyroid artery, behind whose trunk it crosses during its descent. The lower a P IV, the more posterior it becomes. These adenomas are revealed by their vascular pedicles, whose origin is found at the middle or upper third of the thyroid lobe. They emerge with simple traction on their pedicle. They are closely related to the recurrent nerve, which may be adherent to their capsule, so that their mobilisation calls for prior identification of the nerve and possibly its dissection. If no gland, normal or abnormal, is discovered, the search should be transferred to the perithyroid visceral sheath, carefully exploring the posterior aspect of the lobe from the trunk of the inferior thyroid artery to the superior thyroid pedicle. Quite particular attention must be devoted to the posterior aspect of the upper pole of the thyroid lobe, where some very flattened adenomas, closely adherent to the surface of the thyroid capsule, may easily pass unnoticed.

If the P IV has not been discovered, the search should be temporarily suspended and transferred to the homolateral parathyroid gland.

THE SEARCH FOR INFERIOR PARATHYROID (P III)

The usual range of position of P III is more extensive than that of P IV (**Fig. 1.9**). The search must be

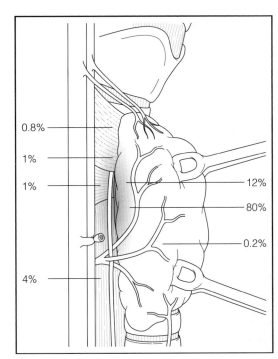

Figure 1.7 • Location of superior parathyroid glands (P IV). The numbers represent the percentages of glands found at different locations in an autopsy study of 503 cases. Adapted from Akerstrom G, Malmaeus J, Bergstrom R. Surgical anatomy of human parathyroid glands. Surgery 1984; 95:14–21.

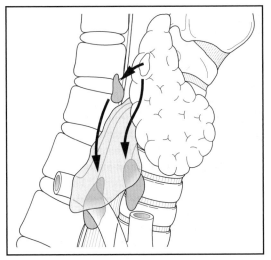

Figure 1.8 • Acquired migration paths of enlarged superior parathyroids (P IV). The enlarged glands tend to migrate posteriorly and downwards.

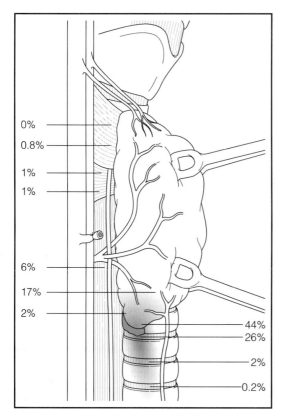

0%
0.8%
1%
1%

6%
17%
2%

44%
26%

2%

0.2%

Figure 1.9 • Location of inferior parathyroid glands (P III). The numbers represent the percentages of glands found at different locations in an autopsy study of 503 cases. Adapted from Akerstrom G, Malmaeus J, Bergstrom R. Surgical anatomy of human parathyroid glands. Surgery 1984; 95:14–21.

made from the inferior thyroid artery to the inferior thyroid pole, and along the thyrothymic ligament. The P III are rarely posterior and become more anterior the lower they are.

The search should first be made at the posterior aspect of the thyroid lobe from the inferior thyroid artery to the lower pole of the lobe. At this site, a normal P III is always situated in front of the recurrent nerve. When it is tumoral its posterior surface may adhere to the nerve. The exploration must be carried all around the inferior pole of the thyroid lobe, checking its lateral, anterior and inferior aspects in turn. During this dissection one must safeguard the thyroid attachments, i.e. the thyrothymic ligament and the inferior thyroid veins. Then the dissection must be carried as low as possible along the thyrothymic ligaments and the thymus. Nearly 25% of P IIIs are situated along the

thyrothymic ligaments or at the upper poles of the thymus.[9–12] Very often they are discovered only after incision of the thymic sheath.

At this stage of the operation, if P III has not been identified, the search should be abandoned and transferred to exploration of the other side. This attitude is justified by the risks of a more aggressive dissection, which may cause devascularisation of a hitherto unperceived normal P III. Similarly, the thymus and thyrothymic ligament must be safeguarded.

Exploration of the second side is made in the same order. The surgeon is favoured by the natural symmetry, though this is somewhat relative (60% of cases).[13]

EVALUATION OF THE INITIAL BILATERAL EXPLORATION

At the end of this bilateral exploration, the surgeon must decide whether to continue the procedure or not in the light of the number of glands discovered and their pathological or normal appearance.

The exploration must be **abandoned in two circumstances:**

1. **The four glands have been discovered and one or more are abnormal.** Routine search for a supernumerary gland is justified only in cases of familial hyperparathyroidism.
2. **One gland is pathological, the other gland(s) identified are normal, but fewer than four glands have been discovered.** Except in case of familial hyperparathyroidism the low risk of multiglandular disease that might pass unnoticed does not justify obstinate pursuit of an exploration that risks proving more dangerous than beneficial for the patient. The diagnosis of a solitary adenoma becomes more likely as the number of normal glands found approaches three.

The exploration should be **pursued in three circumstances:**

1. **No gland or fewer than four glands have been discovered and none is pathological.** A probable adenoma remains to be discovered.
2. **Fewer than four glands have been discovered and at least two of these are enlarged.** The surgeon is dealing with a multiglandular disease

(MGD). The missing gland(s) must be identified.

3. **All four glands have been discovered but all are normal.** The surgeon must remain convinced of his or her diagnosis and consider the possibility of a probable ectopic supernumerary adenoma.

CONTINUATION OF THE EXPLORATION

The surgeon must keep in mind that: (i) congenital ectopias, in the neck or in the anterior mediastinum, respectively caused by defective or excessive embryological migration, are related to P III

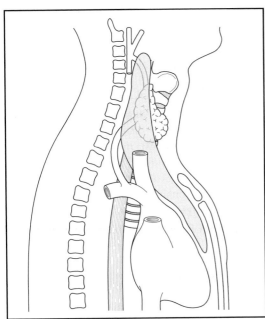

Figure 1.10 • The embryonic migration of the inferior parathyroid gland (P III)-thymus complex results in an extensive area of dispersal of the normal P III from the angle of the mandible to the pericardium.

(**Fig. 1.10**); and (ii) acquired ectopias in the posterior mediastinum caused by migration affected by gravity, secondary to adenomatous pathology, are essentially related to P IV (**Fig. 1.8**) (**Table 1.3**).[14] Therefore, it is essential to know whether the missing gland is a P IV or a P III.

If a P IV is absent:

1. Re-explore the juxta-oesophageal regions, as far down as possible in the posterior mediastinum.
2. Remember the defective migration of P IV and explore the superior thyroid pedicle region.
3. Ligate the superior thyroid pedicle and mobilise the upper pole of the lobe for scrupulous dissection of its posteromedial aspect.
4. Carefully palpate the thyroid lobe to seek an intraparenchymatous parathyroid adenoma.

If a P III is absent:

1. Remember that migration of P III may be excessive and extend the dissection downwards by performing a thymectomy by the cervical route. The exploration must be made, not by endeavouring to progress downwards, since the space between the manubrium and the trachea is very narrow, but by bringing the thymic lobe upwards by gentle progressive traction, which requires ligation of several veins. The thymus may thus be exteriorised over 8 to 10 cm. The elevated thymic lobe must then be dissected since some adenomas are deeply embedded in its substance.
2. Remember the defective migration of P III (undescended gland)[15] and explore the carotid sheath up to the angle of the mandible.
3. Digitally explore the thyroid lobe.

Table 1.3 • Sites, mechanisms and incidence of major ectopias of parathyroid glands III and IV

Site	Parathyroid concerned	Mechanism of ectopia	Incidence (%)
High ectopia in the neck	P III	Embryological: failure of migration	1–2
Anterosuperior mediastinum	P III	Embryological: excessive migration	3.9–5
Posterosuperior mediastinum	P IV	Acquired migration: gravity	4.8
Middle mediastinum	P V*	Embryological: premature fragmentation(?)	0.19–0.3
Intrathyroid	P III, IV, V	Embryological	0.5–3.5

*PV refers to a supernumerary gland.

Truly intrathyroid parathyroid adenomas are rare.[14,16] Most of these so-called intrathyroid adenomas are more or less deeply embedded in a crevice of the thyroid parenchyma. Some other adenomas are hidden just beneath the thyroid capsule and may be revealed by a localised discoloration of the surface of the thyroid, which darkens progressively. Simple incision of the thyroid capsule then allows their dislodgement from their thyroid resting place. Thyroid excision is the last available procedure, but is only indicated when the preoperative investigations suggest an intrathyroid location. Intraoperative ultrasound may be very helpful here.

At the very end of the exploration, and if the abnormal parathyroid sought is still missing, it is very probable that it is not in the neck but in the mediastinum and forms part of the l–2% of mediastinal adenomas, which are virtually inaccessible from the cervical route. This probability will be the greater if four normal parathyroids have been identified in the neck. Median sternotomy should not be done at the same operation for three reasons:

1. The diagnosis should be confirmed.
2. The adenoma should be precisely localised.
3. Left thoracoscopy[17,18] or anterior mediastinotomy via an incision over and removal of the second costal cartilage[19] can be less invasive alternative approaches.

The operation should be halted at the cervical exploration, but one cannot spend too much time dissecting the neck carefully at the first operation.

The parathyroidectomy

According to the number of glands discovered and the number of abnormal or normal glands, several typical scenarios can be envisaged.

SOLITARY PARATHYROID ADENOMA
(Fig. 1.11, see also Plate 5, facing p. 212)

One gland is enlarged and the other gland(s) discovered are normal. This is the commonest situation. The diagnostic test of a single adenoma being one of exclusion, it is the normal appearance of the other glands that leads to the diagnosis of

Figure 1.11 • Conventional open parathyroidectomy: left superior parathyroid adenoma and normal inferior parathyroid gland.

solitary adenoma. The adenoma must be excised, and normal glands preserved.

SPORADIC MULTIGLANDULAR DISEASE

When two glands are enlarged and the two other glands are normal the distinction between double adenoma and hyperplasia may be impossible during the operation. Excision of both enlarged glands is called for, biopsy of the other two grossly normal glands is questionable considering the major risks of hypoparathyroidism due to traumatic biopsies.

When three glands are enlarged, the diagnosis of hyperplasia must be maintained. Cases of triple adenomas coexisting with a fourth normal gland are doubtful. The fourth normal gland should be preserved.

When all four glands are enlarged (Fig. 1.12, see also Plate 6, facing p. 212), in addition to excision of three glands, the fourth, if possible the smallest, should be reduced so as to leave in place a fragment of a weight estimated as identical to that of a normal gland, i.e. around 40–60 mg.

In rare cases of water-clear-cell hyperplasia, revealed at operation by the presence of unusually large, chocolate-brown glands, it is advised to save a larger fragment (100–150 mg) because the parathyroid tissue in this entity functions poorly.[20]

The choice of gland to be left in place may, however, be dictated by relations with the recurrent nerve. It is preferable to leave the fragment from the gland farthest from the nerve. The excision should always begin by exposure of the fragment intended to be left in situ. If the fragment appears non-viable,

Figure 1.12 • Multiglandular disease: four-gland hyperplasia.

it should be totally resected and the same operation should be done on another gland. Two fragments of smaller size may be left to limit the risks of necrosis and hypoparathyroidism.

FAMILIAL HYPERPARATHYROIDISM

Familial hyperparathyroidism most commonly occurs as a component of multiple endocrine neoplasia type 1 (MEN 1) or type 2A (MEN 2A). It is known to occur also in the absence of other endocrinopathies, and is apparently unassociated with MEN. These hereditary variants are more difficult to treat than sporadic forms. The glands most often exhibit varying degrees of histopathological disease and the underlying genetic abnormality may be responsible for recurrence in spite of apparently adequate initial surgery.

Primary hyperparathyroidism in MEN 1

The basic principles of surgery in patients with MEN 1 and hyperparathyroidism include:

1. Obtaining and maintaining normocalcaemia for the longest time possible, avoiding persistent/recurrent hypercalcaemia.
2. Avoiding surgically induced hypocalcaemia.
3. Facilitating future surgery for recurrent disease.

Two approaches have been described as the best practice for patients with hyperparathyroidism in MEN 1:

- subtotal parathyroidectomy, leaving a remnant of no more than 60 mg in the neck;
- total parathyroidectomy with immediate autotransplantation of 10–20 1-mm^3 pieces of parathyroid tissue.[21]

Both approaches should be combined with efforts to exclude supernumerary glands and ectopic parathyroid tissue by including resection of fatty tissue from the central neck compartment and thymectomy in all patients.

In a small group of MEN 1 patients with clinically apparent unigland disease, it has been proposed to limit excision of parathyroid tissue from the side of the neck with the enlarged gland.[22]

Surgery for hyperparathyroidism in MEN 1 is effectively a palliative procedure for the majority of patients. The underlying disease process predisposes patients to persistent or recurrent disease. Total parathyroidectomy has been reported to have a higher initial 'cure' rate than subtotal resection. However, this should not be the case if a systematic search is made for supernumerary glands. Total parathyroidectomy does carry an increased risk of hypoparathyroidism, of up to 47%.[23,24] Cryopreservation of parathyroid tissue should therefore be performed after total parathyroidectomy and is also recommended after subtotal parathyroidectomy. Delayed autotransplantation using cryopreserved parathyroid can be useful in case of persistent hypoparathyroidism.

A large series of re-operations for persistent and recurrent hyperparathyroidism in MEN 1 patients has been reported.[25] Neck exploration resulted in normocalcaemia in 91% of patients, with a rate of 2.1% of permanent injury to the recurrent laryngeal nerve (RLN). Autograft removal was more problematic and resulted in normocalcaemia in 58% of patients. The use of parathyroid autografts does not always simplify subsequent treatment.[26]

Primary hyperparathyroidism in MEN 2A

Before treating hyperparathyroidism in patients with MEN 2A one must rule out a possible coexistent phaeochromocytoma. Hyperparathyroidism in MEN 2A patients is less aggressive than in MEN 1 patients. The main risk of parathyroid surgery in these patients is hypoparathyroidism. Although MEN 2A patients should be considered to have multiglandular disease, most often not all glands are enlarged and aggressive resections are not recommended. Identification of four glands and excision of only macroscopically enlarged glands is associated with a low rate of persistent or recurrent hyperparathyroidism and avoids postoperative hypoparathyroidism.[27] If they look normal, superior glands should be preserved in preference to inferior. Normal inferior glands (which are at higher risk of necrosis during thyroidectomy for medullary carcinoma, lymph node resection and thymectomy) may be preferably autotransplanted. Some authors recommend total parathyroidectomy with autotransplantation in the forearm.[28] The surgeon must bear in mind that permanent hypoparathyroidism can be a worse disease than mild hyperparathyroidism.

PARATHYROID CARCINOMA

Surgery remains the sole therapy for parathyroid carcinoma. The treatment is conditioned by two quite different situations:

The diagnosis has been established or seriously considered at the first operation. Severe hypercalcaemia with very high parathyroid hormone (PTH) levels in a patient with a palpable neck tumour are the classic 'at risk' signs to suggest malignancy. At operation the tumour appears as a grey enlarged parathyroid, often of hard consistency, with a thick capsule with adherence to the sur-

rounding structures. The surgeon must proceed to an en bloc excision of the parathyroid tumour, the thyroid lobe, the other ipsilateral parathyroid and the recurrent, jugulocarotid and pretracheal lymph nodes. The diagnosis by frozen section is facilitated by this monobloc resection, which will give some idea of the extent of local invasion. Some surgeons remove the lymph nodes only if they are clinically invaded or seen to be so on frozen section. If the recurrent nerve is invaded it should be sacrificed.[29,30] The contralateral parathyroids are routinely explored.

The diagnosis is only made postoperatively, from the definitive paraffin section histology. The initial operation will usually have been a simple removal of the tumour. It is advisable to re-operate as soon as possible and to resect the structures adjacent to the tumour, especially if there has been persistent postoperative hypercalcaemia.[30]

Rarely, no obvious evidence of malignancy is found and only the development of recurrences or metastases reveals the true nature of the tumour.

Parathyroid carcinomas are relatively slow growing and should be followed up for life, essentially by clinical evaluation and blood-calcium levels. Local recurrences develop in up to 50% of patients. Distant metastases can be expected in 30% of patients.[31] Most authors advocate, wherever possible, an aggressive surgical policy towards recurrences and metastases.[32,33] Residual tumoral tissue in the neck must be removed en bloc, if necessary together with invaded neighbouring organs such as the trachea or muscular wall of the oesophagus.[30] Distant metastases are most often found in the lungs and bones and may or may not be associated with local recurrence. Any subsequent operations are rarely curative. Disease-free survival of 20–70% and overall survival of 13–70% can be expected 10 years following initial resection.[31] The threat to life is related to the degree of hypercalcaemia, so that long-term survival is possible in the presence of metastases if biochemical control is adequate.[33]

PARATHYROIDECTOMY ASSOCIATED WITH THYROID EXCISIONS

Explorations combining thyroidectomy and parathyroidectomy are frequent. Primary parathyroid exploration is recommended first. Indeed, excision of the thyroid lobe first would lead to section of all the landmarks and moorings used by the surgeon to direct his search for parathyroid tissue. It may also be responsible for an accidental parathyroidectomy, which may pass unnoticed. In cases of a benign thyroid lesion, there should be no hesitation in preserving a layer of thyroid parenchyma so as not to compromise the vascularisation of a normal parathyroid. Excluding MEN 2A patients, definitive hypoparathyroidism is observed in 4.3% of patients who undergo concomitant thyroidectomy and parathyroidectomy.[34]

Overall results of conventional open parathyroidectomy

The immediate operative outcome is usually very straightforward. The plasma calcium returns to normal in 24–48 hours. Nowadays so few patients have bone involvement to a severe degree that significant postoperative hypocalcaemia is relatively uncommon. Preventive treatment for hypocalcaemia is not justified. Apart from hypocalcaemia, the morbidity of parathyroidectomy is mainly represented by laryngeal nerve palsy and haematomas, but this is now reported in only 1% or less of cases.[1] The mortality of parathyroidectomy is very low, close to zero.

PTH levels decrease and are almost undetectable 4 hours after surgery, then begin to return within the normal range on day 1.[35] One month after surgery elevated serum PTH levels are observed in up to 30% of patients despite normalisation of serum calcium levels. In some cases elevated PTH levels are an adaptive reaction to renal dysfunction or vitamin D deficiency.[35] It has also been recently demonstrated that patients operated on for primary hyperparathyroidism (PHP) show decreased peripheral sensitivity to PTH.[36]

When conventional open parathyroidectomy is done by an expert surgeon, 95–98% of patients become normocalcaemic.[1] With MGD the results are less satisfactory than with solitary adenomas. A multicentric study showed that 20% of MEN 1 patients were still hypercalcaemic immediately after surgery.[37] Therefore patients with familial PHP must be managed in specialised centres.

MINIMALLY INVASIVE PARATHYROIDECTOMY (MIP)

In recent years, several new minimally invasive techniques for parathyroidectomy have been developed. These techniques have two common threads:

1. They all have a limited incision when compared with classic open transverse cervical incision.
2. The surgery is targeted on one specific parathyroid gland. In most cases the exploration of other glands is not performed or is limited.

The concept of these limited explorations is based on the fact that 85% of patients will have single-gland disease. Limited parathyroid surgery has been made possible by improvement in preoperative localisation techniques using sestamibi scanning and/or ultrasonography. Nevertheless, whether localisation study results can rule out multi-glandular disease (MGD) is questionable, and for most surgeons the risk of missing MGD during a limited parathyroid exploration justifies the systematic use of the quick parathyroid hormone assay (QPTH) assay.

Patients suspected of MGD on imaging studies or patients with familial hyperparathyroidism are not eligible for limited procedures. Therefore, MIP should be proposed only for patients with sporadic hyperparathyroidism in whom a single adenoma has been clearly localised by means of sonography and sestamibi scanning. In addition evidence of associated nodular goitre and history of previous neck operations may contraindicate MIP. Finally suspicion of parathyroid carcinoma is an absolute contraindication for MIP since these tumours require an extensive en bloc excision.

A recent survey from the International Association of Endocrine Surgeons showed that more than half the surgeons responding now performed MIP.[38] Most of these procedures can be performed either under general or regional anaesthesia.

Unilateral neck exploration

Initially the concept of unilateral exploration was based on finding an enlarged gland and an ipsilateral normal gland.[39–41] Since the introduction of QPTH assay, attempts to identify the ipsilateral gland are no longer made,[42,43] and in most cases unilateral exploration is focused on one gland alone.

Open minimally invasive parathyroidectomy (OMIP)

This procedure is suitable for day-case surgery.[44,45] Accurate preoperative localisation is a prerequisite condition for OMIP. The procedure is carried out through a 2–4 cm incision. For upper adenomas, the incision is made on the anterior border of the sternocleidomastoid muscle (SCM) and a postero-lateral, or 'back-door', approach is used to reach the retrothyroid space. For anterior lower adenomas the incision is made at the suprasternal notch level. This technique when compared with bilateral neck exploration has shown less overall complications (1.2% vs. 3.0%), a 50% reduction in operating time, and a substantial reduction in postoperative stay.[46,47]

Minimally invasive radioguided parathyroidectomy (MIRP)

MIRP is characterised by the use of an intraoperative gamma-probe to direct the dissection according to the level of radioactivity.[48] The operation must be carried out within 3.5 h of the radiopharmaceutical injection. The incision (2–3 cm) is placed according to the expected location of the adenoma as deter-mined by both sestamibi scanning and measure-ment of gamma emissions on the skin. There is no need to use QPTH measurements.[49] The operation is complete if the excised adenoma has more than 20% of background activity. Gratifying results have been obtained from this technique.[50]

Endoscopic parathyroidectomy

Endoscopic techniques are particularly suitable for parathyroid surgery for several reasons:

1. They are the only ablative procedures that do not require any elaborate surgical reconstruction.

2. Most parathyroid tumours are small and benign.
3. Reduction in the length of the scar to about 10–15 mm is appealing to many patients.

The first endoscopic removal of enlarged parathyroid glands was from the mediastinum. Thoracoscopy has successfully allowed excision of mediastinal parathyroid adenomas located deep in the anterior mediastinum or in the midde mediastinum.[17,18]

The three endoscopic neck procedures in most widespread use are:

1. **The pure endoscopic parathyroidectomy.**[51] This technique includes constant gas insufflation and four trocars. A large subplatysmal space is created by blunt dissection. Then the midline is opened and the strap muscles retracted in order to expose the thyroid lobes. A bilateral parathyroid exploration is possible.

2. **Minimally invasive video-assisted parathyroidectomy (MIVAP).**[52] A 15-mm skin incision is made at the suprasternal notch. The cervical midline is opened, and complete dissection of the thyroid lobe is obtained by blunt dissection under endoscopic vision. Small conventional retractors maintain the operative space. This gasless procedure is carried out only through the midline incision and also permits a bilateral exploration.

3. **Endoscopic parathyroidectomy by lateral approach.**[53] A 15-mm transverse skin incision is made on the anterior border of the SCM and a back-door approach is used to reach the retrothyroid space. Three trocars (one 10 mm and two 2–3 mm) are inserted on the line of the anterior border of the SCM (**Fig. 1.13**, see also Plate 7, facing p. 212). The working space is maintained with low-pressure CO_2 at 8 mmHg. During this unilateral exploration, one can identify both the adenoma and the ipsilateral parathyroid gland. The lateral approach is applicable in all cases where the parathyroid lesions are located posteriorly.

Other endoscopic techniques, avoiding scars in the neck area, have been proposed but are less commonly used: axillary approach[54] and anterior chest approach.[55,56]

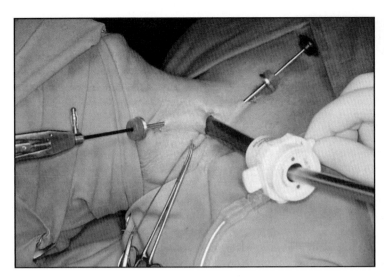

Figure 1.13 • Endoscopic parathyroidectomy by lateral approach – trocar position.

Depending on the type of access employed, conversion to conventional parathyroidectomy is necessary in 8–15% of cases.[57–59] The main causes for conversion include difficulties of dissection, capsular ruptures of large adenomas, false-positive results of imaging studies and MGD not detected by preoperative imaging but correctly predicted by QPTH assay results. In experienced hands endoscopic parathyroid techniques are as safe as the standard open procedure. There is no mortality. The incidence of recurrent nerve palsy is less than 1%. Insufflation is harmless as long as the procedure is performed under low pressure. Endoscopic operations can be completed in less than one hour and the operating time improves dramatically after the first few procedures.[57–59] Nevertheless, these operations are technically more challenging than standard cervical exploration. Endoscopic techniques have the main advantage of offering a magnified view that permits a precise and careful dissection with minimal risks (**Fig. 1.14**, see also Plate 8, facing p. 212). By direct vision through mini-incisions it is probably more difficult to get an adequate view of structures, and optimal conditions for exploration are not met even if surgeons use frontal lamps and surgical loops.

 Two studies comparing conventional parathyroid surgery with endoscopic techniques have shown a diminution of postoperative pain and better cosmetic results with endoscopic techniques[60,61] (**Fig. 1.15**).

Figure 1.14• Endoscopic parathyroidectomy by left lateral approach: recurrent laryngeal nerve and superior parathyroid adenoma.

MIVAP is also associated with a shorter operative time.[60] Those benefits await confirmation by further randomised studies.

MIP in the broader context

After MIP 95–100% of patients are normo-calcaemic.[43,46,48,57–59] However, it should be kept in mind that these excellent results are obtained in a group of carefully selected patients. In addition the risk of persistent PHP is minimised by the use of intraoperative QPTH assessment.

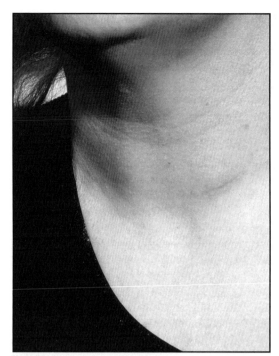

Figure 1.15 Endoscopic parathyroidectomy by lateral approach. Cervical scar after 1 week.

In contrast to open surgery, the MIP surgeon depends on multiple technologies:

1. The adenoma should be clearly localised before the operation. If the lesion is unique and confirmed by imaging studies, a MIP can be proposed. One can choose a lateral or central approach depending on whether the lesion has a posterior or anterior location.
2. The availability of the QPTH assay is of utmost importance. The overall accuracy of intraoperative QPTH monitoring is reported to be 97%.[62] This test may be especially useful when localisation studies are less certain.
3. MIP, and particularly endoscopic techniques, require dedicated instruments.

Demonstrating the advantages of minimally invasive techniques for parathyroid surgery is not easy. Whether MIP is actually less costly than conventional parathyroidectomy is difficult to quantify. The true advantages of MIP to the patient in terms of comfort and cosmetic results are especially impressive on the first postoperative days.[46,50,60,61]

MIP should not replace or be opposed to conventional parathyroidectomy. These operations will probably turn out to be complementary to each other in the future. A longer follow-up is needed before one can evaluate the real risk of recurrent PHP following minimally invasive techniques.

RE-OPERATION FOR PERSISTENT OR RECURRENT PRIMARY HYPERPARATHYROIDISM (PHP)

Persistent PHP is defined as the persistence of hypercalcaemia due to hyperparathyroidism in the 6 months following the initial operation. Recurrent PHP refers to the reappearance of hypercalcaemia after 6 months of normocalcaemia.

Analysis of causes of failure

Before undertaking a second exploration of the neck for PHP it is essential to understand the causes of failure of the initial operation. Persistent PHP may be due to a negative exploration or an excision that is inadequate or inappropriate to the lesions discovered. Thus, persistent PHP is nearly always due to technical error during the first operation. Very rarely, failure is virtually inevitable during the first operation, due to supernumerary glands and major ectopia.

Recurrent PHP constitutes a more complex and controversial problem. The significance of a normocalcaemic interval of at least 6 months between the first operation and the reappearance of hypercalcaemia is debatable. The question is whether this is a true cure of the PHP or a persistent PHP masked by transient return to normal calcaemia.[63,64] Recurrences may develop after normocalcaemic intervals of several years. In most cases they are seen in patients initially operated on for MGD. The development of a second adenoma in a normal gland, which has been checked at the first operation, is uncommon. Persistent PHP is much more commonly observed than recurrent PHP: 80–90% vs. 10–20%.[64]

Carcinoma has a special place among the causes of failed parathyroid surgery. It may be responsible for persistent as well as recurrent PHP. In some

Table 1.4 • Re-operation for persistent-recurrent primary hyperparathyroidism: information supplied from study of case records and surgical implications

Information	Procedure indicated
Familial hyperparathyroidism MEN 1 or MEN 2A	Complete exploration of all residual parathyroid tissue Adapt resection to type of familial hyperparathyroidism
Multiglandular lesions	Complete exploration of all residual parathyroid tissue
Three normal glands	Adenoma not found. Re-operation guided by preoperative localisation studies
P III identified (thymus) P IV identified	Search for homolateral P IV Search for homolateral P III
Four normal glands in neck; experienced surgeon	Adenoma in major ectopic site: mediastinal site very probable
Cancer suspected or atypical adenoma	Suspect local recurrence and look for visceral or bony metastases
Several normal glands removed	Arrange for cryopreservation

cases the recurrence of the carcinoma allows correction of an initial misdiagnosis of a benign adenoma. Recurrences in situ, probably due to capsular rupture and local spread, are due to carcinomas in most of cases but can be seen after removal of a benign lesion (parathyromatosis).

Finally, recurrences have been reported as occurring in grafts of adenomas or hyperplastic glands implanted in the brachioradialis muscle after total parathyroidectomy. It is not the volume of the implanted tissue that is responsible for the recurrence but its uncontrollable hyperfunctional nature, due either to its autonomy or to the effect of local stimulating factors.

Management

CONFIRMATION OF THE DIAGNOSIS

The diagnosis of PHP can only be raised again after elimination of other causes of hypercalcaemia and fresh confirmation of the biochemical syndrome. Among the many causes of persistent hypercalcaemia after unsuccessful parathyroidectomy, thought should be given to the syndrome of familial hypocalciuric hypercalcaemia (FHH).[65] A few patients have been documented as having non-parathyroid tumours that make pure PTH.[66]

CASE HISTORY

The sporadic or familial nature of the PHP should be determined by searching for a family history or another associated endocrinopathy that may fit into the picture of a MEN 1 or 2A. Study of the operation notes is vital to gain details of the operative and histology reports from previous operations. This will supply the surgeon with information that is helpful in planning operative tactics (**Table 1.4**).

PREOPERATIVE LOCALISATION

While preoperative localisation studies may not seem essential, or even desirable, in the case of a primary bilateral exploration most authors consider that ultrasonography and sestamibi scan should be performed routinely in the work-up for any persistent or recurrent PHP. CT scan and MRI should be reserved for patients in whom the former imaging techniques have failed or when a mediastinal location is strongly suspected. Invasive procedures, including selective venous sampling of PTH or selective angiography, should be performed only if non-invasive procedures are inconclusive. Sometimes, image-guided fine-needle aspiration (FNA) may help distinguish a parathyroid tumour from other structures.

The topographic diagnosis should ideally be established by convergence of the results of at least two different investigations. When used together, imaging techniques correctly identify abnormal glands in nearly 95% of cases.[67–73]

METHODS OF RE-OPERATION

Once the diagnosis has been confirmed, the indications for operation must be discussed. Not every patient needs to be re-operated on. The risks

Figure 1.16 Secondary hyperparathyroidism: four-gland hyperplasia.

of doing so should be assessed and balanced against those of leaving the patient with PHP. When available, intraoperative ultrasound and gamma-probe may be helpful here. Most surgeons consider that QPTH monitoring is mandatory in these patients. The increased rate of recurrent nerve damage in these re-operations calls for precise preoperative assessment of the state of the vocal cords.[74]

According to the case history and the results of localisation studies the surgeon must clearly establish if there is or is not a suspicion of MGD (**Fig. 1.16**, see also Plate 9, facing p. 212). If the lesion sought is a solitary adenoma, an open focused approach can be proposed. Conversely, if there is confirmation or strong suspicion of MGD, revision of the transverse cervicotomy is recommended.

The posterolateral approach ('back-door' approach)

This focused approach should be considered when the adenoma sought has been visualised in a posterocervical site: the missing adenoma is probably a P IV. The previous transverse incision is enlarged laterally on the anterior border of the sternocleidomastoid. The approach is behind the muscles and the thyroid, in a zone that is intact or little affected by the previous operation. Search for P IV is made as already described.

The thyrothymic approach ('front-door' approach)

This approach should be considered when the adenoma sought has been visualised anteriorly at the lower pole of the thyroid or along the thyrothymic axis. The missing adenoma is probably a P III. A transverse skin incision is used along the previous cervical incision. The infrahyoid muscles are divided as low as possible allowing direct access to the thyrothymic ligaments. This manoeuvre avoids any dissection between the prethyroid muscles and the thyroid capsule. Search for P III is made as already described.

Revision of the transverse cervicotomy

This long and difficult re-operation is indicated when there is confirmation or strong suspicion of MGD. Search for P IV and P III is made as already described. Ideally all the glands must be identified and assessed. This also involves a search for accessory glands and a bilateral thymectomy. QPTH monitoring and cryopreservation are particularly recommended.

Mediastinal approaches

Most mediastinal adenomas located in the posterior mediastinum or in the anterior mediastinum above the aortic arch can be excised through the neck.[67–73] Only adenomas located deep in the anterior mediastinum or in the middle mediastinum require a thoracic approach. The appropriate approach will be dependent upon careful consideration of localising studies and the depth of the lesion in the mediastinum. Precise localisation can allow a less invasive approach than sternal split: anterior mediastinotomy[19] or left thoracoscopy[17,18] may be preferable to partial or total sternotomy.

Other focused approaches

These approaches concern glands located in a major ectopic cervical area and not accessible via the previous cervicotomy. The skin incision is placed according to the expected location of the adenoma as determined by imaging studies: undescended glands;[15,75] within the carotid sheath in association with the vagus nerve;[75] lateral to the jugulocarotid axis.[76]

ASSOCIATED PROCEDURES

Immediate autotransplantation is debatable, since the hyperfunctional grafts may interfere with assessment of the results of parathyroidectomy. In the presence of persistent PHP it may not be clear whether the source of recurrence is the autograft or residual cervical or mediastinal tissue. Therefore, routine immediate autotransplantation is not recommended.[77–79]

Cryopreservation and secondary autotransplantation are essential adjuncts to re-operation for PHP. In cases of postoperative hypocalcaemia, secondary autotransplantation should not be done too soon. Some hypocalcaemic patients do not spontaneously regain normocalcaemia until after a year.[79] This is the delay that seems advisable before considering secondary autotransplantation.

Graft recurrences must be proven before re-operation on the graft site. Tumoral grafts are sometimes palpable, or may be located by ultrasound or sestamibi scan. In every case, the possibility of recurrence in residual cervical or mediastinal tissue must be eliminated before re-operating on the arm, and Casanova's test may be very helpful.[80]

Results

With experienced parathyroid surgeons, the success rate of re-operations can be as high as 95%.[67–73,81–83] The overall perioperative morbidity, on average 20%, is much higher than in cases of primary neck exploration. There is a dramatically increased risk of permanent recurrent laryngeal nerve paralysis (up to 10%) compared with initial parathyroid surgery. In up to 20% of cases permanent hypoparathyroidism may result. Transplantation of hyperfunctional tissue can result in recurrent disease in 7–17% of patients. Grafts may fail to function in 6–50% of transplanted tissue, with failure occurring more frequently when using cryopreserved tissue.

SECONDARY HYPERPARATHYROIDISM (SHP)

Hyperparathyroidism secondary to uraemia

Secondary hyperparathyroidism (SHP) is present in most, if not all, patients undergoing long-term haemodialysis. Most of them can be managed by prophylaxis and medical therapy. However, between 2.5% and 28% of these patients require surgery because of severe reactive renal hyperparathyroidism, i.e. uncontrolled hypercalcaemia, hyperphosphataemia, high levels of PTH (>500 pg/mL), bone erosions and osteitis fibrosa.

SURGICAL STRATEGIES

The surgical treatment can be considered palliative in nature. Surgery is indicated to treat and prevent the complications of SHP. The underlying disease process, i.e., chronic renal failure, predisposes patients to recurrent disease. Surgery performed in these patients should therefore aim to:

- obtain and maintain correction of hyperparathyroidism for the longest time possible, avoiding persistent disease;
- avoid surgically induced severe hypocalcaemia;
- facilitate future surgery for recurrent disease.

Localisation diagnosis is often considered unnecessary because patients will systematically undergo bilateral neck exploration. However, imaging studies may be performed for two reasons: (i) to reduce the operation time;[84] and (ii) to detect supernumerary and ectopic glands, of which the incidence (6.5–25%) is increased due to the ongoing stimulation of renal failure.[85,86]

The surgical treatment of SHP is performed by using one of two main techniques:

1. **Subtotal parathyroidectomy (SPTX).**[87] This involves identifying four glands and removing at least three but leaving a parathyroid remnant in the neck (approximately 50 mg). The most diffusely hyperplastic gland should be selected. The main disadvantage of this approach is that

a second cervical exploration would be needed if persistent or recurrent SHP occurs.

2. **Total parathyroidectomy + autotransplantation (TPTX + AT).**[88] This involves the resection of at least four glands combined with the transplantation of 10–20 1-mm³ pieces of parathyroid tissue into individual pockets created in the brachioradialis muscle of the forearm, principally to aid future surgery under local anaesthetic for recurrent disease.

The glands may be markedly enlarged. They are often pale and hard, with fibrosis and calcifications, and may be difficult to distinguish from thyroid tissue or lymph nodes (**Fig. 1.16**).

To exclude supernumerary glands resection of fatty tissue from the central neck compartment and bilateral thymectomy should also be performed in both techniques.

Theoretically, there should be no difference in outcome in terms of persistent or recurrent hypercalcaemia between these two approaches, as both involve the controlled excision of all parathyroid tissue, but for a remnant in the neck or as grafts in the arm.

The intraoperative selection of the tissue to be left in the neck or the forearm is of particular importance. Neck-remnant or graft-dependent recurrences are observed most often in patients with nodular tissue at initial surgery.[89–91] In practice, this intraoperative tissue selection is easier to perform ex vivo prior to autotransplantation rather than during the parathyroidectomy.

Because parathyroid remnants or grafts can undergo ischaemic necrosis and result in permanent hypoparathyroidism, cryopreservation of parathyroid tissue should be performed whenever facilities are available.

Both techniques have advantages and disadvantages (**Table 1.5**), and no definitive answer can be given to the question of which method is superior.[92–94] Total parathyroidectomy is recommended for patients with four markedly enlarged glands and for patients who are not transplant candidates.[92–93] Subtotal parathyroidectomy is favoured for children, for patients scheduled to receive a renal transplant, and for patients with any normal-sized parathyroid detected at surgery. Total parathyroidectomy alone, without autotransplantation, may be proposed in frail patients with many risk factors who are not candidates for future renal transplant, or in patients with calciphylaxis. These patients will require permanent therapy with oral calcium and vitamin D postoperatively.

PERIOPERATIVE CARE

Patients may receive oral calcitriol before operation to decrease the severity and the duration of postoperative hypocalcaemia. They should undergo dialysis within one day of operation and then 48 hours postoperatively or as needed. The risk of bleeding is increased as heparin is used during haemodialysis. Hypocalcaemia is found after subtotal and total parathyroidectomy with autotransplantation in 6.3% and 1.4% respectively.[93] Hypocalcaemia may be severe in patients who have

Table 1.5 • Advantages and disadvantages of subtotal parathyroidectomy (SPTX) and total parathyroidectomy + autotransplantation (TPTX + AT) in patients with secondary hyperparathyroidism

Surgical procedure	Advantages	Disadvantages
SPTX	Short or no period of hypocalcaemia postoperatively	Tissue selection not always possible Morbidity of cervical re-operation
TPTX + AT	Tissue selection possible Low morbidity of re-operations on the autografts	Longer period of hypocalcaemia postoperatively Problems in localising the hyperactive tissue: autografts or supernumerary gland? Identification and resection of autografts not always easy (seeding in the muscle)
Both procedures		Do not avoid persistent/recurrent disease due to ectopic supernumerary gland

marked bone disease, and this may require intra-venous calcium. Prolonged hypocalcaemia should be treated with calcitriol (1–4 µg/day) and oral calcium.

Delayed autotransplantation of cryopreserved tissue may be helpful in correcting hypoparathyroidism but should not be performed within 6 months following surgery. However, the functional results are less good than after immediate auto-transplantation of fresh parathyroid tissue.[95,96]

PERSISTENT AND RECURRENT SHP

Persistent or recurrent SHP is encountered in 2–12% of patients. The causes are multiple. First, the initial parathyroidectomy may have been incomplete. It must be expected that an initial resection of no more than three glands will prove to be insufficient. Likewise, the parathyroidectomy may be inadequate if the remnant is too large – more than 60 mg. In both cases, surgical failure accounts for persistent SHP. Recurrent SHP may also be observed after successful subtotal or total parathyroidectomy. Further hyperplasia of para-thyroid tissue can occur in the remnant left in the neck or in autografted fragments in the forearm.

It is known that up to 15% of haemodialysis patients have a supernumerary parathyroid gland in the neck or mediastinum.[11,85,86,97] After removal of four parathyroids, these supernumerary 'missed' glands are capable of causing persistent or recurrent SHP and represent a third cause of surgical failure. During the initial operation, they are usually small and often appear to be embryological rests of para-thyroid cells. Most of these glands are associated with the thymus, either in the mediastinum or the neck. Usually without physiological importance, they can develop functional significance because of long-term stimulation over many years in patients with chronic renal failure.

Another cause of recurrent SHP is para-thyromatosis, in which capsular rupture of the pathological gland causes spillage and inadvertent autotransplantation of cells in the operative site. This tissue will grow and lead to recurrent disease.

In persistent/recurrent SHP, all patients who require re-operation should undergo localisation studies. After TPTX + AT it must be kept in mind that recurrences can occur not only on the grafts but also on supernumerary glands in the neck or the mediastinum. The Casanova test[80] can be used to evaluate whether the origin of recurrence is a residual gland or grafted tissue. The incidence of persistent/recurrent SHP is similar after SPTX and TPTX + AT, namely 5.8% and 6.6% respectively.[93] Cervical re-operations in this setting are more invasive, require greater surgical expertise, and are associated with a higher morbidity than the excision of an autograft in the forearm.

Nevertheless, re-operations on autografted para-thyroid fragments are not always technically simple. Not all the grafts grow in the same way. Some become hypertrophic whereas others stay hypotrophic. Attempts to locate them precisely are difficult because they are embedded in the muscle at varying depths. The volume of the tissue that has to be removed or left is difficult to evaluate. This is particularly true when there is exuberant pseudo-invasive overgrowth that sometimes requires repeated graft resections. In these cases some surgeons prefer to remove all the transplanted tissue as completely as possible.[98] In some cases the problem of persistent or recurrent SHP is no easier to solve after TPTX + AT than after SPTX.[99] Cryopreservation of parathyroid tissue is strongly recommended in re-operations.[96]

Lithium-induced hyperparathyroidism

Approximately 10–15% of lithium-treated patients become hypercalcaemic. This condition is often reversible if lithium is withdrawn. Lithium-induced hyperparathyroidism was first reported in 1973.[100] Hypercalcaemia is generally mild with slight elevation of PTH. It has been suggested that lithium stimulates the entire parathyroid tissue, resulting in hyperplasia,[101] but the literature does not support this proposition, with 33 of 49 reported cases showing a single adenoma as the cause of hyperparathyroidism.[102] Alternatively, it has been suggested that lithium may unmask underlying PHP.[102] For patients who require ongoing treatment with lithium, surgery is indicated.[101–103] The incidence of MGD in this setting contraindicates minimally invasive surgery. Excision should be limited to evidently enlarged glands.

TERTIARY HYPERPARATHYROIDISM

Tertiary hyperparathyroidism is a persistent autonomous hypercalcaemic hyperparathyroidism occurring after kidney transplantation. After renal transplant the hypercalcaemia resolves in 50% of patients in the first month, in 85% in the first 6 months, and in 95% after 6 months. However, elevated PTH and abnormal bone biopsy persist in up to 70% of patients with long-term grafts.[104]

Several factors may prevent the involution of the hyperplastic gland after the primary stimulus, i.e. kidney failure, has been removed:

- impaired renal graft function;
- non-suppressible PTH secretion;
- autonomy or slow involution of parathyroid glands;
- insufficient calcitriol conversion by the kidney.[105–107]

Only 0.2–0.3% of all patients with kidney transplants are reported to require parathyroid surgery.[108] Indications for parathyroidectomy are: subacute severe hypercalcaemia (>3 mmol/L) and symptomatic persistent (>2 years) hypercalcaemia. Transplant patients rarely develop recurrent hyperparathyroidism.

Key points

- Bilateral neck exploration is the gold standard in parathyroid surgery.
- In sporadic primary hyperparathyroidism surgical excision is based on macroscopic evaluation: enlarged glands should be removed, normal glands should be preserved.
- In MEN 1 patients subtotal parathyroidectomy or total parathyroidectomy with autotransplantation should be combined with efforts to exclude supernumerary glands.
- In MEN 2A patients the main risk of parathyroid surgery is hypoparathyroidism.
- In patients with parathyroid carcinoma extensive en bloc surgery is recommended at initial operation and in cases of local recurrence or metastasis.
- In primary hyperparathyroidism, 1 month after successful parathyroidectomy, up to 30% of patients have elevated serum PTH levels despite normalisation of serum calcium levels.
- Minimally invasive parathyroidectomy should be proposed only for patients with sporadic primary hyperparathyroidism in whom a single adenoma has been clearly localised by imaging studies.
- The diagnosis of persistent or recurrent primary hyperparathyroidism can only be raised again after elimination of other causes of hypercalcaemia and confirmation of the biochemical syndrome.
- The sporadic or familial nature of primary hyperparathyroidism should be determined for any re-operation for persistent or recurrent hyperparathyroidism.
- In persistent or recurrent primary or secondary hyperparathyroidism, all patients who require re-operation should undergo localisation studies.
- In patients with secondary hyperparathyroidism the key to a successful operation is to locate all parathyroid glands (supernumerary glands included) and leave 40–60 mg of viable tissue as a remnant in the neck or as an autotransplant in the forearm.
- After total parathyroidectomy + autotransplantation it must be remembered that recurrences are possible not only in the autografts but also in supernumerary glands in the neck or the mediastinum.

REFERENCES

1. Van Heerden JA, Grant CS. Surgical treatment of primary hyperparathyroidism: An institutional perspective. World J Surg 1991; 15:688–92.

2. Cope O. Hyperparathyroidism: diagnosis and management. Am J Surg 1960; 99:394–7.

3. Badder EM, Graham WP, Harrison TS. Functional insignificance of microscopic parathyroid hyperplasia. Surg Gynecol Obstet 1977; 145:863–8.

4. Harrison TS, Duarte B, Reitz RE et al. Primary hyperparathyroidism: four to eight year postoperative follow-up demonstrating persistent functional insignificance of microscopic parathyroid hyperplasia and decreased autonomy of parathyroid hormone release. Ann Surg 1981; 194:429–37.

5. Edis AJ, Beahrs OH, Van Heerden JA. "Conservative" versus "liberal" approach to parathyroid neck exploration. Surgery 1977; 82:446–73.

6. Kaplan EL, Bartlett S, Sugimoto J. Relation of postoperative hypocalcemia to operative techniques. Deleterious effect of excessive use of parathyroid biopsy. Surgery 1982; 92:827–34.

7. Lo Gerfo P, Kim LJ. Technique for regional anesthesia: thyroidectomy and parathyroidectomy. In: Van Heerden JA, Farley DR (eds) Operative technique in general surgery. Surgical exploration for hyperparathyroidism. Philadelphia: WB Saunders, 1999; pp. 95–102.

8. Meurisse M, Hamoir E, Defechereux T. Bilateral neck exploration under hypnosedation. A new standard of care in primary hyperparathyroidism. Ann Surg 1999; 229:401–8.

9. Wang CA. The anatomic basis of parathyroid surgery. Ann Surg 1976; 183:271–5.

10. Gilmour JR. The gross anatomy of the parathyroid glands. J Pathol Bact 1938; 46:133–49.

11. Akerstrom G, Malmaeus J, Bergstrom R. Surgical anatomy of human parathyroid glands. Surgery 1984; 95:14–21.

12. Thompson NW. The techniques of initial parathyroid exploration and reoperative parathyroidectomy. In: Thompson NW, Vinik AI (eds) Endocrine surgery update. New York: Grune & Stratton, 1983; pp. 365–83.

13. Delattre JF, Flament JB, Palot JP. Les variations des parathyroïdes. J Chir 1982; 119:633–41.

14. Henry JF, Denizot A. Anatomic and embryologic aspects of primary hyperparathyroidism. In: Barbier J, Henry JF (eds) Primary hyperparathyroidism. Paris: Springer-Verlag, 1992; pp. 5–18.

15. Fraker DL, Doppman JL, Shawker TH et al. Undescended parathyroid adenoma: An important etiology for failed operations for primary hyperparathyroidism. World J Surg 1990; 14: 342–8.

16. Wheeler MH, Williams ED, Wade JSH. The hyperfunctioning intrathyroid parathyroid gland: a potential pitfall in parathyroid surgery. World J Surg 1987; 11: 110–14.

17. Prinz RA, Lonchina V, Carnaille B et al. Thoracoscopic excision of enlarged mediastinal parathyroid glands. Surgery 1994; 116:999–1005.

18. Ishikawa T, Onoda N, Ogawa Y et al. Thoracoscopic excision for ectopic mediastinal parathyroid tumor. Biomed Pharmacother 2002; 56:34–6.

19. Schinkert RT, Whitaker MD, Argueta R. Resection of select mediastinal parathyroid adenomas through an anterior mediastinotomy. Mayo Clin Proc 1991; 66:1110–13.

20. Tisell L, Hedman J, Hanson G. Clinical characteristics and surgical results in hyperparathyroidism caused by water-clear cell hyperplasia. World J Surg 1981; 5:565–72.

21. Wells SA, Ellis GJ, Gunnels JC et al. Parathyroid autotransplantation in primary parathyroid hyperplasia. N Engl J Med 1976; 295:57–62.

22. Kraimps JL, Duh QY, Demeure M et al. Hyperparathyroidism in multiple endocrine neoplasia syndrome. Surgery 1992; 112:1080–8.

23. O'Riordain DS, O'Brien T, Grant CS et al. Surgical management of primary hyperparathyroidism in multiple endocrine neoplasia type 1 and 2. Surgery 1993; 114:1031–9.

24. Hellman P, Skogseid B, Oberg K et al. Primary and reoperative operations in parathyroid operations in hyperparathyroidism of multiple endocrine neoplasia type 1. Surgery 1998; 124:993–9.

25. Kivlen MH, Bartlett DL, Libutti SK et al. Reoperation for hyperparathyroidism in multiple endocrine neoplasia type 1 (MEN 1). Surgery 2001; 130:991–8.

26. Hubbard JGH, Sebag F, Maweja S et al. Primary hyperparathyroidism in MEN I – how radical should surgery be? Langenbeck's Arch Surg 2002; 368:553–7.

27. Dralle H, Scheumann GFW, Kotzerke J et al. Surgical management of MEN-2. Rec Res Cancer Res 1992; 125:167–95.

28. Wells SA, Farndon JR, Dale JK et al. Long term evaluation of patients with primary parathyroid hyperplasia managed by total parathyroidectomy and heterotopic autotransplantation. Ann Surg 1980; 192:451–8.

29. Sandelin K. Parathyroid carcinoma. In: Clark OH, Duh QY (eds) Textbook of endocrine surgery. Philadelphia: WB Saunders, 1997; pp. 439–43.

30. Obara T, Fujimoto Y. Diagnosis and treatment of patients with parathyroid carcinoma: an update and review. World J Surg 1991; 15:738–44.

31. Sandelin K, Auer G, Bondeson L et al. Prognostic factors in parathyroid cancer: a review of 95 cases. World J Surg 1992; 16:724–31.

32. Obara T, Okamoto T, Ito Y et al. Surgical and medical management of patients with pulmonary metastasis from parathyroid carcinoma. Surgery 1993; 114:1040–8.

33. Sandelin K, Tullgren O, Farnebo LO. Clinical course of metastatic parathyroid cancer. World J Surg 1994; 18:594–8.

34. Henry JF, Denizot A. Initial surgery for primary hyperparathyroidism. In: Barbier J, Henry JF (eds) Primary hyperparathyroidism. Paris: Springer-Verlag, 1992; pp. 87–109.

35. Denizot A, Pucini M, Chagnaud C et al. Normo-calcaemia with elevated parathormone levels after surgical treatment of primary hyperparathyroidism. Am J Surg 2001; 182:15–19.

36. Nordenstrom E, Westerdahl J, Isaksson A. Patients with elevated serum parathyroid hormone levels after parathyroidectomy showing signs of decreased peripheral parathyroid hormone sensitivity. World J Surg 2003; 27:212–15.

37. Goudet P, Cougard P, Vergès B et al. Hyper-parathyroidism in multiple endocrine neoplasia type 1: surgical trends and results of a 256-patient series from Group d'Etude des Néoplasies Endocriniennes Multiples study group. World J Surg 2001; 25:886–90.

38. Sackett WR, Barraclough B, Reeve TS et al. Worldwide trends in the surgical treatment of primary hyperparathyroidism in the era of minimally invasive parathyroidectomy. Arch Surg 2002; 137:1055–9.

39. Roth SI, Wang CA, Pott JT. The team approach to primary hyperparathyroidism. Hum Pathol 1975; 6:645–52.

40. Tibblin SA, Bondeson AG, Ljunberg O. Unilateral parathyroidectomy in hyperparathyroidism due to single adenoma. Ann Surg 1982; 195:245–52.

41. Russel CF, Laird JD, Fergusson WR. Scan-directed unilateral cervical exploration for parathyroid adenoma: a legitimate approach? World J Surg 1990; 14:406–9.

42. Chapuis Y, Richard B, Fulla Y et al. Chirurgie de l'hyperparathyroïdie primaire par abord unilatéral sous anesthésie locale et dosage per opératoire de la PTH 1–84. Chirurgie 1993–1994, 119:121–4.

43. Inabnet WB, Fulla Y, Richard B. Unilateral neck exploration under local anaesthesia: the approach of choice for asymptomatic primary hyper-parathyroidism. Surgery 1999; 126:1004–10.

44. Chen H, Sokoll L, Udelsman R. Outpatient minimally invasive parathyroidectomy: a combination of sestamibi-SPECT localization, cervical block anaesthesia, and intraoperative parathyroid hormone assay. Surgery 1999; 126:1016–22.

45. Gurnell EM, Poultsidis A, McFarlane I et al. Pilot study of minimally invasive parathyroid surgery, with intraoperative parathyroid hormone measurement, as a day-case procedure. Br J Surg 2002; 89:1332–3.

46. Udelsman R, Donovan PI, Sokoll LJ. One hundred consecutive minimally invasive parathyroid explorations. Ann Surg 2000; 232:331–9.

47. Udelsman R. Six hundred fifty-six consecutive explorations for primary hyperparathyroidism. Ann Surg 2002; 235:665–72.

48. Norman J, Chheda H. Minimally invasive para-thyroidectomy facilitated by intraoperative nuclear mapping. Surgery 1997; 122:998–1004.

49. Norman J, Murphy C. Minimally invasive radio-guided parathyroidectomy. In: Van Heerden JA, Farley DR (eds) Operative technique in general surgery. Surgical exploration for hyper-parathyroidism. Philadelphia: WB Saunders, 1999; pp. 28–33.

50. Goldstein RE, Blevins L, Delbeke D et al. Effect of minimally invasive radioguided parathyroidectomy on efficacy, length of stay, and costs in management of primary hyperparathyroidism. Ann Surg 2000; 231:732–42.

51. Gagner M, Rubino F. Endoscopic parathyroidectomy. In: Schwartz AE, Pertsemlidis D, Gagner M (eds) Endocrine surgery. New York: Marcel Dekker, 2004; pp. 289–96.

52. Miccoli P, Bendinelli C, Conte M. Endoscopic parathyroidectomy by a gasless approach. J Laparoendosc Adv Surg Tech A 1998; 8:189–94.

53. Henry JF. Endoscopic exploration. In: Van Heerden JA, Farley DR (eds) Operative technique in general surgery. Surgical exploration for hyper-parathyroidism. Philadelphia: WB Saunders, 1999; pp. 49–61.

54. Ikeda Y, Takami H, Sasaki Y et al. Endoscopic neck surgery by the axillary approach. J Am Coll Surg 2000; 191:336–40.

55. Okido M, Shimizu S, Kuroki S et al. Video-assisted parathyroidectomy for primary hyperparathyroidism: an approach involving a skin-lifting method. Surg Endosc 2001; 15:1120–3.

56. Ikeda Y, Takami H, Tajima G et al. Total endoscopic parathyroidectomy. Biomed Pharmacother 2002; 56(suppl. 1):22s–25s.

57. Miccoli P, Berti P, Conte M et al. Minimally invasive video-assisted parathyroidectomy: lesson

learned from 137 cases. J Am Coll Surg 2000; 191:613–18.

58. Cougard P, Goudet P, Bilosi M et al. Exérèse vidéoendoscopique des adénomes parathyroïdiens: résultats à propos d'une série prospective de 100 patients. Ann Chirur 2001; 126:314–19.

59. Henry JF, Iacobone M, Mirallié E et al. Indications and results of video-assisted parathyroidectomy by a lateral approach in patients with primary hyper-parathyroidism. Surgery 2001; 130:999–1004.

60. Miccoli P, Bendinelli C, Berti P et al. Video-assisted versus conventional parathyroidectomy in primary hyperparathyroidism: a prospective randomized study. Surgery 1999; 126:1117–22.

61. Henry JF, Raffaelli M, Iacobone M et al. Video-assisted parathyroidectomy via lateral approach versus conventional surgery in the treatment of sporadic primary hyperparathyroidism. Results of a case–control study. Surg Endosc 2001; 15:1116–19.

62. Irvin GL, Carneiro DM. Rapid parathyroid hormone assay guided exploration. In: Van Heerden JA, Farley DR (eds) Operative technique in general surgery. Surgical exploration for hyper-parathyroidism. Philadelphia: WB Saunders, 1999; pp. 18–27.

63. Muller H. True recurrence of hyperparathyroidism: proposed criteria of recurrence. Br J Surg 1975; 62:556–9.

64. Akerstrom G, Juhlin C. Reoperation in primary hyperparathyroidism. In: Akerstrom G (ed.) Current controversy in parathyroid operation and reoperation. Austin TX: RG Landes Company, 1994; pp. 131–65.

65. Heath H III. Familial benign hypercalcemia – from clinical description to molecular genetics. West J Med 1994; 164:554–62.

66. Strewler GH, Budayr AA, Clark OH et al. Production of parathyroid hormone by a malignant non-parathyroid tumor in a hypercalcemic patient. J Clin Endocrinol Metab 1993; 76:1373–6.

67. Carty SE, Norton JA. Management of patients with persistent or recurrent primary hyperparathyroidism. World J Surg 1991; 15: 716–23.

68. Rodriguez JM, Tezelman S, Siperstein AE et al. Localization procedures in patients with persistent or recurrent hyperparathyroidism. Arch Surg 1994; 129:870–5.

69. Shen W, Duren M, Morita E et al. Reoperation for persistent or recurrent hyperparathyroidism. Arch Surg 1996; 131:861–9.

70. Jaskowiak N, Norton JA, Alexander HT et al. A prospective trial evaluating a standard approach to reoperation for missed parathyroid adenoma. Ann Surg 1996; 224:308–22.

71. Thompson GB, Grant CS, Perrier ND et al. Reoperative parathyroid surgery in the era of sestamibi scanning and intraoperative parathyroid hormone monitoring. Arch Surg 1999; 134:699–704.

72. Wadstrom C, Zedenius J, Guinea A et al. Reoperative surgery for recurrent or persistent primary hyperparathyroidism. Aust NZ J Surg 1998; 68:103–7.

73. Mariette C, Pellissier L, Combemale F et al. Reoperation for persistent or recurrent primary hyperparathyroidism. Langenbeck's Arch Surg 1998; 383:174–9.

74. Patow CA, Norton JA, Brennan MF. Vocal cord paralysis and reoperative parathyroidectomy. Ann Surg 1986; 203:282–5.

75. Chan TJ, Libutti SK, McCart JA et al. Persistent primary hyperparathyroidism caused by adenomas identified in pharyngeal or adjacent structures. World J Surg 2003; 27:675–9.

76. Udekwu AO, Kaplan EL, Wu TC et al. Ectopic parathyroid adenoma of the lateral triangle of the neck: report of two cases. Surgery 1987; 101:114–18.

77. Brennan MF, Norton JA. Reoperation for persistent and recurrent hyperparathyroidism. Ann Surg 1985; 201:40–4.

78. Saxe AW, Brennan MF. Strategy and technique of reoperative parathyroid surgery. Surgery 1981; 89:417–23.

79. Saxe AW, Brennan MF. Reoperative parathyroid surgery for primary hyperparathyroidism caused by multiple-gland disease: total parathyroidectomy and autotransplantation with cryopreserved tissue. Surgery 1982; 91:616–21.

80. Casanova D, Sarfati E, De Francisco A et al. Secondary hyperparathyroidism: Diagnosis of site or recurrence. World J Surg 1991; 15:546–54.

81. Weber CJ, Sewell CW, Mc Garity WC. Persistent and recurrent sporadic primary hyperparathyroidism: histopathology, complications, and results of reoperation. Surgery 1994; 116:991–98.

82. Lo CY, Van Heerden JA. Parathyroid reoperations. In: Clark OH, Duh QY (eds) Textbook of endocrine surgery. Philadelphia: WB Saunders, 1997; pp. 411–17.

83. Norton JA. Reoperation for missed parathyroid adenoma. Adv Surg 1997; 31:273–8.

84. Tanaka Y, Tominaga Y, Funahashi H et al. Pre-operative localization studies in secondary hyper-plasia. Acta Chir Austriaca 1996; 28(suppl. 124): 14–16.

85. Edis AJ, Levitt MD. Supernumerary parathyroid glands: implications for the surgical treatment of secondary hyperparathyroidism. World J Surg 1987; 11: 398–401.

86. Hibi Y, Tominaga Y, Sato T et al. Reoperation for renal hyperparathyroidism. World J Surg 2002; 26:1301–7.

87. Stanbury SW, Lumb GA, Nicholson WF. Elective subtotal parathyroidectomy for autonomous hyperparathyroidism. Lancet 1960, 1:793–8.

88. Wells SA, Gunnels JC, Shelbourne JD et al. Transplantation of the parathyroid glands in man: Clinical indications and results. Surgery 1975; 78:34–44.

89. Tanaka Y, Seo H, Tominaga Y et al. Factors related to the recurrent hyperfunction of autografts after total parathyroidectomy in patients with severe secondary hyperparathyroidism. Jpn J Surg 1993; 23:220–5.

90. Ohta K, Manabe T, Katagiri M et al. Expression of proliferating cell nuclear antigens in parathyroid glands of renal hyperparathyroidism. World J Surg 1994; 18:625–9.

91. Tominaga Y, Tanaka Y, Sato K et al. DNA studies in graft-dependent hyperparathyroidism. Acta Chir Austriaca 1996; 28(suppl. 124):65–8.

92. Takagi H, Tominaga Y, Uchida K et al. Subtotal versus total parathyroidectomy with forearm autograft for secondary hyperparathyroidism in chronic renal failure. Ann Surg 1984; 200:18–23.

93. Rothmund M, Wagner PK, Schark C. Subtotal parathyroidectomy versus total parathyroidectomy and autotransplantation in secondary hyperparathyroidism: A randomized trial. World J Surg 1991; 15:745–50.

94. Gagne ER, Urena P, Leite-Silva S et al. Short and long-term efficacy of total parathyroidectomy with immediate autografting compared with subtotal parathyroidectomy in hemodialysis patients. J Am Soc Nephrol 1992; 3:1008–17.

95. Tanaka Y, Funahashi H, Imai T et al. Functional and morphometric study of cryopreserved human parathyroid tissue transplanted into nude mice. World J Surg 1996; 20:692–9.

96. Niederle B. The technique of parathyroid cryopreservation and the results of delayed autotransplantation. A review. Acta Chir Austriaca 1996; 28(suppl. 124):68–71.

97. Numano M, Tominaga Y, Uchida K et al. Surgical significance of supernumerary parathyroid glands in renal hyperparathyroidism. World J Surg 1998; 22:1098–103.

98. Dubost C, Kracht M, Assens P et al. Reoperation for secondary hyperparathyroidism in hemodialysis patients. World J Surg 1986; 10:654–60.

99. Henry JF, Denizot A, Audiffret J et al. Results of reoperations for persistent or recurrent secondary hyperparathyroidism in hemodialysis patients. World J Surg 1990; 14: 303–7.

100. Garfinkel PE, Ezrin C, Stancer HC. Hypothyroidism and hyperparathyroidism associated with lithium. Lancet 1973; 2:331–2.

101. McHenry CR, Racke F, Meister M et al. Lithium effects on dispersed bovine parathyroid cells grown in tissue culture. Surgery 1991; 110:1061–6.

102. Awad SS, Miskulin J, Thompson NW. Parathyroid adenomas versus four-gland hyperplasia as the cause of primary hyperparathyroidism in patients with prolonged lithium therapy. World J Surg 2003; 27:486–8.

103. Nordenstrom J, Strigard K, Perkeck L et al. Hyperparathyroidism associated with treatment of manic-depressive disorders by lithium. Eur J Surg 1992; 158:207–11.

104. Sitges-Serra A, Esteller E, Ricart MJ et al. Indications and late results of subtotal parathyroidectomy for hyperparathyroidism after renal transplantation. World J Surg 1984; 8:534–9.

105. Saha HH, Salmela KT, Ahonen PJ et al. Sequential changes in vitamin D and calcium metabolism after successful renal transplantation. Scand J Urol Nephrol 1994; 28:21–5.

106. Straffen AM, Carmichael DJ, Fainety A et al. Calcium metabolism following renal transplantation. Ann Clin Biochem 1994; 31:125–9.

107. Sancho JJ, Stiges-Serra A. Metabolic complications for patients with secondary hyperparathyroidism. In: Clark OH, Duh QY (eds) Textbook of endocrine surgery. Philadelphia: WB Saunders, 1997; pp. 394–401.

108. Fassbinder W, Brunner FP, Brynger H et al. Combined report on regular dialysis and transplantation in Europe. Nephrol Dial Transplant 1991; 6(suppl.):28–32.

CHAPTER

Two

The thyroid gland

Gregory P. Sadler

ANATOMY AND EMBRYOLOGY

The thyroid gland is formed by two lobes, one either side of the trachea. A short isthmus connects the lobes across the front of the trachea. Each lobe derives its blood supply from two main arteries. The superior thyroid artery (a branch of the external carotid) enters the superior pole on the anterior surface. The inferior thyroid artery (from the thyrocervical branch of the subclavian artery) enters the lobe midway down the lateral border. Venous drainage is variable but is usually threefold: a middle thyroid vein directly to the internal jugular, superior thyroid veins (running with the superior thyroid artery), and a plexus of veins draining from the inferior aspect of the lower pole. Lymphatic drainage is to local nodes located in the central compartment and thence to the anterior cervical chain.

Embryologically the gland is derived from the median thyroid diverticulum in the floor of the pharynx. It grows downwards between the ventral ends of the first and second pharyngeal arches, the stalk of the diverticulum elongating to become the thyroglossal duct. This duct (later obliterated) extends from the foramen caecum at the base of the tongue to the isthmus, its distal part remaining as the pyramidal lobe of the thyroid. The ultimobranchial bodies, arising from the fourth pharyngeal pouch

on each side, become applied to the lateral portion of each thyroid lobe and contribute the parafollicular cells, or C-cells. These cells of neural crest origin become secondarily involved with the thyroid, produce calcitonin and may later assume clinical importance as the cells giving rise to medullary thyroid carcinoma.

INVESTIGATION OF THYROID FUNCTION

Thyroid hormones and thyroid-stimulating hormone (TSH)

Control of synthesis and release of the thyroid hormones is provided by thyroid-stimulating hormone (TSH). This regulatory hormone is released from the anterior pituitary and is the primary hormone measured when assessing thyroid status. TSH release is regulated via a negative-feedback loop provided by the thyroid hormones thyroxine (T_4) and triiodothyronine (T_3). The higher the levels of T_4 and/or T_3 the lower the level of TSH. In contrast, the lower the levels of T_4 and/or T_3 the higher the level of TSH.

TSH concentration can be measured precisely by a sensitive immunochemiluminometric assay (normal range 0–5 mU/L). Increased TSH concentrations are found in primary hypothyroidism (e.g. autoimmune thyroiditis) and after treatment of thyrotoxicosis by surgery or radioiodine. Suppressed TSH concentrations occur in hyperthyroidism. Thus measurement of TSH is usually all that is needed to establish a biochemically euthyroid state.

The thyroid hormones (T_4 and T_3) are stored in the thyroid gland in thyroid colloid. They are bound to thyroglobulin and released in response to TSH. In circulation the hormones are bound to thyroxine-binding globulin (TBG), thyroxine-binding prealbumin (TBPA) and albumin.

The principal metabolic effects of the thyroid hormones are exerted by unbound free T_4 and T_3 (0.03–0.04% and 0.2–0.5% of the total circulating hormones respectively). Because almost all T_4 and T_3 is protein bound, measurement of total hormone concentrations is influenced by conditions that change the serum concentrations of thyroxine-binding proteins. For example, increased concentrations are found in pregnancy and in women taking oral contraceptives, and low concentrations occur in the nephrotic syndrome. Drugs such as salicylates and some antibiotics compete with T_4 and T_3 for protein binding.

Radioimmunoassays for free T_4 and T_3 are now readily available and give a precise assessment of thyroid function. T_3 is the more active physiological hormone, with 80% being produced in the periphery by monodeiodination of T_4. Measurement of T_3 is particularly important in T_3 toxicosis, when there is a clinical picture of thyrotoxicosis with normal serum T_4 concentrations.

Thyroid antibodies

THYROGLOBULIN

Antibodies to thyroglobulin, the major constituent of colloid and precursor of thyroid hormones, are found in most people with Graves' disease and virtually 100% of those with Hashimoto's thyroiditis.[1] Measurement of thyroglobulin levels has now become standard in the long-term follow-up and monitoring of patients who have undergone total thyroidectomy and radioiodine ablation therapy for differentiated thyroid cancer.[2]

THYROID PEROXIDASE

Antibodies to thyroid peroxidase (TPO), previously known as thyroid microsomal antigen, are found in most patients with Graves' disease or Hashimoto's thyroiditis.[3] Raised titres are also detected in patients with postpartum thyroiditis and non-organ-specific autoimmune diseases such as rheumatoid arthritis.

TSH RECEPTOR AUTOANTIBODIES

Most TSH receptor autoantibodies (TRAbs) have a stimulatory action, but in some instances antibodies bind to the receptor and block activity. Measurement of TRAbs is especially valuable in the diagnosis of Graves' disease, being detected in approximately 90% of patients.[4] Neonatal hyperthyroidism may result from transplacental passage of TRAbs.

Calcitonin

Increased serum levels of calcitonin (from the parafollicular cells) are found in patients with medullary thyroid carcinoma (MTC).[5]

Measurement of basal or stimulated calcitonin concentrations is employed to assess the completeness of surgical resection of MTC and is valuable in the follow-up and detection of metastases after thyroidectomy. Screening for the detection of familial MTC, usually as part of the multiple endocrine neoplasia type 2A (MEN 2A) or type 2B (MEN 2B) syndrome, no longer depends on measurement of stimulated calcitonin concentrations.

Identification of germ-line mutations in the RET proto-oncogene on chromosome 10 means that families can be directly tested for the germ-line mutation (replacing biochemical screening)[6] (see Chapter 4).

Carcinoembryonic antigen

Though carcinoembryonic antigen (CEA) is not a direct tumour marker in MTC, when present it is suggestive of a poor prognostic tumour.

Thyroid isotope scanning

Scanning the thyroid gland with either radioactive ^{123}I or technetium pertechnetate (^{99m}Tc) in an attempt to provide a differential diagnosis in euthyroid patients with a solitary nodule should be discouraged. Fine-needle aspiration cytology is the

Figure 2.1 • ^{123}I scan of 'cold' thyroid nodule.

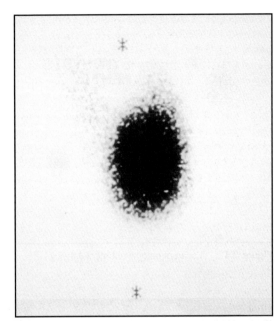

Figure 2.2 • Toxic autonomous thyroid nodule.

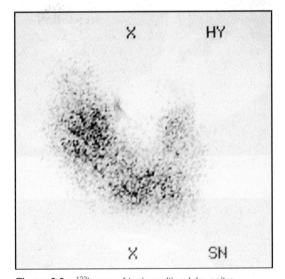

Figure 2.3 • ^{123}I scan of toxic multinodular goitre.

accepted investigation of choice in this group of patients.

When scanning is performed nodules are characterised into those that are non-functioning 'cold' (**Fig. 2.1**), normally functioning 'warm' and hyperfunctioning 'hot'. Although the finding of a hot nodule is usually consistent with benign pathology, more than 80% of nodules are cold and only 20% of these will be malignant. Iodine scanning is therefore not helpful in the diagnosis of malignancy and has no significant role in the investigation of euthyroid patients with a solitary nodule. Discrepant imaging is well documented, with hot ^{99m}Tc images being cold on ^{123}I scanning.[7] It has therefore been suggested that all ^{99m}Tc hot scans should be re-evaluated with ^{123}I.

Isotope scanning is most useful in the investigation of the solitary autonomous toxic nodule (**Fig. 2.2**) or toxic multinodular goitre (**Fig. 2.3**). Iodine scanning is also helpful in the evaluation of patients with metastatic thyroid tumours and in the localisation of ectopic thyroid tissue (**Fig. 2.4**). Other isotopes previously used in the evaluation of patients with MTC – pentavalent dimercaptosuccinic acid (DMSA),[8] thallium[9] and meta-iodobenzyl guanidine (MIBG)[10] – have now been largely superseded by magnetic resonance imaging (MRI) and positron emission tomography (PET) scanning.

Radioiodine uptake

Radioactive ^{123}I is taken into the thyroid gland in a manner identical to inorganic iodine. Measurement of the uptake of an administered dose after 4 and 48 hours is useful in assessing patients with thyrotoxicosis. Increased uptake is seen in most forms of the disorder, with the notable exceptions of thyrotoxicosis due to subacute thyroiditis and after excessive T_4 intake.

Ultrasonography

This technique is operator dependent but capable of identifying impalpable nodules as small as 0.3 mm in diameter. Ultrasonography also discriminates

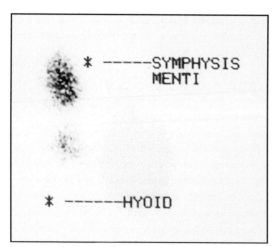

Figure 2.4 • ¹²³I scan of ectopic submental thyroid.

cystic lesions from solid lesions but is not reliable in distinguishing benign disease from malignant disease. Cystic nodules constitute 15–25%[11] of all thyroid nodules and when 4 cm or more in diameter may have a malignancy rate of approximately 20% (**Fig. 2.5**).[12]

CT and MRI

Computed tomography (CT) and magnetic resonance imaging (MRI) play an increasingly important part in the investigation of thyroid disease, particularly in the evaluation of retrosternal goitres and glands producing major pressure effects and distortion of adjacent structures (**Fig. 2.6a,b**).

Figure 2.5 • Ultrasound scan of mixed thyroid nodule with cystic and solid component.

(a)

(b)

Figure 2.6 • **(a)** CT scan showing a large retrosternal goitre extending below the level of the aortic arch. **(b)** Extensive retrosternal goitre, narrowing the trachea and pushing it well across to the left. The patient presented with significant stridor.

Fine-needle aspiration cytology (FNAC)

Fine-needle aspiration cytology (FNAC) employs a fine-gauge (21 or 23) needle to obtain a thyroid sample suitable for cytological assessment. First used in Scandinavia in the early 1950s,[13] it is now universally accepted as being a highly accurate cost-effective method with low morbidity and good patient compliance. In experienced hands the high diagnostic accuracy is such that the method can diagnose colloid nodules, thyroiditis, papillary carcinoma, medullary carcinoma, anaplastic carcinoma and lymphoma.

The major limitation of FNAC is the inability to distinguish benign from malignant follicular neoplasms,[14] this distinction being dependent on the histological criteria of capsular and vascular invasion.

Recently guidelines have been issued such that thyroid cytology should now be reported in a similar fashion to breast cytology. The five cytological categories are summarised in **Table 2.1**.

Lowhagen et al. reported no false-positive results with respect to malignancy and a false-negative rate of 2.2%, which later decreased to zero.[14]

Grant et al. found a false-negative rate of only 0.7% in 439 patients studied and concluded that FNAC was a safe, reliable and accurate means of discriminating between benign and malignant lesions.[15]

Suspicious lesions are mostly the follicular tumours, and because of the inability of the technique to provide histological details all such lesions should be resected. An inadequate sample rate of

Table 2.1 • Classification of FNA cytology

FNAC category	Cytology
THY 1	Insufficient material
THY 2	Benign (nodular goitre)
THY 3	Suspicious of neoplasm (follicular)
THY 4	Suspicious of malignancy (papillary/medullary/lymphoma)
THY 5	Definite malignancy

15% is not uncommon, but such a result should not be regarded as being from a benign lesion but is an indication for repeat aspiration.

Needle core biopsy

A cutting needle biopsy yields a cylinder or core of tissue suitable for histological examination; this has high diagnostic accuracy but has the disadvantages of being a painful procedure. Potential complications include haematoma, tracheal puncture and recurrent laryngeal nerve damage, and lesions less than 3 cm in size may not be amenable to this technique. All of these complications can be minimised by ultrasound guidance. The technique is most useful in establishing the diagnosis where lymphoma is suspected following FNAC, thus saving the need for an open biopsy. Any risk of seeding malignancy along the needle tract has been greatly exaggerated.

DEVELOPMENTAL ABNORMALITIES OF THE THYROID

Thyroglossal cyst

This condition results from persistence of part of the thyroglossal duct and is usually found as a midline cyst (occasionally more laterally) just below the hyoid bone or above the thyroid cartilage. Less commonly the cyst is found at a higher level above the hyoid bone. The essential diagnostic feature is that of upward movement on swallowing, and because of the attachment of the thyroglossal tract to the foramen caecum, the cyst rises on protrusion of the tongue. These cysts are prone to infection and therefore should be excised. The most appropriate and successful operation is the Sistrunk procedure, with excision of the central portion of the hyoid bone. Malignancy, usually of a papillary type, can occur within the thyroglossal cyst as a primary phenomenon.[16]

Thyroglossal fistula

This results from infection or inadequate removal of a thyroglossal cyst, the opening usually being at a lower level in the neck than the original cyst. Careful tracing of the tract to the foramen caecum and excision of the central portion of the hyoid bone achieves complete excision of the fistula.

Lingual thyroid

When the thyroid gland fails to descend it may be found in the back of the tongue close to the foramen caecum. If large it can result in respiratory or swallowing difficulties and haemorrhage. Diagnosis is confirmed by radioiodine scanning, and treatment with T_4 should result in shrinkage. Therapeutic radioactive iodine is an alternative treatment measure and excision is rarely necessary.

Ectopic thyroid

Arrested descent of the thyroid results in the gland being found at any point along the line of the thyroglossal tract. In these circumstances this may be the only thyroid tissue present. If excision is carried out, full replacement T_4 dosage is required.

GOITRE

The term goitre, derived from the Latin 'guttur', meaning throat, is used as a non-specific term to indicate diffuse enlargement of the thyroid gland. A classification of goitre is shown in **Table 2.2**.

Simple goitre

Simple goitre is the result of TSH stimulation, usually secondary to inadequate concentrations of circulating thyroid hormones. In these circumstances, TSH stimulation causes diffuse glandular hyperplasia and an increase in hormone output. Iodine deficiency is a key factor in simple endemic goitre, associated with a low iodine content of water and food.[17] There are 5 to 10 mg of iodine in the thyroid pool, with a turnover rate of 1% daily. The minimum daily dietary requirements of iodine are therefore small, about 50 to 100 µg. Endemic goitrous areas are mountainous regions such as the Alps, Andes and Himalayas. In Britain, recognised regions include the Chilterns, Cotswolds, Derbyshire and South Wales.

Table 2.2 • Classification of goitre

Simple goitre (endemic or sporadic)	Diffuse hyperplastic goitre Nodular goitre
Toxic goitre	Diffuse (Graves' disease) Toxic multinodular goitre Toxic solitary nodule
Neoplastic goitre	Benign Malignant
Thyroiditis	Subacute (granulomatous): de Quervain's Autoimmune (Hashimoto's) Riedel's Acute suppurative
Miscellaneous	Chronic bacterial infection (e.g. tuberculosis or syphilis) Actinomycosis Amyloidosis Dyshormonogenesis

Iodine deficiency in its most extreme form is associated with cretinism, congenital hypothyroidism and various degrees of mental impairment. Usually an endemic goitre commences as a soft diffuse enlargement appearing in childhood, which can evolve into a colloid goitre at a later stage when TSH stimulation has diminished. Times of physiological stress, such as puberty and pregnancy, result in increased demands for T_4 and are accompanied by TSH stimulation of the thyroid and diffuse hyperplasia.

The natural history of thyroid stimulation by TSH is such that there are varying levels of cellular stimulation throughout the gland, where active and inactive lobules coexist. With high TSH levels nodules form, and throughout the thyroid there follow changes of hyperplasia, cystic degeneration, haemorrhage, colloid-filled follicles, fibrosis and later calcification. Simple goitre occurring during adulthood in a non-endemic area is usually described as sporadic; the nodules of endemic goitre appear earlier in life. All types of simple goitre occur more often in women.

Environmental factors such as the dietary goitrogen thiocyanate in cassava or vegetables of the brassica family may cause thyroid enlargement.[18] The interaction of environmental goitrogens and iodine deficiency may explain some of the differences in the prevalence of endemic goitre seen in areas with similar degrees of iodine deficiency. Other agents, including calcium and drugs such as the antithyroid agent carbimazole, are capable of acting at various sites within the thyroid gland, and by interfering with the process of hormone synthesis lead to hyperplasia with goitre formation. Paradoxically, excess iodine intake can inhibit proteolysis and release of thyroid hormones leading to goitre and hypothyroidism.

Deficiency of one or more of the enzymes in the thyroid responsible for T_4 synthesis may be the cause of sporadic goitre. These deficiencies, either complete or partial, are usually genetic and are well illustrated by the dyshormonogenic Pendred's syndrome, in which thyroid enlargement progresses to nodular goitre with associated deafness. Severe forms of dyshormonogenesis result in hypo-thyroidism and cretinism in the infant. Treatment consists of T_4 and thyroidectomy if the goitre produces pressure symptoms or cosmetic concerns.

Prevention and treatment

Prevention of the development of simple endemic goitre can be achieved by the addition of iodine to the diet as, for example, in table salt. At a prenodular stage a hyperplastic goitre can be made to regress in size by giving T_4 0.1–0.15 mg daily, often over several years. Thyroidectomy may be indicated for cosmetic reasons or because of pressure effects if the gland does not regress.

THYROID NODULE

Thyroid nodules are common, being a feature of many different thyroid diseases. In a non-goitrous area, the prevalence of palpable thyroid nodules in a population aged 30 to 59 years was 4.2%.[19]

At adult autopsy the prevalence of thyroid nodules (many less than 1 cm in diameter and impalpable) is much greater, perhaps even as high as 50%.[20] Although the majority of thyroid nodules are benign and include colloid lesions, follicular adenomas, nodular thyroiditis and degenerative cysts, the essential clinical problem, particularly when the lesion is solitary, remains the distinction between benign and malignant diseases.

Clinical assessment

HISTORY

Most thyroid nodules are asymptomatic but the acute development of a painful swelling in the thyroid is usually due to haemorrhage into a pre-existing colloid nodule. This is an important condition to recognise as spontaneous resolution, sometimes aided by aspiration, occurs in a few weeks without intervention. Rapid growth of an existing nodule, with discomfort radiating into the face or jaw, may be due to malignancy but this presentation tends to be seen in elderly people with an anaplastic carcinoma. Often malignant nodules may be slow growing and be present for many years before a diagnosis is made.

Thyroid nodules (like most thyroid conditions) occur more often in women, thus a solitary nodule in a man carries a greater risk of malignancy. Young people are particularly at risk for malignancy. A solitary nodule is likely to be malignant in 50% of children under 14 years of age.[21,22] A family history of thyroid or other endocrine disease may be relevant to the diagnosis of MTC in MEN 2A, MEN 2B and non-MEN familial syndromes (see Chapter 4).

Several key environmental and geographical factors require consideration. The incidence of follicular cancer is increased in endemic goitrous areas,[23] for example, whereas iodine-rich regions such as Iceland have an increased incidence of papillary cancer.[24]

Although the association between thyroid carcinoma and a history of head and neck irradiation in children was first recorded in 1950,[25] the true magnitude of the problem was only identified by DeGroot and Paloyan in the Chicago area in 1973.[26] Irradiation also increases the incidence of benign thyroid nodules but the reported risk of malignancy in a palpable nodule found in a previously irradiated thyroid ranges from 20 to 50%. Age at exposure is a significant factor, with the very young being particularly at risk (as demonstrated by the Chernobyl nuclear reactor accident).

High-dose external irradiation to the neck for conditions such as Hodgkin's lymphoma may also increase the risk of thyroid malignancy.[27] The latent period for developing post-irradiation tumours ranges from 6 to 35 years. Therapeutic radioiodine used in the treatment of Graves' disease and the administration of diagnostic isotopes are not associated with any increased risk of malignancy.

EXAMINATION

A preliminary clinical examination of the patient is directed towards assessment of thyroid status, although most patients with a solitary thyroid nodule will be euthyroid. A nodule in a hyperthyroid patient is highly unlikely to be malignant. Previously much emphasis was placed on the distinction between a clinically solitary nodule and a multinodular gland in the mistaken belief that multinodular goitres were unlikely to contain a malignancy. When a dominant lesion is present within a multinodular gland, the malignancy rate may be virtually identical to that of the true solitary nodule.

A hard, fixed nodule is likely to be malignant, but it is not uncommon for papillary lesions to be cystic and follicular lesions to be soft as a result of haemorrhage. A very hard lesion may be an entirely benign calcified colloid nodule. Lymphadenopathy, either in the central paratracheal groups or in the lateral deep cervical region, is a common finding in papillary and medullary carcinomas and when noted should be treated with a very high index of suspicion clinically.

Although voice change and hoarseness may be non-specific findings, a proven recurrent laryngeal nerve palsy on the side of a palpable thyroid nodule is likely to indicate malignant infiltration. Rarely, direct pressure from a benign lesion can also produce vocal cord paralysis. Although the presence of pressure symptoms and clinical identification of tracheal deviation or retrosternal extension does not aid the distinction of a malignant from a benign lesion, these features nevertheless will be major considerations in the selection of patients for surgery.

Following this careful clinical assessment, the clinician will have formed an opinion as to the likelihood of malignancy. Further supportive and diagnostic tests are now appropriate. The thyroid status will be confirmed by measurement of T_4 and TSH. Chest X-ray may demonstrate a retrosternal goitre or airway distortion or show evidence of macroscopic metastases. Most calcified thyroid nodules are benign, but some papillary and medullary neoplasms have a characteristic fine stippled or punctate calcification.

The measurement of serum calcitonin concentration is not routinely indicated in the work-up of a goitre. Hypercalcitonaemia is not absolutely specific for medullary thyroid tumours, in that increased concentrations may be seen in patients with carcinoma of the breast, pancreas or lung, or in those with carcinoid tumours, phaeochromocytoma and bony metastases. Thyroglobulin measurement, although valuable in the follow-up of patients with malignant tumours, has no value in their initial diagnosis.

FNAC

FNAC is now considered mandatory in the investigation of the solitary thyroid nodule. This highly accurate and cost-effective technique is the method of choice for achieving a precise diagnosis in most patients with thyroid nodular disease. When a conservative approach to the management of the thyroid nodule is contemplated a second FNAC some weeks following the initial visit has been shown to increase diagnostic accuracy and reduce the incidence of missed malignancies.[28] Delbridge et al. have shown that proton magnetic resonance spectroscopy (PMRS) analysis of FNAC specimens helps to make the distinction between benign and malignant lesions and thereby reduces unnecessary surgery for patients with benign follicular neoplasms.[29]

ULTRASONOGRAPHY

Ultrasonography (US) has limited diagnostic value in the assessment of thyroid nodules but allows a clear delineation of multinodularity. An apparently solitary nodule may be shown on ultrasonography to be surrounded by small impalpable nodules. US may also be useful in demonstrating the presence of enlarged, non-palpable cervical nodes, and used to target biopsies.

ISOTOPE SCANNING

Unless the patient has thyrotoxicosis, scintigraphy of the thyroid, either with ^{123}I or technetium pertechnetate (^{99m}Tc), has little value in the investigation of the patient with a thyroid nodule.

Treatment

THYROID HORMONE ADMINISTRATION

There is little evidence that the administration of T_4 is capable of reducing the size of benign nodules. The possibility of reducing the size of an incorrectly diagnosed malignant nodule by T_4 is clearly a potential pitfall.

SUMMARY OF INDICATIONS FOR SURGERY

Patients in whom there is a suspicion of malignancy (based on clinical features or FNAC) should be considered for surgery. When malignancy is not an issue, surgery should be offered to patients with symptoms of pressure (dyspnoea, choking and dysphagia). Occasionally patients with no pressure symptoms may require surgery on cosmetic grounds. A scheme of management for patients with solitary thyroid nodular disease is shown in **Fig. 2.7**. Clinical features such as characteristics of nodule, lymphadenopathy, recurrent laryngeal nerve palsy, family history and history of irradiation may override cytological findings in the decision for surgery.

SURGERY FOR THYROID NODULES

The minimum surgical procedure for adequate treatment of the solitary thyroid nodule is a unilateral **total** lobectomy with removal of the isthmus and pyramidal lobe. In experienced hands this is a relatively safe operation with minimal risk of damaging either the parathyroids or the recurrent laryngeal nerve. A full histological examination of the nodule is permitted with no risk of tumour spillage in the operative field. This surgical procedure completely obviates the need to re-operate on the same side and remove a posterior thyroid lobe remnant if the definitive histology should be returned as malignant or if there should be any benign nodule recurrence at a later date. These are significant and important benefits compared with the outmoded procedure of unilateral **subtotal** lobectomy.

Frozen-section histology is useful where papillary or medullary thyroid cancer is suspected as confirmation may indicate the need for total thyroidectomy at the same operation. Ideally, however, a preoperative biopsy will have been achieved. Frozen-section histology is not advocated for follicular lesions (diagnosis of malignancy in this situation is often difficult).[30]

THYROID CYSTS

Confirmation of the diagnosis of a thyroid cyst is usually made by fine-needle aspiration, and this simple technique can be both diagnostic and therapeutic (**Fig. 2.8**). A full cytological assessment usually requires sampling thyroid tissue adjacent to the cyst to avoid missing a carcinoma in the cyst wall. If a cyst refills it is appropriate to re-aspirate but after two or three attempts surgery is likely to be indicated. A large cyst (>4 cm in diameter), a significantly blood-stained aspirate, cytological findings of neoplasia or a history of irradiation are all indications for surgery.

MULTINODULAR GOITRE

The usual indications for surgery are cosmesis, local pressure symptoms, a dominant nodule increasing in size or showing cytological features that raise the possibility of malignancy, thyrotoxicosis or retrosternal extension (**Fig. 2.9**). The surgical procedure will be tailored to the situation found at operation. Often asymmetrical nodularity is present, with one lobe significantly larger than the other; in this situation a unilateral total lobectomy with a subtotal procedure on the opposite side may be indicated.

 More recently, however, there is an increasing trend amongst endocrine surgeons to perform a total thyroidectomy for multinodular goitre, leaving no thyroid tissue in situ.[31]

RETROSTERNAL GOITRE

Almost all retrosternal goitres arise from growth of the lower half of the thyroid lobes, extending down into a substernal position. The degree of descent of the gland is variable, but when palpable in the neck it is usually classified as substernal whereas a gland entirely within the chest is intrathoracic. Not infrequently a retrosternal goitre may be asymptomatic and found as a coincidental observation on a chest radiograph (**Fig. 2.10**). However, many patients are symptomatic, with problems of

52

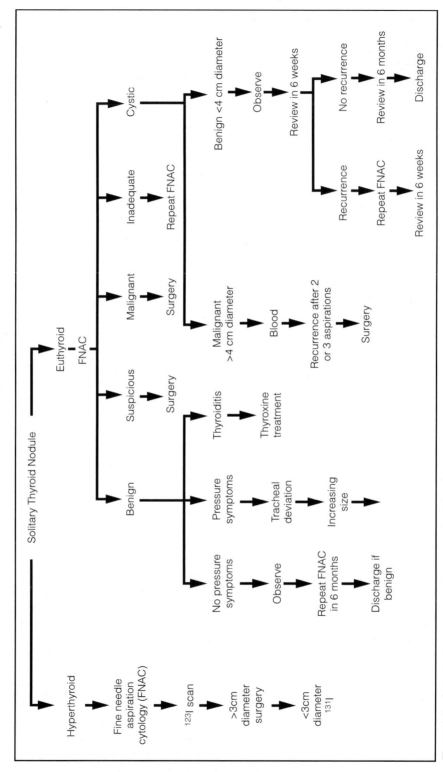

Figure 2.7 • Scheme of management for solitary thyroid nodule.

Figure 2.8 • Aspiration of cystic thyroid nodule demonstrating therapeutic as well as diagnostic value of fine-needle aspiraiton.

airway compression, 'asthma', dysphagia and even thyrotoxicosis. Rarely, patients may present with hoarseness of the voice from a vocal cord palsy (a direct effect of pressure from a benign lesion on the recurrent laryngeal nerve). More dramatic pressure effects can lead to superior vena cava compression syndrome (**Fig. 2.11**). The incidence of malignancy in retrosternal glands is probably no different to that of other nodular goitres, but of course a gland behind the sternum is not amenable to palpation or FNAC for diagnosis.

Confirmation of the diagnosis can be made by a combination of plain radiographs and either CT or MRI. The last two investigations will give precise information concerning airway compromise. Respiratory function tests with flow loop studies are also helpful in patient assessment.

The diagnosis of a retrosternal goitre is usually an indication for surgery (**Fig. 2.12**, see also Plate 10,

facing p. 212), both to obtain a precise histological diagnosis and to remove the significant risk of progressive airway obstruction resulting from growth of the gland or from haemorrhage into a benign colloid lesion.

THYROID CANCER

Thyroid cancer is rare (3.7–4.7 per 100 000 population), accounting for less than 1% of all malignancies and 0.5% of all cancer deaths.[32–34] Thyroid cancer constitutes an extremely heterogeneous group of tumours, with a wide spectrum of biological behaviour. In most instances, if it is treated appropriately there is a high survival rate. Disappointingly, because of the lack of long-term follow-up studies or large randomised trials comparing various procedures, the optimal management for many of these tumours remains controversial.

Molecular biology of thyroid cancer

Thyroid cancer results from complex alterations and disorders in the genetic content of a single cell, which is subsequently inherited by its daughter cells. Several genetic aberrations have been investigated and shown to be implicated in thyroid tumorigenesis.

Oncogenes when activated stimulate tumour growth.[35] Members of the *RAS* family of oncogenes play an important role in thyroid tumour development.[36] In addition growth factors, such as epidermal growth factor (EGF)[37] (and its receptor EGFR), insulin-like growth factor 1 (IGF-1), fibroblast growth factor (FGF) and TSH, as well as the *Gsα* gene and the *RET* proto-oncogene (see section on Medullary carcinoma) are implicated in tumour growth. Recently *RAS* mutations have been identified in some aggressive thyroid cancers. This finding raises the possibility that they may be useful as markers of poor prognosis.[38]

Tumour suppressor genes, especially *p53*,[39] exert an influence on thyroid cell growth by inhibiting tumorigenesis. Mutations in *p53* can lead to its inactivation, which may be important in thyroid tumour initiation and progression, especially leading to anaplastic change.

54

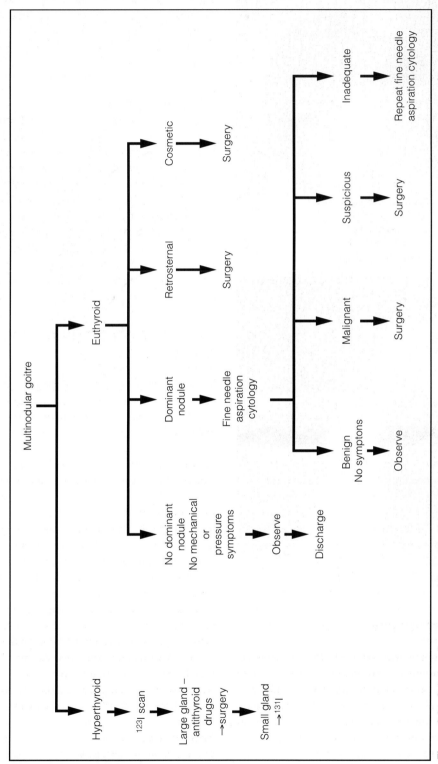

Figure 2.9 • Scheme of management for multinodular goitre.

Figure 2.10 • Chest X-ray revealing the incidental finding of a deviated trachea secondary to a previously undiagnosed retrosternal goitre.

Figure 2.11 • Venogram of a patient with retrosternal goitre producing obstruction of the superior vena cava.

Papillary carcinoma

This is the commonest thyroid malignancy, accounting for approximately 70–80% of cancers. It more commonly affects children and young adults and has an increased incidence in iodine-rich areas. Exposure to ionising radiation (as experienced in Chernobyl) or direct irradiation of the neck, particularly in young people, may predispose to thyroid cancer, and approximately 85% of such irradiation-

Figure 2.12 • Large retrosternal goitre causing respiratory distress. Specimen resected without the need of a sternotomy.

induced tumours are papillary.[26] A rare familial form of the disease has also been described.[40]

PATHOLOGY

Macroscopically the tumours tend to appear as a hard whitish nodule infiltrating the thyroid gland. Papillary cancer is often multifocal (though this is often a microscopic finding and not apparent at surgery). Encapsulation of tumours is unusual (though when present this is thought to be a good prognostic factor). The tumour has a propensity for early lymphatic spread both within the thyroid and to the paratracheal and cervical lymph nodes. Blood-borne spread to lungs and bones is usually a late feature. Tumours can be divided into three main types based on their size and extent.

Micropapillary cancer

These lesions by definition are less than 1 cm in diameter and usually not clinically obvious. They are most frequently reported as incidental findings following thyroidectomy for other conditions. They rarely metastasise to regional lymph nodes and are a common finding at autopsy, being detected in 6–13% of thyroid glands of patients dying from causes other than thyroid disease.

Though the primary tumour is not usually clinically apparent, spread to local cervical nodes may be the presenting feature (the so-called lateral aberrant thyroid). Distant metastatic disease is rare, though deaths have been reported.

 The Mayo Clinic group described four deaths in 396 patients with tumours 1.5 cm or less in diameter,[41] and Noguchi et al. documented two deaths in 867 patients.[42]

Intrathyroidal

These lesions are larger than the micropapillary tumours (i.e. >1 cm) and are situated totally within the thyroid. They have a less favourable prognosis than microcancers.

Extrathyroidal

These tumours are locally advanced, extending through the thyroid capsule and often involving adjacent structures such as the trachea, oesophagus and recurrent laryngeal nerve. The prognosis of this disease type is the least favourable.

HISTOLOGY

The typical lesion has a mixture of papillary projections and follicular structures. The cuboidal cells with pale abundant cytoplasm have intranuclear cytoplasmic inclusions, nuclear overlapping and grooves (Orphan Annie cells). Psammoma bodies occur and are associated with a high incidence of lymphatic spread. The presence of involved lymph nodes, however, does not seem to adversely affect the prognosis. Follicular, encapsulated, diffuse sclerosing and tall-cell varieties of papillary carcinoma have been described and are associated with a poorer long-term prognosis.

CLINICAL PRESENTATION

Clinically, papillary carcinoma usually presents as a hard solitary nodule. Locally enlarged cervical nodes may be present (particularly in children and younger patients). Cystic degeneration of the primary tumour (or metastases) occasionally leads to the mistaken diagnosis of simple thyroid cyst (or branchial cyst in the case of nodal metastases).

Local invasion of the recurrent laryngeal nerve can result in vocal cord palsy, airway symptoms (because of tracheal involvement) and/or dysphagia as a result of oesophageal invasion. Less than 1% of patients at the time of initial presentation will show features of distant metastases. The highest frequency of metastases at initial presentation is seen in children, but ultimately up to 20% of patients develop distant spread.[43]

Follicular carcinoma

This malignancy accounts for 15–20% of thyroid cancers and has a higher incidence in iodine-deficient areas (associated with chronic TSH stimulation). It can also be caused by previous irradiation. The disease has a female to male ratio of 3:1, affecting an older age group than papillary carcinoma (mean age 50 years). A rare familial form also exists (**Fig. 2.13**).[44]

PATHOLOGY

Follicular carcinoma is usually encapsulated, solitary and frequently exhibits vascular invasion. Metastatic spread is via the bloodstream. In contrast to papillary tumours, lymphatic spread is usually a late phenomenon, seen with advanced tumours. Follicular carcinoma is classified into two types according to histopathological features.

Minimally invasive cancer

This type is the most common follicular malignancy. Tumours exhibit either only slight invasion into the capsule or occasionally just through the capsule but not widely into the surrounding thyroid. Invasion into capsular blood vessels may also be present.

Widely invasive cancer

This is far less common than minimally invasive cancer. However, it is a more aggressive tumour whose diagnosis depends on histological confirmation of capsular and angioinvasive features. At surgery, venous extension into the middle thyroid and internal jugular veins may be present. Although most well-differentiated tumours have a well-formed

Figure 2.13 • Patient with longstanding multinodular goitre and coexisting follicular thyroid carcinoma.

follicular structure, the oxyphilic Hürthle cell lesion is composed mainly of cells with eosinophilic granular cytoplasm, large clear nuclei and trabecular architecture. Some consider this variety to be a particularly aggressive form of follicular carcinoma, with a greater propensity for multifocality and lymph node metastases.[45] Furthermore, therapeutic options in Hürthle cell tumours are limited by the inability of the lesion to concentrate radioactive iodine. They do, however, synthesise thyroglobulin.

CLINICAL FEATURES

Follicular thyroid cancer presents as a discrete solitary thyroid nodule increasing in size. Tumours are usually firm but may be softened by haemorrhage within the lesion. Metastatic disease may already be present at the time of diagnosis, with bone and lung involvement. Cervical lymphadenopathy is not usually present at initial presentation.

In contrast to papillary thyroid carcinoma (where FNAC has a high specificity and sensitivity), follicular carcinoma cannot be diagnosed precisely by FNAC. The cytology report will describe a follicular tumour and only 20% of these will subsequently be identified as follicular carcinoma.

Treatment of differentiated thyroid cancer

There is universal agreement that thyroidectomy is the treatment of choice for patients with thyroid cancer. The precise extent of the procedure, however, depends upon the type of cancer present and remains controversial.[46] The introduction of guidelines on the management of thyroid cancer in the UK has been demonstrated to increase the number of patients treated in specialist centres and to decrease the size of the thyroid remnant following thyroid surgery. The treatment goals in the management of thyroid cancer are listed in **Box 2.1**.

Patients with papillary carcinoma can be separated into high- and low-risk groups with regard to risk for recurrence and long-term survival. Several sophisticated prognostic scoring systems have been introduced to identify patients with high-risk tumours and aid comparison between different surgical therapies. The AGES scoring system from the Mayo Clinic considers: Age of patients, histological Grade and Extent and Size of tumour.[47] Most patients being assessed by the scoring system fit into the low-risk group, with an excellent long-term prognosis. Other scoring systems include AMES (Age, Metastasis and Extent and Size) and MACIS (Metastasis, Age, Completeness of resection, Invasion and Size).

Total thyroidectomy has been advocated for the treatment of differentiated thyroid cancer. This is because of its ability to treat multifocal tumour,

Box 2.1 • Treatment goals in thyroid cancer

- Eradicate the primary tumour
- Reduce the incidence of distant or local recurrence
- Facilitate treatment of metastases
- Cure the maximum number of patients
- Achieve all of these objectives with minimal morbidity

decrease local recurrence, decrease distant recurrence, reduce the risk of anaplastic change in remaining remnants, facilitate treatment with ^{131}I and permit postoperative measurements of thyroglobulin concentration for monitoring the patient's subsequent progress.

Papillary carcinoma is usually multifocal, thus unilateral or even near total thyroidectomy may not necessarily remove all disease. It is likely, however, that many small foci of microscopic tumour remaining after less than total thyroidectomy stay dormant and do not necessarily progress and achieve clinical importance. Nevertheless, local tumour recurrence is an extremely serious event, carrying a risk of death.

Retrospective studies of patients undergoing thyroidectomy have demonstrated a reduced local recurrence rate with total thyroidectomy compared with a subtotal resection.[48]

With respect to mortality risk, it has been shown that high-risk patients have a lower mortality rate at 25 years when treated by bilateral resection than by ipsilateral lobectomy.[45] The rare but life-threatening complication of anaplastic transformation in an inadequately resected papillary carcinoma can be avoided by initial total thyroid clearance.

Most patients with differentiated thyroid cancer present with a unilateral thyroid nodule. In this situation, the minimum primary procedure performed should be total lobectomy on the side of the lesion, isthmusectomy and removal of the pyramidal lobe. If papillary carcinoma is (or has been) confirmed by intraoperative frozen section or preoperative FNAC, a total thyroidectomy is the most appropriate surgical treatment for both intrathyroidal and extrathyroidal tumours.

Thyroidectomy must always include clearance of any involved pretracheal and paratracheal lymph nodes. The thymus should not be disturbed to avoid devascularising the inferior parathyroids, often situated within the superior thymic horns. Lymph nodes in the lateral carotid chain group are biopsied and, if they give a positive result on frozen-section histology, should be cleared by a modified neck dissection, leaving the internal jugular vein and sternomastoid muscle intact (**Fig 2.14**, see also Plate 11, facing p. 212). There is no evidence to

Figure 2.14 • Total thyroidectomy for papillary thyroid cancer with right-sided modified neck dissection to remove involved cervical nodes.

support the use of the more extensive and mutilating classic block dissection of the neck. More extensive extrathyroidal papillary carcinomas, however, may require radical excision of adjacent structures, even including part of the trachea with construction of a temporary tracheostomy.

Recently, the concept of sentinel node assessment has been applied to the operative management of patients with differentiated thyroid cancer, although the precise role of this technique has yet to be defined.

A unilateral total lobectomy and isthmusectomy is adequate for minimal (<1 cm) lesions and the rare encapsulated papillary cancers, which generally have an excellent prognosis. The recurrent laryngeal nerve must be identified throughout its course in all of these procedures so that damage may be avoided. Rarely is it necessary to sacrifice the nerve to achieve tumour clearance. The incidence of permanent postoperative hypoparathyroidism should be no more than 3%, care being taken to identify the parathyroid glands and leave their blood supply intact.

Follicular tumours that cannot be diagnosed on FNAC are treated by total lobectomy, isthmusectomy and removal of the pyramidal lobe. Frozen section is usually unhelpful, failing to demonstrate capsular or vascular invasion, because of sampling difficulties. If the definitive histology is returned as a minimal carcinoma, then a unilateral procedure may be all that is required, if the tumour is <1 cm. A lesion shown to be frankly invasive requires a total thyroidectomy, either performed within a few days of the initial lobectomy or after a period of 3–4 months. Lymph node dissection is not routinely performed for follicular tumours.

Hürthle cell lesions, considered by some to have a bad prognosis, should be treated by total thyroidectomy and central neck node dissection[43] to remove enlarged or involved nodes.

POSTOPERATIVE TREATMENT

Thyroxine (T$_4$)

Any patient who has undergone total thyroidectomy requires replacement treatment with T$_4$, and in patients with differentiated thyroid cancer there is compelling evidence for prescribing T$_4$ to suppress TSH concentrations, which may influence the biological behaviour of any metastatic tumour.

Thyroglobulin

Measurement of thyroglobulin concentration is a sensitive indicator of residual or recurrent differentiated thyroid cancer after total thyroidectomy and when the patient is on full replacement/suppressive T$_4$ dosage.[2] It should be measured routinely at each postoperative clinic visit and has markedly reduced the need for routine serial radio-iodine scanning.

Measurement of thyroglobulin concentration may be difficult when there are circulating autoantibodies to thyroglobulin (TgAb). In these circumstances there is the potential to underestimate the risk or likelihood of metastatic malignancy.[49]

Radioactive iodine (^{131}I)

Radioactive iodine is a most useful means of detecting metastatic disease when total thyroidectomy has been performed. However, the metastases in approximately 20% of patients older than 50 years of age with papillary cancer cannot concentrate ^{131}I.[46] Most metastases from follicular carcinomas, with the exception of the Hürthle cell variety, can be imaged by radioiodine. If total thyroidectomy has been performed for differentiated cancer, postoperatively patients are initially given T$_3$ 20 µg t.d.s. and have a ^{131}I scan approximately 6 weeks later. T$_3$ is discontinued 2 weeks before the scan to allow an increase in TSH concentration, which stimulates any thyroid epithelial cells to become iodine avid before administering a therapeutic dose of 150–200 mCi ^{131}I. If there are no metastases or residual remnants of thyroid, the uptake at 24 hours should be less than 1%. It is also useful to obtain a baseline thyroglobulin level when the initial dose of radioiodine is administered.

Patients are then placed back onto T$_3$ and a second diagnostic radioiodine scan using 1–2 mCi ^{131}I is obtained 3 months later. If this subsequent scan is clear then patients can be converted to T$_4$ 150 µg/day (this is then titrated until the TSH level is suppressed below 0.1iU).

If the second scan is not clear, repeated therapeutic doses of ^{131}I are given as necessary until all residual uptake is ablated. The maximum cumulative dose of ^{131}I should be no greater than 800–1000 mCi. Patients whose metastases are visible only on radioiodine scanning despite negative results on chest radiography or tomography have an excellent prognosis.[50] Once the patient is stable and disease free, follow-up is achieved by a combination of clinical examination and measurement of serum thyroglobulin concentration. Ultrasound examination has also been shown to be a sensitive tool in assessing whether cervical lymphadenopathy is present in the postoperative follow-up of patients.[51] PET scanning may be useful in patients suspected of having recurrent or persistent differentiated thyroid cancer but who fail to demonstrate evidence of disease on radioiodine scanning.[52]

Local radiotherapy and retinoic acid

Radiotherapy may be useful in controlling locally advanced differentiated thyroid cancer, where microscopic or gross disease persists following surgical resection.[53] Similarly, radiotherapy has a role in controlling pain from distant bony metastases. Recently attention has been focused on the possibility of 'redifferentiating' tumours that fail to take up radioiodine by administering retinoic acid. Initial studies appear promising but whether this therapy proves to be effective remains to be seen. Haugen et al. have identified retinoic acid receptor isoforms in some thyroid cancers. This offers the possibility of identifying which tumours may respond well to retinoic acid therapy.[54]

Medullary carcinoma

This tumour arises from the thyroid C-cells (derived from neural ectoderm). It accounts for approximately 8% of malignant thyroid tumours. In 1959 Hazard described the tumour as a solid, non-follicular carcinoma with coexisting amyloid.[55] In 1966 Williams, while further defining the histology of the tumour, proposed that the disease arose from the parafollicular or C-cells, later shown to secrete calcitonin, a peptide capable of lowering the blood calcium concentration and amenable to measurement by radioimmunoassay.[56,57] Medullary thyroid cancer (MTC) is a sporadic tumour in 80% of patients and familial in 20%. The familial syndromes, which are inherited in an autosomal dominant manner with almost complete penetrance but variable expressivity, consist of the MEN 2A and MEN 2B syndromes (**Fig. 2.15**) and the rarer non-MEN familial form.

PATHOLOGY

MTC is a solid tumour usually occurring in the upper two-thirds of the thyroid (where the C-cells are concentrated). It is often multicentric and bilateral (particularly in the familial form). The typical histological picture is one of infiltrating neo-plastic cells invading the thyroid, forming glandular and solid areas with an amyloid stroma. The tumour grows locally but readily spreads by lymphatics to regional nodes (**Fig. 2.16**) and via the bloodstream to distant sites such as liver, lungs and bones. The tumour synthesises and secretes calcitonin, which proves to be a most valuable biochemical and histochemical marker. CEA and calcitonin gene-related peptide (CGRP) are also produced by C-cells, but they have little clinical value as tumour markers, though raised CEA levels are thought to be associated with a poorer long-term prognosis.

Figure 2.15 • Tongue of patient with multiple endocrine neoplasia type 2B syndrome showing ganglioneuromas.

Figure 2.16 • MRI scan demonstrating right-sided cervical lymphadenopathy in a patient with medullary thyroid cancer.

CLINICAL FEATURES

As with most thyroid tumours, the disease typically presents as a mass in the neck, often with enlarged cervical and mediastinal lymph nodes. Involvement of adjacent organs and the recurrent laryngeal nerve may cause respiratory or swallowing difficulties and voice changes. Sporadic disease has a peak incidence at 40–50 years of age whereas inherited familial disease is usually seen at a younger age. Diarrhoea is often a prominent clinical feature, but the ability of this tumour to secrete a range of hormones and peptides, including calcitonin, prostaglandins, 5-hydroxytryptamine and adreno-corticotropic hormone, can give rise to a range of clinical syndromes, which may include Cushing's syndrome.

Although the familial varieties of the disease can present in an identical clinical manner to sporadic disease, genetic screening for *RET* mutations allows detection of the inherited condition at a preclinical stage before there is histological or macroscopic evidence of the disease.

DIAGNOSIS

Clinical assessment and the taking of a careful family history are fundamental to establishing a precise diagnosis. When there is a high index of suspicion FNAC and measurement of serum calcitonin concentration usually provides confirmation. Though the diagnosis of MTC may be secure it is important to distinguish the sporadic from the familial variety. Because of the close association of phaeochromocytoma and MTC in the MEN familial forms, it is considered mandatory in all patients to measure the 24-hour urinary catecholamine and metanephrine concentrations before progressing to any invasive procedure such as surgery. A thyroidectomy performed on a patient with an undiagnosed, untreated phaeochromocytoma is likely to have disastrous physiological and clinical consequences.

TREATMENT

Total thyroidectomy is the appropriate procedure to adequately treat multicentric and bilateral disease. The central and paratracheal lymph nodes are cleared from the level of the thyroid cartilage to the upper mediastinum, including thymectomy. The lateral nodes in the carotid sheath are sampled and, if involved with tumour, a modified radical node dissection is performed, preserving the internal jugular vein, sternomastoid muscle and spinal accessory nerve. Even when the primary tumour is extensive, the recurrent laryngeal nerve can usually be preserved. Because of the multifocal nature of familial tumours, a bilateral lymph node clearance is advised in this setting. However, when more than one lymph node compartment is involved with metastatic disease there is little chance of normalisation of calcitonin.[58]

PROGNOSIS

The presence or absence of distant metastases and lymph node positivity are major factors in determining the ultimate prognosis. Excellent 10-year survival figures of approximately 90% have recently been reported,[59] but when lymph node metastases are present this survival rate is reduced to 45%. Sporadic disease and MEN 2B tumours are associated with the worst prognosis. A better outlook is seen in patients with non-MEN familial and MEN 2A syndromes.

FOLLOW-UP

After surgery, regular clinical and biochemical follow-up is carried out with measurement of calcitonin and CEA concentrations. When increased concentrations of these tumour markers persist after thyroidectomy or develop subsequently this may signify persistent or recurrent disease. Ultrasonography, CT, MRI and scanning with MIBG, octreotide or DMSA can be utilised to detect this disease (**Fig. 2.17**). For occult disease, selective venous catheterisation and sampling for calcitonin concentration has been used.[60] Laparoscopic assessment of the liver may detect small metastases not

Figure 2.17 • CT scan demonstrating laryngeal metastatic deposit from medullary thyroid carcinoma. Patient treated by hemilaryngectomy.

visible by conventional scanning. A proportion of these patients can be helped by re-operative surgery, but the benefits of radical re-operative surgery remain controversial. External irradiation can occasionally produce some benefit, and chemotherapy with doxorubicin is toxic and response rates are disappointing.

Anaplastic carcinoma

This tumour has a peak incidence between 60 and 70 years of age, occurs slightly more often in women, and has a higher incidence in endemic goitrous areas. The tumour rapidly infiltrates local structures and metastasises via the bloodstream and lymphatics. The frequent finding of foci of papillary or follicular carcinoma in anaplastic tumours gives rise to the view that this disease originates in an unrecognised or untreated differentiated tumour.[61] The clinical findings are typically those of an elderly woman, often with a long history of goitre that suddenly starts to grow rapidly. Involvement of adjacent structures results in hoarseness, dysphonia, dysphagia and a compromised airway.

Although the clinical findings are virtually diagnostic, confirmation should be obtained by FNAC, the aspirate showing bizarre giant multinucleated and pleomorphic tumour cells. Resection of the thyroid is rarely possible because of the local extent of disease. Incision biopsy for diagnostic purposes should be avoided for fear of initiating uncontrollable local spread of the disease. If surgery is possible, it should be to relieve an obstructed airway by excision of the isthmus. Radiotherapy and doxorubicin are the main modalities of treatment, but invariably the tumour rapidly progresses usually leading to death of the patient within 6 months.

Malignant lymphoma

Thyroid lymphoma, usually of the non-Hodgkin's B-cell type, can develop as part of a generalised lymphomatous process involving other viscera, but the disease is usually confined as a primary tumour to the thyroid (**Fig 2.18**). The majority of such lymphomas arise in a background of longstanding autoimmune Hashimoto's thyroiditis,[62] although it must be emphasised that only a very small number

Figure 2.18 • CT scan showing a small lymphoma confined to the right thyroid lobe. No local lymphadenopathy is seen.

of patients with this relatively common disorder ultimately go on to develop lymphoma.

These tumours infiltrate throughout lymphatics and blood vessels, spreading directly into adjacent tissue and involving cervical nodes.

As in the case of anaplastic carcinoma, this is primarily a disease of elderly women, a typical patient presenting with a painless firm thyroid mass, rapidly increasing in size. There may be a history of goitre or autoimmune disease, and some patients will be frankly hypothyroid or already receiving T_4. This tumour grows to involve adjacent cervical structures, and lymphadenopathy is invariably present. FNAC usually raises a high degree of suspicion but full characterisation of the lymphoma requires histological assessment. In most patients this is possible by a needle core biopsy. Radiotherapy and chemotherapy are the main treatment modalities. Chemotherapy is of most value for extrathyroidal and disseminated disease. Surgery may be necessary to free the trachea when there is impending obstruction. Although a 5-year survival of 85% has been reported,[63] the overall prognosis of the disease is significantly influenced by the histopathological grade of the lesion and the presence of locally extensive or disseminated disease.

Squamous cell carcinoma

This is a rare tumour, distinct from the squamous metaplasia often seen in papillary carcinomas. It is an aggressive disease with a clinical course similar to that of anaplastic carcinoma. Most squamous cell tumours are unresectable.

Metastatic carcinoma of the thyroid

The thyroid gland can be the site of metastatic spread from tumours such as breast and kidney. Careful clinical assessment may suggest the correct diagnosis but confirmation is usually obtained by FNAC. In some instances resection of the thyroid gland is indicated if the primary disease is otherwise well controlled.

HYPERTHYROIDISM

Hyperthyroidism has a prevalence in the UK of approximately 27 per 1000 women and 2.3 per 1000 men.[64] Although Graves' disease is the most common cause of hyperthyroidism, there is an extensive list of other causes that require consideration (**Box 2.2**).

Graves' disease (diffuse toxic goitre) is an immunological disorder in which thyroid-stimulating antibodies (TsAbs) of the IgG type bind to the TSH receptor and stimulate the thyroid cell to produce and secrete an excess of thyroid hormones. Human leucocyte antigen (HLA) studies demonstrate that patients positive for HLA B8 and HLA DR3 have an increased susceptibility to the disease. The thyroid gland hypertrophies, producing diffuse enlargement, although nodular varieties of the condition are recognised. An important subgroup is that of internodular hyperplasia in a background of multinodular goitre. Histologically there is acinar hyperplasia, high columnar epithelium, increased vascularity and often lymphoid infiltration.

Clinical features

Most of the symptoms and signs of thyrotoxicosis (**Box 2.3**) result from excess thyroid hormones stimulating metabolism, heat production and oxygen consumption. Cardiac features are caused by beta-adrenergic sympathetic activity. Although Graves' disease can occur at any age, it is especially common in young women between 20 and 40 years

Box 2.2 • Causes of thyrotoxicosis

Common
• Diffuse toxic goitre (Graves' disease)
• Toxic multinodular goitre (Plummer's disease)
• Toxic solitary nodule
• Toxic multinodular goitre with internodular hyperplasia
• Nodular goitre with hyperthyroidism due to exogenous iodine
• Exogenous thyroid hormone excess (factitious)
• Thyroiditis (subacute and autoimmune) – transient
Rare
• Diffuse thyroid autonomy
• Metastatic thyroid carcinoma
• Struma ovarii
• Pituitary tumour secreting thyroid-stimulating hormone
• Choriocarcinoma and hydatidiform mole
• Neonatal thyrotoxicosis
• Postpartum hyperthyroidism
• After ^{131}I therapy

Figure 2.19 • A patient with Graves' disease.

of age (**Fig. 2.19**). The onset may be gradual or abrupt, with an extremely variable subsequent course often characterised by exacerbations and remissions. Clinical features due to hypermetabolism tend to predominate, although in elderly people the cardiovascular and neurological features usually

Box 2.3 • Clinical features of thyrotoxicosis (see also Fig. 2.19)

- Palpitations, tachycardia, cardiac arrhythmias, cardiac failure
- Sweating
- Tremor
- Hyperkinetic movements
- Nervousness
- Myopathy
- Tiredness and lethargy
- Weight loss (occasional weight gain due to increased appetite)
- Heat intolerance
- Diarrhoea
- Vomiting
- Irritability
- Emotional disturbance
- Behavioural abnormalities
- Ophthalmic signs
- Irregular menstruation and amenorrhoea
- Pretibial myxoedema
- Thyroid acropathy
- Vitiligo
- Alopecia

Figure 2.20 • CT scan of orbit in Graves' disease ophthalmopathy demonstrating marked infiltration of the extraocular muscles.

Although the ophthalmopathy is usually bilateral, it may affect only one eye. Diplopia, particularly on upward outward gaze, results from weakening and paralysis of the external ocular muscles. The cornea is vulnerable to damage, and in extreme cases ulceration may occur. Papilloedema, retinal haemorrhage and optic nerve damage (malignant exophthalmos) can progress to blindness (**Fig. 2.20**).

Investigation

Measurement of free T_4, T_3 and TSH concentrations will confirm the diagnosis (in T_3 toxicosis, T_4 concentrations will be normal whereas concentrations of T_3 will be increased and TSH suppressed). A radioactive iodine or technetium scan is not essential in the diagnosis of Graves' disease, although it is necessary in the assessment of toxic solitary and multinodular goitre to determine the site of nodular overactivity. Radioactive iodine uptake studies are particularly appropriate when a diagnosis of thyroiditis or factitious hyperthyroidism is being considered.

In Graves' disease there are three treatment options that can be used either alone or in combination to restore the euthyroid state:

- antithyroid drugs
- radioactive iodine
- surgery

dominate. Hyperthyroidism may be severe and even fatal. In children the condition often causes growth abnormalities.

The immunological changes in Graves' disease are complex and undoubtedly cause many of the ophthalmic symptoms and signs. The ophthalmopathy has two major components:

1. **Non-infiltrative ophthalmopathy** – resulting from increased sympathetic activity leading to upper lid retraction, a stare and infrequent blinking.
2. **Infiltrative ophthalmopathy** – causing oedema of the orbital contents, lids and periorbital tissues, cellular infiltration and deposition of mucopolysaccharide material within the orbit.

Each of these treatments has an important role, but for each patient all factors – medical, personal and social – are carefully considered to produce a treatment plan individualised for each patient.

Medical treatment

ANTITHYROID DRUGS: PROPYLTHIOURACIL, CARBIMAZOLE AND METHIMAZOLE

These drugs interfere with the incorporation of iodine into tyrosine residues and prevent the coupling of iodotyrosines into iodothyronines. Carbimazole may also have some immuno-suppressive action on TsAb production. Medical treatment with thionamides has two principal roles:

1. Treatment of patients with a new diagnosis of Graves' disease in the hope of inducing a permanent remission.
2. To render the toxic patient euthyroid in preparation for surgery.

Although most patients can be rendered euthyroid with antithyroid drugs there is a less than optimum remission rate after an 'adequate' course of medication. A relapse rate of approximately 43% is seen in the first year after stopping drugs, and approximately 20% of the remaining patients relapse in each of the subsequent 5 years.[66] Antithyroid drugs are therefore only a satisfactory long-term solution to the problems of hyperthyroidism for less than 50% of patients. Carbimazole is prescribed in a dose of 10–15 mg 8-hourly, reducing to 5 mg 8-hourly once the euthyroid state has been achieved. Iatrogenic hypothyroidism may be prevented by the administration of a small dose of T_4 in a so-called blocking/replacement regimen. Patients must be followed-up carefully, with regular clinical assessment and measurement of thyroid function tests. All patients should be warned concerning side effects, particularly those relating to effects on the bone marrow resulting in leucopenia, agranulocytosis and aplastic anaemia. Instructions are given to discontinue carbimazole and seek medical advice immediately should buccal ulceration or a sore throat develop. Other side effects include rashes, pruritus, arthritis and nausea.

Propylthiouracil is more widely used in the USA than elsewhere and can be used effectively if **mild** side effects have occurred with carbimazole. The other major indication for administration of antithyroid drugs is to render the patient euthyroid once a decision has been made to proceed with surgery.

BETA-ADRENERGIC BLOCKERS

Many of the manifestations of hyperthyroidism, particularly those relating to the cardiovascular system, can be ameliorated by the administration of beta-blockers, such as propranolol. This agent also reduces peripheral conversion of T_4 to T_3. Beta-blockers are usually used in combination with one of the thionamides, particularly in patients who are severely toxic and in those being prepared for surgery. The usual dose of propranolol is 20–40 mg 8-hourly. Long-acting beta-blockers can be administered once daily. Beta-blockers are absolutely contraindicated in patients with asthma. When used as preoperative preparation, propranolol must not be omitted on the morning of surgery and must be continued for at least 5 days postoperatively because of the 8-day half-life of circulating T_4.

RADIOACTIVE IODINE

[131]I can be used to control thyrotoxicosis by destruction of overactive thyroid tissue. There would seem to be no adverse effects of ^{131}I treatment with respect to leukaemia, thyroid carcinoma, fetal damage or genetic mutation, and in the USA the therapy is even given to children. [131]I (555 MBq) is administered as an ablative dose and the patient covered with carbimazole 10 mg t.d.s. started 3 days after the administration and continued for approximately 1 month to counter the effects of thyroid hormone release, which might precipitate a thyroid crisis.

Although some patients require additional doses of ^{131}I as a result of an inadequate initial response, most patients will be cured of toxicity. An ablative dose (555 MBq) renders more than 60% of patients hypothyroid in 1 year.[66] Regular long-term surveillance is required and T_4 replacement given as necessary. Thyroid eye disease may worsen after radioactive iodine treatment. Glucocorticoids can be given to attempt to reduce this risk.

Surgery

Thyroidectomy in patients with Graves' disease is safe and rapidly renders the patient euthyroid. The principal indications for surgery are:

I. Relapse after an adequate course of antithyroid drugs.
2. Severe thyrotoxicosis with a large goitre.
3. Difficulty in controlling toxicity with antithyroid drugs (including poor compliance).
4. High T_4 concentrations (>70 pmol/L).

Surgery would be offered to most patients under 40 years of age fulfilling the above criteria.

OPERATIVE STRATEGY

Details of thyroidectomy are covered in the section dealing specifically with surgical technique (see p. 69). Two surgical options are available, bilateral subtotal thyroidectomy (leaving a 3–4 g posterior remnant of thyroid tissue on each side of the trachea) or total thyroidectomy. Increasingly many endocrine surgeons seem to favour total thyroid-ectomy as a treatment for Graves' disease. This approach removes the possibility of recurrent disease, appears to improve the outlook for patients with significant eye disease, and eliminates annual thyroid function tests to assess remnant function.

Special circumstances in Graves' disease

REACTION TO ANTITHYROID DRUGS

Thyrotoxic patients who have demonstrated an adverse reaction to antithyroid drugs may be prepared for surgery by the use of beta-blockers. However, in patients who have asthma or where anti-thyroid drugs have not rendered the patient completely euthyroid, Lugol's iodine or potassium iodide tablets (60 mg t.d.s.) is an extremely useful alternative (the so-called 'thyroid stun').

CHILDREN

Treatment should be started with antithyroid drugs and continued for no more than 12–18 months. When treatment is discontinued, relapse may follow in up to 50% of patients. Such children are usually candidates for surgery, and the resection must be more radical than in adults because remnant growth and recurrent hyperthyroidism are more likely.

PREGNANCY

Hyperthyroidism occurring in pregnancy poses a difficult management problem.[67] Radioactive iodine is absolutely contraindicated. Antithyroid drugs are used, propylthiouracil being the drug of choice as it crosses the placenta less readily than carbimazole. Once control of thyrotoxicosis has been achieved, the dose of antithyroid drugs should be reduced as far as possible and the thyroid status of the mother carefully measured. A blocking/replacement regimen must not be used, as T_4 does not cross the placenta in sufficient amounts to avoid fetal hypothyroidism. In a patient still requiring high doses of antithyroid drugs or in whom hyperthyroidism is difficult to control, surgery may be safely performed in the second trimester.

RECURRENT HYPERTHYROIDISM AFTER SURGERY

Further surgery is hazardous as it is likely to be unsuccessful and carries a significant risk of damage to recurrent laryngeal nerves and parathyroid glands. In patients over the age of 40, ^{131}I is the treatment of choice, whereas under 40 years of age, antithyroid drugs are prescribed in the hope of achieving lasting remission.

NEONATAL HYPERTHYROIDISM

TsAbs crossing the placenta may stimulate the fetal thyroid to produce transient hyperthyroidism.[68] Active supportive treatment with antithyroid drugs is necessary and the whole process is usually self-limiting within a period of 1–2 months.

OPHTHALMIC GRAVES' DISEASE

The effect of surgery on this condition is somewhat unpredictable, although in the past total thyroid-ectomy has been advocated in an attempt to arrest the progress of the eye disease. Patients must be warned that effective treatment of the thyrotoxicosis is not a guarantee that ophthalmopathy will regress. Mild symptoms can be treated by the administration of methylcellulose eye drops, but more severe disease may require steroids, lateral tarsorrhaphy or even orbital decompression.

TOXIC MULTINODULAR GOITRE

Antithyroid drugs are of no value as a long-term treatment in the younger patient because toxicity is due to autonomy of the nodules and will recur once any medication is discontinued. However, in the older patient who is unsuitable for surgery, long-term treatment with carbimazole may be appropriate. ^{131}I can be used for small goitres, but usually a total thyroidectomy is most appropriate after achievement of the euthyroid state with antithyroid drugs.

TOXIC SOLITARY NODULE

This condition is caused by a single autonomous thyroid nodule. Patients with a nodule greater than 3–4 cm are more commonly treated by thyroid lobectomy, tumours below this size can successfully be managed by ^{131}I (the normal thyroid gland being protected from iodine uptake as it is suppressed).

Follow-up

Because of the risk of developing postoperative hypothyroidism, patients who have undergone any form of treatment for hyperthyroidism must be followed-up on a long-term basis, with regular clinical and biochemical assessment.

THYROIDITIS

The thyroid gland may be subject to inflammatory change in a variety of conditions, which may be focal or diffuse and are often associated with thyroid dysfunction.

Subacute thyroiditis

This condition, often called granulomatous thyroiditis or de Quervain's thyroiditis, is probably of viral origin. It is characterised by painful swelling of one or both thyroid lobes, with associated malaise and fever. Often there is a preceding history of sore throat or viral infection a week or two before the onset of thyroid symptoms. Approximately one-third of patients are asymptomatic apart from enlargement of the thyroid gland, but 10–15% have a more acute illness with symptoms and signs of hyperthyroidism resulting from the outpouring of thyroid hormones into the circulation from the damaged inflamed thyroid. Thyroid hormone concentrations are increased but, in contrast to Graves' disease, there is low uptake of radioactive iodine on scintigraphy. The erythrocyte sedimentation rate and other markers of acute inflammation are invariably raised. The disease process is usually self-limiting, with resolution of local symptoms and thyroid dysfunction. A few patients, however, pass through a mild hypothyroid phase. Local symptoms can be controlled with aspirin but, if these are severe and prolonged, a course of corticosteroids can be helpful. The transient hyperthyroidism does not require treatment with antithyroid drugs.

Autoimmune thyroiditis (Hashimoto's thyroiditis)

Focal thyroiditis is often seen in association with other thyroid disease, particularly Graves' hyperthyroidism, and is a common finding in autopsy studies. A condition of lymphomatous thyroiditis was described by Hashimoto, and occurs as a diffuse process throughout the gland, which usually enlarges to several times normal size. Although classically the gland enlargement is diffuse, there may be nodularity and lobulation making it difficult to distinguish from simple multinodular goitre or even malignant disease.

Histologically there is infiltration of the thyroid by lymphocytes and plasma cells, and frequently secondary lymphoid nodules and adjacent stromal fibrosis. The condition is due to an immunological disorder characterised by thyroid antibodies – anti-thyroglobulin and anti-thyroid peroxidase (anti-TPO, or antimicrosomal) – in the serum. A positive family history of other autoimmune disease such as pernicious anaemia, gastritis, vitiligo, diabetes mellitus, Addison's disease, autoimmune liver disease and thyrotoxicosis is often obtained.[69] As a result of destructive changes within the infiltrated thyroid, hypothyroidism usually ensues, and when present requires treatment with T_4. This medication suppresses TSH and leads to shrinkage of the thyroid gland with relief of any local symptoms. Pressure symptoms and involvement of adjacent structures are rare and surgery is usually not required. The risk of developing lymphoma of the thyroid, although small, is increased several times in the presence of Hashimoto's thyroiditis.[54] When a gland that is involved with autoimmune disease is seen to enlarge rapidly or develop a firm asymmetrical nodular area, exclusion of lymphoma by FNAC or core biopsy is required.

Riedel's thyroiditis

This condition, sometimes called invasive fibrous thyroiditis, is characterised by a dense fibrous inflammatory infiltrate throughout the gland, sometimes extending through the capsule to involve adjacent structures. The condition is rare but is important because the clinical picture mimics thyroid malignancy. Sclerosing cholangitis and retroperitoneal, mediastinal and retro-orbital fibrosis may coexist. Needle biopsy is likely to be uninformative, and often an open incision biopsy is required to establish a precise diagnosis. Surgical resection of the isthmus will be required to free a compromised airway.

Acute suppurative thyroiditis

The thyroid gland can be affected by a variety of bacterial or fungal agents, producing clinical features of an acute, painfully inflamed organ. Confirmation of diagnosis and bacteriology is obtained by needle aspiration, and appropriate antibiotics are administered. The condition is rare in Western practice.

Postpartum thyroiditis

Postpartum thyroiditis is now recognised more often and is characterised by an early thyrotoxic phase usually with mild symptoms and transient dysfunction.[70,71] There is a later hypothyroid phase, sometimes requiring treatment with T_4; long-term hypothyroidism occurs in up to 25% of patients.

HYPOTHYROIDISM

Hypothyroidism is a clinical state resulting from insufficient thyroid hormone or more rarely a resistance of the tissues to T_4. Causes can be classified as congenital (cretinism) or acquired (adult type). Retardation of growth and impaired mental development are the serious features of hypothyroidism in the infant. The child fails to thrive, is constipated and displays the classical physical signs of a puffy face, large tongue and protuberant abdomen. In adults the extreme presentation is that of myxoedema, characterised by weight gain, facial puffiness and pallor, dry skin, hair loss, hoarseness of the voice, declining intellect and, in extreme cases, psychiatric disturbance and even coma. The causes of hypothyroidism are listed in **Box 2.4**.

Hypothyroidism is confirmed by measurement of TSH, which is raised. Free T_4 and T_3 concentrations will be low in primary hypothyroidism. Treatment is with thyroxine. Caution must be exercised in starting therapy in myxoedematous and elderly patients (who may already be suffering from heart disease). Initially a low dose of thyroxine is administered (0.025 mg) increasing gradually to full replacement level.

Box 2.4 • Causes of hypothyroidism

Primary hypothyroidism
• Thyroid agenesis
Disorders of thyroid hormone synthesis
• Iodine deficiency
• Dyshormonogenesis
• Antithyroid drugs
Thyroid gland damage
• Hashimoto's thyroiditis
• Surgical resection of the thyroid
• Radioactive iodine ablation
• Post-subacute thyroiditis
Secondary hypothyroidism (pituitary)
• Pituitary tumour
• Autoimmune hypophysitis
Tertiary hypothyroidism (hypothalamic)
• Hypothalamic tumour
• Generalised or peripheral thyroid hormone resistance

THYROIDECTOMY

The term 'thyroidectomy' embraces a variety of surgical procedures but the precise procedure should be tailored to the existing pathology (**Table 2.3**).

Unilateral total thyroid lobectomy

Informed consent should be obtained from all patients. Preoperative examination of the vocal cords (by indirect laryngoscopy) is now considered advisable. This procedure will exclude an unsuspected pre-existing unilateral nerve palsy, which is particularly important if the patient has undergone previous thyroid surgery.

General anaesthesia, with endotracheal intubation and muscle relaxation, is used and the patient is placed supine on an operating table tilted 15° upwards at the head end to reduce venous engorgement. A small degree of neck extension aids access to the thyroid but care must be taken not to extend the neck too much (this may result in cervical trauma, particularly in the elderly patient).

A skin incision should be marked out to lie in a suitable skin crease above the sternal notch. The length of the incision will depend on the degree of thyroid enlargement and whether further procedures (such as modified neck dissection are contemplated).

The incision is deepened through the platysma, and upper and lower skin flaps are raised by a combination of sharp and blunt dissection in the plane superficial to the anterior jugular vessels. The upper flap is freed to the level of the thyroid notch and the lower flap to the suprasternal notch. These skin flaps are held apart with a suitable self-retaining retractor and a midline incision is made through the fascia over the thyroid. It is the length of this vertical incision that determines access to the thyroid. The strap muscles will be separated, dissected from the thyroid and retracted laterally. These muscles are not routinely divided. If greater exposure is required to gain safe access to a large or vascular goitre, the strap muscles may be divided.

The thyroid lobe is dislocated and delivered forwards by the insertion of the index finger between the thyroid lobe and strap muscles. The middle thyroid veins, if apparent at this stage,

Table 2.3 • Thyroid surgery

Procedures	Indications
Unilateral total lobectomy, including pyramidal lobe and isthmus	Solitary nodules Unilateral multinodular disease
Bilateral subtotal thyroidectomy (unilateral lobectomy and contralateral resection)	Diffuse toxic goitre of Graves' disease Bilateral non-toxic and toxic multinodular goitre Hashimoto's disease
Total thyroidectomy	Most cases of papillary, follicular and medullary carcinoma
Excision of isthmus	May be only procedure possible in anaplastic carcinoma or lymphoma to free airway Riedel's thyroiditis

should be ligated and divided. Any adhesions lateral to the thyroid lobe are divided by a combination of sharp and blunt dissection and the thyroid lobe retracted further medially, usually with a gauze swab between the operator's thumb and the gland. Tissue forceps must not be placed on the thyroid when performing surgery for a solitary nodule, in case the lesion should prove to be malignant and cell spillage occur.

Full mobilisation of the thyroid lobe is achieved by ligation and division of the superior thyroid vessels at the upper pole. To gain access to these vessels it is often helpful to pass a finger upwards in the plane behind the vessels, breaking down adhesions; then with gentle downward traction on the thyroid the vessels come clearly into view. The space medial to the superior thyroid artery is carefully opened with a pledget or artery forceps to expose the external branch of the superior laryngeal nerve (ESLN). This may be identified on the inferior pharyngeal constrictor before entering the cricothyroid muscle. A non-toothed forceps is then passed under the vascular pedicle to lift the vessels forwards. The branches of the superior thyroid artery and vein must be tied close to the thyroid gland to avoid damage to the ESLN. In approximately 20% of patients, this nerve may pass between the branches of the vessels and is in great

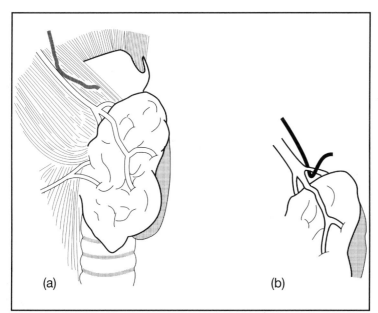

Figure 2.21 • **(a)** The external superior laryngeal nerve (ESLN) passing medial to the superior thyroid artery before entering the cricothyroid muscle. **(b)** The ESLN is in a vulnerable position when passing between branches of the superior thyroid artery.

danger if mass ligation is carried out (**Fig. 2.21**). In a further 20% of patients the nerve runs its distal course through the inferior pharyngeal constrictor muscle, is not visible at surgery and is at no risk of damage.

The recurrent laryngeal nerve (RLN) should now be identified before continuing with dissection of the thyroid lobe. The nerve may run close to the tracheo-oesophageal groove but there is enormous variability of its position, course and relationship to key anatomical structures in the neck. If damage is to be avoided, an accurate knowledge of the normal anatomy and these variations is of paramount importance. Palpation of the RLN as a cordlike structure against the trachea is often a useful initial guide to the nerve's location. The nerve can then be exposed by gentle dissection of the overlying fascial layers with a small artery clip. The nerve often has a small blood vessel running on its surface, aiding in its identification (the vasa nervorum). Vulnerability is somewhat greater on the right than on the left because of the obliquity of the nerve's course in the lower third of the wound. The nerve usually lies deep to the inferior thyroid artery but can be rendered vulnerable by anterior fixation in a fork formed by the glandular branches of this artery (**Fig. 2.22**). Precise definition of the nerve–artery

Figure 2.22 • Recurrent laryngeal nerve held in a vulnerable anterior position by fork of inferior thyroid artery branches.

relationship is most important. A potential pitfall for the unwary exists when the RLN passes superficial to the inferior thyroid artery, appears to pulsate and may therefore be mistaken for a vessel and ligated.

The RLN can be displaced from its usual position by nodules, particularly in the posterior part of the thyroid lobe, and occasionally is displaced anteriorly, close to the lower pole of the thyroid into a dangerous position where it may be ligated and divided with the inferior thyroid veins. Clearly these veins must not be clipped until the nerve has been identified in its lower third. During unilateral lobectomy, the small arterial branches to the thyroid must all be individually clipped and tied close to the gland, staying on the thyroid capsule. The main trunk of the inferior thyroid artery is not ligated, to minimise ischaemic damage to the parathyroids.

The nerve is perhaps in most danger close to its point of entry into the larynx as it passes through Berry's ligament, often adopting a curving, looping course before entering the larynx. To identify the nerve in this region the suspensory fascia must be carefully divided. This manoeuvre is most safely accomplished by staying close to the thyroid and picking up superficial layers one at a time with fine haemostats, being absolutely certain that at each stage only fascia and small arterial branches are included. The nerve is soon seen at a deeper level, glistening, with its fine accompanying arterial blood vessel aiding identification. The inferior cornu of the thyroid cartilage is a most dependable landmark for the point of entry of the RLN into the larynx.

In approximately 1% of patients the nerve on the right is non-recurrent, arising from the vagus and passing medially close to the inferior thyroid artery before turning to ascend and enter the larynx (**Fig. 2.23**). Ligation of the main trunk of the inferior thyroid artery in these circumstances could result in permanent damage to the nerve. It is well recognised that the RLN can divide into several branches before entering the larynx and therefore clear identification of all divisions is necessary for their preservation.

The parathyroid glands should also be identified. When they are in their usual positions, the inferior gland can be located close to the lower pole of the thyroid anterior to the RLN. The superior gland is

Figure 2.23 • Non-recurrent laryngeal nerve passing in close proximity to the inferior thyroid artery before ascending to the larynx.

usually seen just above the inferior thyroid artery; in more than 90% of patients it is within a 1-cm radius of the junction of the inferior thyroid artery and the RLN. The dissection of the thyroid should continue close to the capsule of the gland, with ligation and division of the individual branches of the inferior thyroid artery, preserving those branches that supply the parathyroid glands. It is possible to tease the parathyroid glands away from the thyroid with their blood supply intact, leaving them free but perfectly viable. It must be remembered that enlargement of the thyroid can carry the parathyroid glands far forwards onto the anterolateral surface of the thyroid, when they may be devascularised or inadvertently excised. In these circumstances they should be diced into 1-mm cubes and autotransplanted into several pockets in the sternomastoid muscle.

It is important to keep diathermy usage to a minimum as heat conduction may damage the RLN, the blood supply to the parathyroids or the delicate joints within the larynx.

The thyroid lobe is now almost completely free and is dissected further medially by dividing the vascular fascia binding it to the trachea and larynx. The division of Berry's ligament is completed, taking care to re-identify the RLN. Small vessels close to the nerve at this point require careful clipping and ligation otherwise troublesome bleeding may obscure the nerve's entry point to the larynx. Indeed, safe thyroidectomy is utterly dependent on careful haemostasis as it is only by this discipline that the RLN and parathyroid glands can be identified and left undamaged.

Mobilisation of the thyroid lobe is now complete, and the resection must include the isthmus and pyramidal lobe. The cut surface of the contralateral thyroid lobe is usually oversewn with Vicryl® to obtain haemostasis. The wound is closed in layers with absorbable material to the muscle layers, and the skin is closed with a subcuticular Prolene suture or skin clips, which can be removed at 3 days, or a synthetic absorbable monofilament suture.

Total thyroidectomy

Total thyroidectomy is usually performed for thyroid cancer but increasingly for gross multi-nodular disease. The opposite lobe is mobilised in a similar manner to that described for unilateral lobectomy. If the procedure is for cancer an appropriate lymph node clearance will also be necessary.

Subtotal thyroidectomy

When subtotal thyroidectomy is performed, perhaps for Graves' disease, the principles of identification of the vital structures are the same as those employed in a unilateral total lobectomy. In Graves' disease a small remnant, usually 3–4 g, of tissue is left in situ on each side of the trachea haemostasis secured by suturing the lateral edge of each remnant, without tension, to the anterior surface of the trachea with Vicryl®. As in unilateral lobectomy,

the main trunk of the inferior thyroid artery is not ligated, but individual small bleeding vessels on the surface of the remnant may require ligation. Unilateral total lobectomy and a contralateral resection leaving a larger single remnant may be an acceptable alternative strategy.

Recently, minimal-access and endoscopic techniques have been adapted to permit thyroidectomy, usually by performing a unilateral lobectomy for benign disease. The precise role and relevance of this technique in the management of thyroid disease remains to be defined.

Retrosternal goitre

Retrosternal goitres derive their blood supply from the superior and inferior thyroid arteries, and these are usually accessible in the neck. Ligation and division of the superior pole vessels is an essential, preliminary step before mobilisation of the gland is attempted. The retrosternal portion can then be delivered from behind the sternum by gentle traction aided by the introduction of a finger alongside the gland. Placement of traction sutures in the thyroid or the gentle introduction of a dessert spoon alongside the gland may also facilitate delivery. Median sternotomy is rarely necessary to remove a retrosternal thyroid.

Recurrent goitre

Surgery for recurrent thyroid disease is particularly hazardous with respect to damage to the RLN and parathyroid gland, as identification of these structures is likely to be impeded by the presence of scar tissue. A lateral approach to the thyroid lobe can be gained by dissecting in the plane between the strap muscles and the anterior border of the sternomastoid (where there may be fewer adhesions).

Complications of thyroidectomy

The most important complications of thyroidectomy are shown in **Box 2.5**. Complications relating to damaged individual structures can be kept to a minimum by operating in a bloodless field and performing a meticulous anatomical dissection.

- Recurrent laryngeal nerve injury
- External superior laryngeal nerve injury
- Hypoparathyroidism
- Laryngeal oedema – airway obstruction
- Bleeding – haematoma
- Hypothyroidism
- Hyperthyroidism
- Wound infection
- Keloid
- Suture granuloma

RECURRENT LARYNGEAL NERVE (RLN)

Damage to the RLN should be extremely rare after routine thyroidectomy, although the risk of damage is increased when performing re-operative thyroid surgery.[72,73] Identification of the RLN at surgery is the fundamental step to avoiding damage. When this policy is employed, any nerve damage is likely to be a transient neuropraxia and recovery will be expected, usually after a period of a few weeks or months. If the nerve has not been identified, then paralysis will be permanent in up to one-third of patients whose nerves have been injured. Extremely low nerve injury rates have been reported, even when performing extensive surgery for thyroid cancer.[74]

EXTERNAL BRANCH OF SUPERIOR LARYNGEAL NERVE (ESLN)

Assessment of damage to the ESLN is difficult, as the changes may be subtle and easily overlooked. Disability results in changes of voice pitch, range and projection. Damage to the ESLN is particularly devastating in singers. The nerve is most likely to be damaged at the time of ligation and division of the superior thyroid vessels.[75] To avoid this complication the arterial branches should be individually ligated close to the thyroid and the nerve identified whenever possible.

HYPOPARATHYROIDISM

Careful identification of the parathyroid glands and preservation of their delicate arterial blood supply can avoid this complication. In bilateral subtotal resection for Graves' disease, the incidence of hypoparathyroidism should be no more than 0.5%. The complication is more common after total thyroidectomy for cancer but even in these circumstances the incidence has been reported within the range of only 1–3%.[71]

HYPOTHYROIDISM

This sequel of thyroidectomy is most likely to occur after surgery for Graves' disease, with an incidence as high as 50%. This is not a true complication but an acceptable feature of the treatment of hyperthyroidism and is easily managed by the administration of T_4.

RECURRENT HYPERTHYROIDISM

If this occurs after surgery for Graves' disease, it represents a failure of the operation. The incidence is approximately 5% and varies depending on the size of the thyroid remnants left in situ, the immunological processes taking place within them and iodine intake.

THYROID CRISIS

This potentially life-threatening condition is rarely seen but classically occurs in the postoperative period. It is usually encountered in patients who have undergone surgery for thyrotoxicosis without adequate preoperative preparation or where a diagnosis of thyrotoxicosis has not been established prior to emergency or elective surgery. Hormones released by gland manipulation result in an acute postoperative thyrotoxicosis. The condition may also result from stress or infection. The clinical picture includes extreme distress, dyspnoea, tachycardia, hyperpyrexia, vomiting, diarrhoea, confusion and/or delirium.

Propylthiouracil (200–250 mg) is given every 4 hours, by nasogastric tube if necessary, and Lugol's or potassium iodide should be given. Adrenergic effects are treated by careful administration of propranolol under ECG-monitored control. General supportive measures consist of rehydration with intravenous fluids, cooling with ice packs, the administration of oxygen, digoxin (if there is evidence of cardiac failure), appropriate sedation and corticosteroids.

HAEMORRHAGE

Bleeding into the wound is a serious complication of thyroidectomy. When the bleeding and haematoma occur deep to the strap muscles, the situation can rapidly develop into a life-threatening emergency because of associated airway obstruction resulting from laryngeal and subglottic oedema.

AIRWAY OBSTRUCTION

Although mortality from thyroidectomy is extremely rare, airway obstruction remains the most potentially dangerous complication. It was once thought that airway obstruction caused by postoperative bleeding was due to compression of the trachea by the expanding haematoma. This is unlikely to be the case except in the rare condition of tracheomalacia. It is subglottic and laryngeal mucosal oedema consequent upon venous and lymphatic obstruction that occludes the airway. It must be appreciated that airway obstruction can occur by this mechanism as a result of operative manipulation of the trachea without any postoperative bleeding or haematoma deep to the strap muscles. It is crucial that early signs of airway obstruction (patient distress and stridor) should be recognised and the immediate suture removal undertaken.

If symptoms are mild and there is no haematoma, conservative measures of humidified oxygen or heliox (a combination of helium and oxygen) and intravenous steroids may suffice. A senior anaesthetist must be consulted immediately. Intubation may prove necessary to restore an occluding airway. If a skilled anaesthetist is not immediately available, the situation can be retrieved by insertion of two or three white needles directly into the trachea. Any obvious haematoma should be evacuated, and this should ideally be performed under general anaesthesia with endotracheal intubation in the operating room. Rarely is it necessary to remove sutures on the ward.

WOUND COMPLICATIONS

The use of absorbable suture material has virtually abolished the complication of suture granuloma after thyroidectomy. Keloid scars may still occur in susceptible individuals.

• **Key points**

- Family history is important in thyroid disease.
- Clinical examination and FNAC are essential in evaluating the thyroid nodule.
- Thyroid nodules in children are more likely to be cancers.
- Smaller intrathyroidal papillary, micropapillary and minimally invasive follicular cancers may be adequately treated by total thyroid lobectomy and TSH suppression.
- Larger intrathyroidal, extrathyroidal and widely invasive follicular cancers should be treated by total thyroidectomy and radioiodine ablation.
- Prophylactic lymph node dissection is not necessary in differentiated thyroid cancer (DTC).
- Overall prognosis in DTC is very good.
- Medullary thyroid cancer requires a more aggressive surgical approach than DTC. Genetic testing should be considered.
- Treatment options in thyrotoxicosis should be tailored to individual patient needs.
- Patients should be fully counselled with regards to the complications of thyroid surgery prior to operation.

REFERENCES

1. Beever K, Bradbury J, Phillips D et al. Highly sensitive assays of autoantibodies to thyroglobulin and to thyroid peroxidase. Clin Chem 1989; 35:1949–54.

2. van Herle AJ, Uller RP. Elevated serum thyroglobulin: a marker of metastases in differentiated thyroid carcinoma. J Clin Invest 1975; 56:270–7.

3. Doullay F, Ruf J, Codaccioni JL et al. Prevalence of autoantibodies to thyroperoxidase in patients with various thyroid and autoimmune diseases. Autoimmunity 1991; 9:237–44.

4. Rees-Smith B, McLachlan SM, Furmaniak J. Autoantibodies to the thyrotropin receptor. Endocr Rev 1988; 9:106–21.

5. Melvin KEW, Tashjian AH. The syndrome of excessive thyrocalcitonin produced by medullary carcinoma of the thyroid. Proc Natl Acad Sci USA 1968; 59:1216–22.

An important biochemical marker in determining the presence of medullary thyroid cancer before operation. Screening for phaeochromocytoma then becomes mandatory prior to surgery.

6. Mulligan LM, Kwok JBJ, Healey CS et al. Germline mutations of the RET proto oncogene in multiple endocrine neoplasia type IIA. Nature 1993; 363:458–60.

7. Turner JW, Spencer RB. Thyroid carcinoma presenting as a pertechnetate hot nodule without ^{131}I uptake. Case report. J Nucl Med 1976; 17:22–3.

8. Ochi H, Yamamoto K, Endo K et al. A new imaging agent for medullary carcinoma of the thyroid. J Nucl Med 1984; 25:323–5.

9. Hoefnagal CA, Delprat CC, Marcuse HR et al. Role of thallium-201 total-body scintigraphy in follow up of thyroid carcinoma. J Nucl Med 1986; 27:1854–7.

10. Clarke SEM, Lazarus CR, Wraight P et al. Pentavalent (^{99m}Tc) DMSA, ^{131}I MIBG, and (^{99m}Tc) MDP. An evaluation of three imaging techniques in patients with medullary carcinoma of the thyroid. J Nucl Med 1988; 29:33–8.

11. Rosen IB, Walfish PG, Miskin M. The ultrasound of thyroid masses. Surg Clin North Am 1979; 59:19–33.

12. Rosen IB, Wallace D, Strawbridge HG et al. Re-evaluation of needle aspiration cytology in detection of thyroid cancer. Surgery 1981; 90:747–56.

13. Soderstrom N. Aspiration biopsy punctures of goitres for aspiration and biopsy. Acta Med Scand 1952; 144:237–44.

14. Lowhagen T, Granberg PO, Lundell G et al. Aspiration biopsy cytology (ABC) in nodules of the thyroid gland suspected to be malignant. Surg Clin North Am 1979; 59:3–18.

15. Grant CS, Hay ID, Gough IR et al. Long term follow up of patients with benign thyroid FNA cytologic diagnosis. Surgery 1989; 106:980–91.

FNAC has become the cornerstone of diagnosis in the thyroid nodule. Both UK and US guidelines state that all patients with a thyroid nodule should have FNAC performed, irrespective of whether ultrasound scan is carried out.

16. Stephenson BM, Wheeler MH. Carcinoma of the thyroglossal duct. Aust NZ J Surg 1994; 64:212.

17. Gaitin E, Nelson NC, Poole GV. Endemic goitre and endemic thyroid disorders. World J Surg 1991; 15:205–15.

18. Gaitin E. Aetiology of benign thyroid disease – environmental aspects. In: Wheeler MH, Lazarus JH (eds) Diseases of the thyroid. Pathophysiology and management. London: Chapman & Hall Medical, 1994; pp. 73–84.

19. Vander JB, Gaston EA, Dawber TR. The significance of non toxic thyroid nodules: final report of a 15 year study of the incidence of thyroid malignancy. Ann Intern Med 1968; 69:537–40.

20. Hellwig CA. Thyroid gland in Kansas. Am J Clin Pathol 1935; 5:103–11.

21. Hayles AB, Johnson LM, Beahrs OH et al. Carcinoma of the thyroid in children. Am J Surg 1963; 106:735–43.

22. Harness JK, Thompson NW, Nishiyama RH. Childhood thyroid carcinoma. Arch Surg 1971; 102:278–84.

23. Cuello C, Correa P, Eisenberg H. Geographic pathology of thyroid carcinoma. Cancer 1969; 23:230–9.

24. Williams ED, Doniach I, Bjarnason O et al. Thyroid cancer in an iodine rich area: a histo-pathological study. Cancer 1977; 39:215–22.

25. Duffy BJ, Fitzgerald PJ. Cancer of the thyroid in children: a report of 28 cases. J Clin Endocrinol Metab 1950; 10:1296–308.

26. DeGroot LJ, Paloyan E. Thyroid carcinoma and radiation: a Chicago endemic. JAMA 1973; 225:487–91.

27. Naunheim KS, Kaplan EL, Straus FH et al. High dose external radiation to the neck and subsequent thyroid carcinoma. In: Kaplan EL (ed.) Surgery of the thyroid and parathyroid glands. Edinburgh: Churchill Livingstone, 1983; pp. 51–62.

28. Henry JF, Denizot A, Porcelli A et al. Thyro-peroxidase immunodetection for the diagnosis of malignancy on fine-needle aspiration of thyroid nodules. World J Surg 1994; 18:529–34.

29. Delbridge L, Lean CL, Russell P et al. Proton magnetic resonance and human thyroid neoplasia II: potential avoidance of surgery for benign follicular neoplasms. World J Surg 1994; 18:512–17.

30. Monzani F, Caraccio N, Iacconi P et al. Prevalence of cancer in follicular thyroid nodules: is there still a role for intraoperative frozen section analysis? Thyroid 2003; 13(4):389–94.

31. Reeve TS, Delbridge L, Cohen A. Total thyroid-ectomy: the preferred option for multinodular goitre. Ann Surg 1987; 206:782–6.

   This treatment option has become increasingly popular amongst surgeons in recent years; it removes the need for dangerous re-operative surgery and the increased risk of damage to the RLN.

32. Thompson NW, Nishiyama RH, Harness JK. Thyroid carcinoma. Current controversies. Curr Probl Surg 1978; 15:1–67.

33. Thompson NW. In: Johnston IDA, Thompson NW (eds) The thyroid nodule: surgical management in endocrine surgery. London: Butterworths, 1983; pp. 14–24.

34. Reeve TS. Operations for non-medullary cancer of the thyroid gland. In: Kaplan EL (ed.) Surgery of the thyroid and parathyroid glands. Edinburgh: Churchill Livingstone, 1983; pp. 63–74.

35. Wynford Thomas D. Molecular basis of epithelial tumorigenesis: the thyroid model. Crit Rev Oncogen 1993; 4:1–23.

36. Lemoine NR, Mayall ES, Wyllie FS et al. High frequency of Ras oncogene activation in all stages of human thyroid tumorigenesis. Oncogene 1989; 4:159–64.

37. Lemoine NR, Hughes CM, Gullick WJ et al. Abnormalities of the EGF receptor system in human thyroid neoplasia. Int J Cancer 1991; 49:558–61.

38. Garcia-Rostan G, Zhao H, Camp RL et al. Ras mutations are associated with aggressive tumor phenotypes and poor prognosis in thyroid cancer. J Clin Oncol 2003; 21(17):3226–35.

39. Fagin JA, Matsuo K, Karmakar A et al. High prevalence of mutations of the p53 gene in poorly differentiated human thyroid carcinomas. J Clin Invest 1993; 91:179–84.

40. Lote K, Anderson K, Nordal E et al. Familial occurrence of papillary thyroid carcinoma. Cancer 1980; 46:1291–7.

41. McConahey WM, Hay ID, Woolner LB et al. Papillary thyroid cancer treated at the Mayo Clinic, 1946 through 1970: initial manifestations, patho-logic findings, therapy and outcome. Mayo Clin Proc 1986; 61:978–96.

42. Noguchi S, Yamashita H, Murakami N et al. Small carcinomas of the thyroid – a long-term follow up of 867 patients. Arch Surg 1996; 131:187–91.

   A comprehensive study, showing that the vast majority of minimal papillary cancers are treated adequately by surgery alone and that the likelihood of death from this tumour is small.

43. Thompson NW. Differentiated thyroid carcinoma. In: Wheeler MH, Lazarus JH (eds) Diseases of the thyroid, pathophysiology and management. London: Chapman & Hall Medical, 1994; pp. 367–77.

44. Ozaki O, Ito K, Kobayashi K et al. Familial occur-rence of differentiated non medullary thyroid carcinoma. World J Surg 1988; 12:565–71.

45. Thompson NW. Total thyroidectomy in the treat-ment of thyroid carcinoma. In: Thompson NW, Vinik AI (eds) Endocrine surgery update. New York: Grune & Stratton, 1983; pp. 71–84.

46. Stephenson BM, Wheeler MH, Clark OH. The role of total thyroidectomy in the management of differentiated thyroid cancer. In: Daly JM (ed.) Current opinion in general surgery. Philadelphia: Current Science, 1994; pp. 53–9.

47. Hay ID, Grant CS, Taylor WF et al. Ipsilateral lobectomy versus bilateral lobe resection in papil-lary thyroid carcinoma: a retrospective analysis of surgical outcome using a novel prognostic scoring system. Surgery 1987; 102:1088–95.

48. Mazzaferri EL, Young RL. Papillary thyroid carcinoma: a 10 year follow up report of the impact of therapy in 576 patients. Am J Med 1981; 70:511–18.

   Keystone study detailing the long-term outcome from using different treatment modalities in papillary thyroid cancer. Forms the basis for TSH suppression in treating thyroid cancer.

49. Spencer CA, Takeuchi M, Kazarosyan M et al. Serum thyroglobulin autoantibodies: prevalence, influence on serum thyroglobulin measurement and prognostic significance in patients with differentiated thyroid carcinoma. J Clin Endocrinol Metab 1998; 83:1121–7.

   Study demonstrating potential errors in following patients with thyroglobulin, and suggests a solution in thyroglobulin antibody measurement. Care should be taken when comparing thyroglobulin results between different labs.

50. Vassilopoulou-Sellin R, Kline MJ, Smith TH et al. Pulmonary metastases in children and young adults with differentiated thyroid cancer. Cancer 1993; 71:1348–52.

51. Kouvaraki MA, Shapiro SE, Fornage BD et al. Role of preoperative ultrasonography in the surgical management of patients with thyroid cancer. Surgery 2003; 134(6):946–54; discussion 954–5.

52. Khan N, Oriuchi N, Higuchi T et al. PET in the follow-up of differentiated thyroid cancer. Br J Radiol 2003; 76(910):690–5.

53. Kebebew E, Clark OH. Locally advanced differentiated thyroid cancer. Surg Oncol 2003; 12(2):91–9.

54. Haugen BR, Larson LL, Pugazhenthi U et al. Retinoic acid and retinoid X receptors are differentially expressed in thyroid cancer and thyroid carcinoma cell lines and predict response to treatment with retinoids. J Clin Endocrinol Metab 2004; 89(1):272–80.

55. Hazard JB, Hawk WA, Crile G. Medullary (solid) carcinoma of the thyroid. A clinico-pathologic entity. J Clin Endocrinol Metab 1959; 19:152–61.

56. Williams ED. Histogenesis of medullary carcinoma of the thyroid. J Clin Pathol 1966; 19:114–18.

57. Tashjian AH, Howland BG, Melvin KEW et al. Immunoassay of human calcitonin: clinical measurement, relation to serum calcium and studies in patients with medullary carcinoma. N Engl J Med 1970; 283:890–5.

58. Machens A, Gimm O, Ukkat J et al. Improved prediction of calcitonin normalization in medullary thyroid carcinoma patients by quantitative lymph node analysis. Cancer 2000; 88(8):1909–15.

59. Pyke CM, Hay ID, Goellner JR et al. Prognostic significance of calcitonin immunoreactivity, amyloid staining and flow cytometric DNA measurements in medullary thyroid carcinoma. Surgery 1991; 110:967–71.

60. Sizemore GW. Medullary carcinoma of the thyroid. Semin Oncol 1987; 14:306–14.

61. Backdahl M, Hamberger B, Lowhagen T et al. Anaplastic giant cell thyroid carcinoma. In: Wheeler MH, Lazams JH (eds) Diseases of the thyroid. Pathophysiology and management. London: Chapman & Hall, 1994; pp. 379–85.

62. Sirota DK, Segal RL. Primary lymphomas of the thyroid gland. JAMA 1979; 242:1743–6.

63. Devine RM, Edis AJ, Banks PM. Primary lymphoma of the thyroid: a review of the Mayo Clinic experience through 1978. World J Surg 1981; 5:33.

64. Tunbridge WMG, Evered DC, Hall R et al. The spectrum of thyroid disease in a community: the Wickham survey. Clin Endocrinol 1977; 7:481–93.

65. Sheldon J, Reid DJ. Thyrotoxicosis: changing trends in treatment. Ann R Coll Surg Engl 1986; 68:283–5.

66. Kendall-Taylor P, Keir MJ, Ross WM. Ablative radioiodine therapy for hyperthyroidism: long term follow up study. BMJ 1984; 289:361–3.

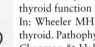

Study detailing the hypothyroid rate with radioiodine and emphasising the need for long-term follow-up with TSH estimation.

67. Masiukiewicz US, Burrow GN. Hyperthyroidism in pregnancy: diagnosis and treatment. Thyroid 1999; 9:647–52.

68. Zimmerman D. Foetal and neonatal hyperthyroidism. Thyroid 1999; 9:727–33.

69. Furmaniak J, Rees-Smith B. Diagnostic tests of thyroid function and structure – thyroid antibodies. In: Wheeler MH, Lazarus JH (eds) Diseases of the thyroid. Pathophysiology and management. London: Chapman & Hall Medical, 1994; pp. 117–30.

70. Lazarus JH, Othman S. Thyroid disease in relation to pregnancy. Clin Endocrinol 1991; 34:91–8.

71. Amino N, Miyai K, Onishi T et al. Transient hypothyroidism after delivery in autoimmune thyroiditis. J Clin Endocrinol Metab 1976; 2:296–301.

72. Wade JSH. Vulnerability of the recurrent laryngeal nerves at thyroidectomy. Br J Surg 1955; 43:164–80.

73. Beahrs OH, Vandertoll DJ. Complications of secondary thyroidectomy. Surg Gynaecol Obstet 1963; 117:535–9.

74. Clark OH. Total thyroidectomy: the treatment of choice for patients with differentiated thyroid cancer. Ann Surg 1982; 196:361–70.

75. Lennquist S, Cahlin C, Smeds S. The superior laryngeal nerve in thyroid surgery. Surgery 1987; 102:999–1008.

Three

The adrenal glands

Richard D. Bliss and
Tom W.J. Lennard

ANATOMY

The two adrenal glands have a characteristic golden colour due to the cholesterol in the cortex and are both retroperitoneal structures, weighing approximately 5–7 g in the adult male. Their positions and shapes are slightly different from each other. The right gland is pyramidal in shape and lies at the upper pole of the right kidney, between the right crus of the diaphragm and the inferior vena cava. The left adrenal gland is crescentic and lies on the upper part of the medial aspect of the left kidney. The tail of the pancreas may lie over the inferior part of the left adrenal and the left crus of the diaphragm lies behind this gland. Each gland consists of two distinct parts, which have different structures and functions – the outer cortex and the inner medulla.

Blood supply

The blood supply is similar for both glands, although there are a few differences due to the embryology of the major vessels. Classically, there are three arteries and a single vein for each gland. The arteries include branches from the inferior phrenic arteries, the renal arteries and direct branches from the aorta. In practice, the major vessels often divide before entering the glands to enter as a leach of vessels.

The adrenal vein is most commonly a single vessel that drains into the left renal vein on the left and directly into the inferior vena cava on the right. The right vein is therefore extremely short and is a major landmark for the surgeon. The veins drain from the medulla and therefore the venous return from the cortex flows through the medulla. This is relevant in that an enzyme involved in the synthesis of catecholamines (phenylethanolamine N-methyltransferase) is influenced by the levels of glucocorticoid hormones secreted by the cortex.

Lymph drainage

There are two lymphatic plexuses, one in the medulla and one under the capsule of the gland. As expected, the lymphatics follow the arterial supply to the pre-aortic nodes, then to the para-aortic and paracaval nodes and on to the thoracic duct.

Nerve supply

The gland has a rich nerve supply primarily to the adrenal medulla. The cortex has a few vasomotor nerve fibres but the rest supply the medulla and are derived from the splanchnic nerves (T5–9). The medulla itself should be regarded as a collection of modified postganglionic nerve fibres where the axon has degenerated and been replaced with innumerable granules containing either adrenaline or noradrenaline. The preganglionic sympathetic nerve fibres pass through the hilum of the adrenal to synapse with the phaeochromocytes in the medulla.

Microscopic anatomy

As mentioned above, the adrenal gland should be considered as two separate glands with distinct macroscopic and microscopic appearances. The medulla accounts for only 15% of the volume of the adrenal gland and consists of eosinophilic cells known as phaeochromocytes. They have a variable size and shape to their nuclei and hence the diagnosis of malignancy is difficult for the pathologist without the presence of invasion. They possess multiple granules in the cytoplasm attached to the membrane of the cell. These are characterised histologically by their reaction to various salts and typically stain brown to dichromate salts, hence they are referred to as chromaffin cells. There are large vascular spaces within the medulla.

The cortex of the adrenal gland is divided into three layers: the outer zona glomerulosa, the zona fasciculata and the innermost zona reticularis. There is a noticeable border between the zona reticularis and the medulla.

The zona glomerulosa produces mineralocorticoids, particularly aldosterone. It consists of an arrangement of columnar cells organised into clusters. There is relatively little cytoplasm compared with the nucleus. The zona fasciculata is the largest of the cortical zones. It occupies approximately 75% of the adrenal cortex and the cells are poorly staining, polyhedral and organised in columns running radially through the zone. It is primarily responsible for the production of glucocorticoids. The zona reticularis is characterised by large clusters of cells and is easily differentiated from both the zona fasciculata and the medulla. It produces the sex hormones, particularly dehydroepiandrosterone (DHEA).

Embryology

The embryological origins of the two layers of the adrenal are completely different. The cortex starts to appear at approximately the fifth week of gestation as two clefts, either side of the embryonic dorsal mesentery. This is mesodermal in origin. It enlarges to form the primitive (or fetal) cortex by the seventh week. At this stage, the developing adrenal gland is invaded by cells migrating from the neural crest (ectodermal in origin) to form the adrenal medulla. At the seventh week, the mesodermal layer produces another group of cells known as the secondary cortex, which becomes the mature adult adrenal cortex. The primary cortex produces large amounts of DHEA, which is made available for conversion to oestrogens by the placenta. The fetal adrenal does not produce cortisol itself until just before delivery.

At birth, the adrenal gland is large and is approximately one-third the size of the kidney. The primary cortex shrinks rapidly after delivery of the baby until it has disappeared after a year or so. It takes until puberty for the adrenal gland to regain the size it had at birth. Prior to delivery, the zona glomerulosa starts to appear, followed after delivery by the inner zona fasciculata and finally the zona reticularis emerges a few months after birth.

Accessory cortical adrenal tissue is often found (up to 50% of neonates) in the tissue around the adrenals or more rarely in relation to structures from the urogenital ridge. This usually disappears but may persist or even enlarge if the adrenals are stimulated. Ectopic medullary tissue is often found in masses around the aorta or the sympathetic plexus (organ of Zuckerkandl). Phaeochromocytomas may arise in any tissue derived from the neural crest.

PHYSIOLOGY

Adrenal medulla

The adrenal medulla produces adrenaline (epinephrine), noradrenaline (norepinephrine) and dopamine. It is basically a modified sympathetic ganglion, whereby the postganglionic cells have lost their axons and developed secretory functions.

The catecholamines are synthesised from tyrosine via a series of steps, outlined in **Fig. 3.1**. It should be noted that tyrosine hydroxylase controls the rate-limiting step. Cortisol (produced in the cortex) is necessary for the induction of phenylethanolamine N-methyltransferase (PNMT), which converts adrenaline to noradrenaline.

Figure 3.1 • Synthesis of catecholamines.

The catecholamines are released after stimulation of the medulla as the secretory granules fuse with the cell membrane (exocytosis) in a calcium-dependent process.

The majority of the released catecholamines are taken back up into the presynaptic terminals of the chromaffin cells, the rest being transported away from the adrenal into the systemic circulation. The catecholamines taken up by neural tissue are broken down by monoamine oxidase, into hydroxy-methoxy mandelate (HMMA) and homovanillic acid (HVA) (from dopamine). Carboxy-O-methyl transferase produces the deactivation of adrenaline and noradrenaline taken up by extraneural tissue, via metadrenaline and normetadrenaline to VMA.

PHYSIOLOGICAL EFFECTS

Catecholamines affect most tissues in the body but particularly the cardiovascular system and they have several metabolic effects. Basal secretion is quite low and substantial release of preformed catecholamines requires a marked stimulus during special conditions.

The actions are mediated via characteristic cell-membrane-bound receptors, the α- and β-adrenergic receptors, each with their own subclasses. The physiological effects are typified as the flight or fight response, i.e. preparing the organism for optimal performance in times of threat. An increase in heart rate, blood pressure and cardiac output, excitation of the central nervous system, contraction of iris, changes in tone of arterioles depending upon the organ affected – increased blood flow to muscles, decreased to the splanchnic circulation – and a breakdown of lipid, glycogen, and protein to provide metabolic substrate for action all occur.

Adrenal cortex

Each of the three zones of the cortex produces different hormones. The outer zona glomerulosa produces the salt-retaining hormone aldosterone, the zona fasciculata produces cortisol, and the inner-most zona reticularis produces the sex hormones. All are derivatives of cholesterol and have a characteristic molecular shape.

MINERALOCORTICOIDS

Aldosterone is the main mineralocorticoid hormone and causes an increase in resorption of sodium. This leads to an increase in the volume of the extracellular fluid by acting on the epithelium of the distal tubule and collecting duct of the kidney. Aldosterone therefore causes a fall in potassium and hydrogen ions in exchange for sodium. It is produced under the control of renin via angiotensin. A fall in the circulating volume or blood pressure, or an increase in sympathetic output stimulates the secretion of renin from the juxtaglomerular apparatus of the kidney. Renin has a half-life in the circulation of 80 minutes and splits angiotensin I from circulating angiotensinogen. Angiotensin-converting enzyme (ACE) then converts angiotensin I to angiotensin II, mostly in the lungs. This stimulates the secretion of aldosterone from the adrenal cortex. Numerous other stimuli are known to initiate aldosterone secretion, including adreno-corticotropic hormone (ACTH) from the pituitary and a direct stimulatory effect of an elevated plasma potassium.

GLUCOCORTICOIDS

Cortisol is the major glucocorticoid along with corticosterone. Synthesis is via a series of steps as

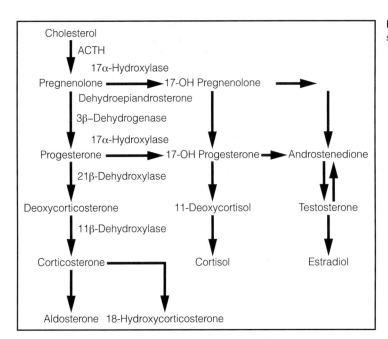

Figure 3.2 • Synthesis of steroids.

outlined in **Fig. 3.2**. The major effects of gluco-corticoids are upon glucose and protein metabolism. They are necessary for maintaining hepatic glycogen stores, they stimulate protein catabolism and lipolysis and cause hyperglycaemia. They also have a weak mineralocorticoid effect. In supraphysiological doses (therapeutic or pathological), skeletal weakening is caused by a decrease in intestinal absorption and increasing urinary excretion of calcium.

Cortisol is secreted under the direct control of ACTH. The cortisol level is continually regulated via a negative-feedback mechanism on both the hypothalamus and pituitary. The hypothalamus secretes corticotropin-releasing hormone (CRH) to stimulate the secretion of ACTH from the anterior pituitary. Serum levels of cortisol show a diurnal rhythm, with the highest levels in the early morning; this is also controlled by the hypothalamus.

Steroids are fat-soluble and enter cells to bind to a receptor. The ligand-receptor complex then diffuses into the nucleus of the cell and there binds to DNA to affect protein synthesis over a relatively long period of time (hours to days).

SEX STEROIDS

Dehydroepiandrosterone (DHEA) and androstenedione are weakly androgenic sex steroids. They are converted in peripheral tissues to testosterone and oestrogens, via the aromatase enzyme system. Corticotropin stimulates the secretion of the adrenal androgens. Tumours producing DHEA, androstenedione and DHEA precursors cause virilisation in women.

CONGENITAL ADRENAL HYPERPLASIA AND ADRENOGENITAL SYNDROMES

Congenital adrenal hyperplasia (CAH) includes a group of conditions that are usually inherited as an autosomal recessive disorder. They are characterised by a block in the synthesis of cortisol. This can occur anywhere on the synthetic pathway from cholesterol, and the clinical effects depend upon the level of the block. Due to failure of the negative-feedback loop, there is an increase in the levels of ACTH secreted by the pituitary and this leads to hyperplasia of the adrenal glands. The adrenogenital syndrome is a subcategory of CAH characterised by abnormalities in the external genitalia.

In all of these syndromes there is a deficiency of the end steroid and overproduction of the steroid intermediary at the level of the enzyme deficiency.

The most common enzyme block is a deficiency of 21-hydroxylase, which accounts for 90% of cases, causing a deficiency of glucocorticoid and mineralocorticoid. Due to the high concentrations of the intermediary prior to 21-hydroxylase, there are high levels of androgens. This deficiency causes ambiguous genitalia in females as the child is masculinised in utero. There is also salt loss and hyperkalaemia, which requires the administration of mineralocorticoid and salt to correct it. All of the congenital adrenal hyperplasia deficiencies are treatable by replacement of glucocorticoid, mineralocorticoid or both. Some also require sex hormone treatment from puberty.

Figure 3.3 • Excised adrenal gland from patient with congenital adrenal hyperplasia. Note nodular appearance caused by high circulating ACTH and large overall size (scale in cm).

Management

The standard treatment for CAH and adrenogenital syndrome includes the replacement of the steroid beyond the enzyme block. This results in restoration of the feedback loop, a subsequent reduction of ACTH and a reduction of the androgens causing the virilisation. The genital effects of androgen excess may require surgical intervention prior to and after puberty.[1]

Treatment may be difficult in some patients as there may be inadequately treated hyperandrogenism and iatrogenic hypercortisolism. Recently, more evidence has emerged indicating that patients with CAH who are proving difficult to manage medically may benefit from bilateral adrenalectomy. This can lead to a further decrease of androgens, and improved control of the signs and symptoms of hypercortisolism (particularly obesity), as the dose of exogenous steroids may be reduced.[2,3] The adrenal gland can become significantly enlarged in these syndromes and may need to be removed for this reason (Fig. 3.3).

CUSHING'S SYNDROME

Cushing's syndrome is characterised by increased levels of circulating glucocorticoids. It is conveniently divided into two types: ACTH-dependent, due to either pituitary or ectopic origin; and ACTH-independent, due to adrenal origin. The most common cause of hypercortisolism is iatrogenic administration of steroids for the treatment of other diseases. The characteristics of the syndrome, however, are identical regardless of the cause.

Features of Cushing's syndrome (Figs 3.4 and 3.5)

Cushing's syndrome is a rare disorder but may be responsible for many symptoms and therefore frequently enters a list of differential diagnoses. It has a prevalence of 10 cases per million per year. The majority of these patients have ACTH-dependent Cushing's syndrome.

The clinical presentation of Cushing's syndrome has numerous and variable features, as outlined in Table 3.1.[4,5]

Aetiology

ACTH-DEPENDENT CUSHING'S

There are two main causes of ACTH-dependent Cushing's syndrome: pituitary adenoma that secretes ACTH or ectopic ACTH secretion.

ACTH-secreting pituitary adenoma

This was the form of Cushing's syndrome described by Harvey Cushing in 1932,[6] and is often referred to as Cushing's disease. These tumours are usually microadenomas (<1 cm), so pituitary magnetic resonance imaging (MRI) is the imaging modality of choice. Nevertheless, very small tumours may not always be detected. Moreover, MRI cannot distinguish between corticotropin adenomas and

Figure 3.4 • Clinical appearance of patient with Cushing's syndrome. Note body habitus.

Figure 3.5 • Cushing's syndrome. Note facial plethora and moon face.

non-functioning pituitary incidentalomas. Therefore, biochemical confirmation is also required to achieve a confident diagnosis.

Ectopic secretion of ACTH

This is usually secondary to small-cell lung cancer and accounts for 10–15% of ACTH-dependent Cushing's syndrome.[7] Clinical examination and/or abnormal chest X-ray (CXR) appearance usually make the diagnosis obvious, without the need to perform specialised imaging. ACTH levels are usually higher than in pituitary disease, resulting in relatively greater prevalence of pigmentation, muscle weakness and hypokalaemia. Most of the remainder are caused by carcinoid tumours, usually of bronchial origin.[8,9] Such tumours may be so small and slow-growing that even high-resolution MRI or spiral CT are not always able to identify them reliably.

ACTH-INDEPENDENT CUSHING'S SYNDROME

Causes of ACTH-independent Cushing's syndrome fall into one of three categories.

Adrenal adenoma and carcinoma

ACTH is usually suppressed by negative feedback, and levels are therefore low. Carcinomas are most reliably identified preoperatively as a result of their size or concomitant hypersecretion of androgens. Postoperative histology can be difficult to interpret as distinguishing between adrenocortical adenomas and carcinomas is rarely possible on histological grounds alone.

Bilateral adrenal hyperplasia

This is a rare condition and may be associated with other symptoms of Carney's syndrome (see Chapter 4) such as myxomas, blue naevi and

Table 3.1 • The symptoms and signs of Cushing's syndrome

Signs and symptoms	Occurrence (%)
Obesity	95
Facial plethora	80
Hirsutism	80
Menstrual disorders	80
Hypertension	75
Muscular weakness	60
Striae	50
Acne	40
Psychological symptoms	40
Congestive heart failure	20
Oedema	20
Headache	10
Hyperpigmentation	10
Back pain	60
Buffalo hump	55
Diabetes	15
Fractures	20
Bruising	40

pigmented lentigines.[10] Note that Cushing's disease can cause nodular hyperplasia of the adrenals secondary to stimulation by high circulating levels of ACTH.[11]

Iatrogenic

Symptoms are usually mild and only after long-term administration of steroids are the gross symptoms and signs of Cushing's syndrome evident.

Diagnosis

Once the diagnosis has been considered and drugs excluded, blood and urine tests are employed to confirm Cushing's syndrome.[12]

1. **24-hour urinary cortisol.** This reflects the average plasma cortisol level. It is reliable, and sensitivities of up to 95% have been recorded although the investigation may need repeating

two or three times.[13] Note that in alcoholics, if alcohol is withdrawn, then the cortisol may well fall to give a false-negative result. Stress may increase the levels of cortisol and give a false-positive result.

2. **Cortisol diurnal rhythm.** An elevated (>50 nmol/L) sleeping midnight cortisol level is said to have 100% sensitivity and specificity in the investigation of Cushing's syndrome. However, this investigation is best performed in a dedicated inpatient investigation unit. Level of noise, disturbance and general patient stress on the average acute medical or surgical ward might be expected to result in loss of cortisol diurnal rhythm even in normal individuals! Loss of diurnal rhythm is also a feature of chronic alcohol abuse and severe depression.

3. **Low-dose dexamethasone suppression test.** A dose of dexamethasone is given to exploit the loss of negative feedback. After administration of dexamethasone (1–2 mg) the night before, the 09.00 cortisol level should be suppressed (<50 nmol/L) in normal people, but it fails to do so in those with Cushing's syndrome. False-positive results may be obtained if the patient is taking drugs that speed up the metabolism of dexamethasone such as phenytoin, carbamazepine and rifampicin.[14]

Once the diagnosis has been established, the cause of the Cushing's syndrome must be established, i.e. is the elevated cortisol ACTH-dependent or not?

• **ACTH measurement.** If the elevated cortisol is ACTH-dependent, then the ACTH will be elevated; if it is ACTH-independent, then the measured ACTH will be low or undetectable. ACTH is measured with a two-site immunometric assay and should be measured on two or three separate occasions to minimise any variability.

ACTH-independent Cushing's syndrome

As mentioned above, if Cushing's is ACTH independent, then it is due to adrenal disease. Imaging of the adrenals is therefore required to localise the site of the adrenal disease.

CT SCAN (Figs 3.6 and 3.7)

A CT scan will reveal an adrenal adenoma or carcinoma. It is impossible to distinguish between the two accurately by CT scan alone, although a size >3.5 cm increases the risk of malignancy. Local invasion or heterogeneity of the tumour all point towards a malignant lesion.[15,16] This risk is also raised if the tumour is secreting multiple hormones, particularly if also virilising hormones (measuring testosterone and DHEA). Note that after prolonged stimulation of the adrenals with high levels of ACTH (ACTH-dependent Cushing's), nodular changes may occur in the adrenals and this may be mistaken for a true adrenal mass.

MRI SCAN (Figs 3.8 and 3.9)

This may help to distinguish between an adenoma and carcinoma because an adenoma has a higher water content than a carcinoma. T2-weighted, both unenhanced and gadolinium-enhanced T1-weighted

Figure 3.8 • T1-weighted MRI scan of right adrenal adenoma.

Figure 3.6 • CT scan of adrenal mass. Suspicion of carcinoma is raised by the irregular outline and non-homogeneous nature suggestive of central necrosis. Carcinoma was later confirmed histologically.

Figure 3.7 • CT scan of adrenal adenoma (arrowed) in contrast to Fig. 3.6.

Figure 3.9 • MRI scan of right adrenal adenoma. Fast spin echo T2-weighted to highlight water. Note bright appearance of adrenal indicating high water content and likelihood of the mass being a benign adenoma. This was subsequently confirmed histologically.

scans and chemical shift studies can be performed. With all of these images, sensitivities of 95% for distinguishing adenoma from carcinoma have been reported.[17]

ACTH-dependent Cushing's syndrome

To make the diagnosis in ACTH dependent Cushing's Syndrome, both bloodwork and imaging will be required.

HIGH-DOSE DEXAMETHASONE SUPPRESSION TEST

This is based on the fact that pituitary tumours usually retain some negative feedback control, but this is lost in patients with an ectopic source of ACTH. Dexamethasone is a synthetic glucocorticoid that binds to the cortisol receptors in the pituitary and so would prevent the normal secretion of ACTH. A dose of 2 mg dexamethasone is given 6-hourly for 2 days. A reduction in serum cortisol to <50% of the baseline value points towards Cushing's being due to pituitary secretion of ACTH. In ACTH-independent Cushing's or ectopic ACTH-dependent Cushing's, then no significant drop in cortisol will be seen.[18]

OVERNIGHT HIGH-DOSE DEXAMETHASONE SUPPRESSION TEST

This involves giving 8 mg dexamethasone, and measuring serum cortisol at 09.00 the next morning and again the morning following this. If plasma cortisol is reduced to less than 32% of baseline, then the sensitivity is 71% and specificity is 100%.[19]

INFERIOR PETROSAL SINUS CATHETERISATION

This directly measures the ACTH produced from the pituitary gland as the pituitary secretions drain into the petrosal sinus via the cavernous sinus.[20] Peripheral blood levels of ACTH must also be measured to detect any concentration gradient. Both sinuses should be sampled as ACTH may only be secreted into a single sinus, and corticotropin-releasing factor (CRF) should be infused to avoid the possibility that the ACTH is being produced in an episodic fashion.[21]

IMAGING

Once the pituitary gland has been identified as the source of the ACTH, it should be imaged. This is achieved by MRI or CT scan, but note that the offending lesion is often a pituitary microadenoma. This means that the pituitary may often appear normal and an adenoma is detected in only 50–60% of patients.[22] CT or MRI of the chest should be used if ectopic ACTH-dependent Cushing's is diagnosed.

Treatment

Surgery is the mainstay of treatment for Cushing's syndrome of both pituitary and adrenal origin. Pituitary surgery will not be dealt with in detail in this book, suffice to say that this is usually performed through the trans-sphenoidal route. Surgery to the adrenal will be discussed in detail at the end of this chapter.

If primary surgery to the pituitary to excise the microadenoma is unsuccessful (which it may be in up to 40%), or if a treatable ectopic source of ACTH is not found, then bilateral adrenalectomy may be indicated to excise the target organ. Other options to treat the pituitary directly include external beam irradiation or complete surgical ablation of the pituitary, which results in the other hormones of the anterior pituitary becoming deficient. If bilateral adrenalectomy is performed, the patient will be left with permanent adrenal failure and will have to take both glucocorticoid and mineralocorticoid replacement to avoid Addisonian crises. The patient should always wear an alert badge and carry a shock pack of glucocorticoids for rapid treatment of stress, such as infection and trauma. The results of bilateral adrenalectomy for the treatment of pituitary ACTH-dependent Cushing's syndrome are encouraging, with a remission rate of 95%. Quality-of-life questionnaires show a less favourable outcome, with several symptoms remaining, and there may be long-term recurrence if adrenal remnants are left.[23,24] A complication of bilateral adrenalectomy after previous pituitary surgery is Nelson's syndrome, which results in marked hyperpigmentation and possible mass effects on the pituitary as the ACTH-secreting tumour enlarges and secretes large quantities of ACTH (with melanocyte-stimulating hormone) due to the lack of negative feedback. The incidence of Nelson's syndrome may be reduced, or at least delayed, by prior radiotherapy to the pituitary.[25]

If the cause of the Cushing's syndrome is localised to a unilateral lesion in the adrenal, then adrenalectomy is indicated. Treatment for these patients needs to be particularly careful, as they are prone to postoperative infections, skin injury, fractures and hypoglycaemia, as complications of the Cushing's syndrome. Prophylactic antibiotics should be given preoperatively, and it is also important to bear in mind that the remaining adrenal gland will be suppressed; therefore steroid replacement will be required until it recovers. This should be confirmed with a Synacthen test before complete withdrawal of steroid supplements (this may take over a year). There is no role for subtotal adrenalectomy or adrenal autotransplantation.[26]

If the cause of the Cushing's is ectopic ACTH production, treatment of the primary tumour is indicated if possible. But this is often impossible,[27] and so controlling the symptoms becomes paramount. This may be achieved medically by the use of ketoconazole, metyrapone, aminoglutethimide or mitotane, which inhibit cortisol production or secretion. However, even in patients with limited life expectancies, bilateral adrenalectomy may still be the best way to achieve good palliation, particularly if this can be achieved laparoscopically.

ADRENOCORTICAL CARCINOMA

Adrenocortical carcinoma is fortunately a rare tumour and has an incidence of 2/million/year. It is, however, one of the most lethal endocrine tumours, with overall survival rates of 20–35% at 5 years.

There is a slight gender bias, with a female:male ratio of 4:3, and it presents at two peak incidences of age, namely the first and fifth decades. Most of the tumours are hormonally functional and commonly present by producing more than one hormone – in particular virilising tumours in women (this may account for the slight sex distribution bias).[28] Approximately a third of adrenocortical carcinomas are biochemically silent, however, and this obviously is highly relevant to the investigation of incidental adrenal masses (see below).

Inherited susceptibility

(see also Chapter 4)

Adrenocortical carcinoma is associated with three named syndromes:

- Multiple endocrine neoplasia type 1 (MEN 1) – pituitary, parathyroid, pancreatic and foregut carcinoid tumours. This has a known mutation on chromosome 11.
- Beckwith–Wiedemann syndrome – affects children and is associated with exophthalmos, macroglossia and nephromegaly. This involves two mutations on chromosome 11: IGF-2 and H19.
- Li–Fraumeni syndrome – affects children and young adults and is characterised by breast carcinomas, osteosarcomas and brain tumours. It is caused by inactivation of the tumour suppressor gene *p53*.

Diagnosis

Diagnosis of adrenocortical carcinoma is usually only made histologically and this can be difficult with the only absolute criterion being the presence of metastases. Like many endocrine tumours, it is impossible to distinguish cytologically between an adrenal adenoma or carcinoma and therefore percutaneous biopsy is not helpful as this may be falsely reassuring and has a relatively high morbidity rate. In addition, seeding of tumour cells in the biopsy track has also been reported, which should increase the concern about requesting this procedure.[29]

Functioning tumours may, as previously mentioned, present by the clinical effects of multiple hormones. If only a single hormone is produced, this is most commonly a virilising tumour, but feminising, cortisol-secreting or, rarely, aldosterone-secreting carcinomas can occur.

In assessing resectability, evidence of invasion of local structures should be sought on CT or MRI scans, and on the right side a venogram may assist in evaluating caval involvement (**Fig. 3.10**).

Suspicion of malignancy may be raised on imaging of the adrenal glands. The likelihood of malignancy increases with increasing size of the adrenal mass: the larger the adrenal tumour, the greater the risk

Figure 3.10 • Venogram indicating invasion of inferior vena cava from a malignant phaeochromocytoma in the right adrenal gland.

and **3.9**). None of these features, however, are diagnostic of malignancy. MRI is particularly useful if invasion of the inferior vena cava is suspected. Scintigraphy with iodocholesterol or 6-β-iodomethylnorcholesterol (NP-59) may be useful in further imaging of the adrenals, as uptake of the isotope is decreased or absent in adrenal carcinomas.[31] Adrenal adenomas and nodular hyperplasia usually produce images in which the gland takes up tracer. However, with scintigraphy the patient is exposed to significant doses of radiation and the scan takes 3 days to complete as it requires the adrenal to metabolise the cholesterol. The cost, availability and duration mean that many medical physics departments may have difficulty and/or reluctance in providing these scans.

Treatment

SURGERY

If a likely diagnosis of malignancy has been made preoperatively, the surgeon should be prepared to deal with a locally advanced tumour and laparoscopic surgery should not be performed electively. Direct access to the major vessels should be easily attainable and radical resection is the best chance of achieving a cure.

A transabdominal approach is the method of choice and this can be extended to include a thoraco-abdominal approach if necessary, particularly on the right side to gain control of the inferior vena cava if needed. The role of laparoscopic surgery in adrenal carcinoma is unknown due in part to few reports of its use, and because port-site recurrences have been reported. Laparoscopic surgery for benign adrenal tumours is the gold standard (see below) but many carcinomas are only diagnosed as malignant on postoperative histology. Surgery may also be needed to treat recurrent disease.

MEDICAL

The first-line medical therapy is mitotane (o'p-DDD). Mitotane inhibits cortisol synthesis and is also cytotoxic, but is still effective in non-functioning adrenal carcinomas. The role of mitotane as adjuvant treatment is unclear but as first-line therapy for adrenal carcinoma a response rate of 30% is reported. Suramin, a polysulphonated naphthylurea, has been used with some effect as a single agent.

of malignancy.[16] Malignancy in adrenal tumours smaller than 5 cm is rare, but has been reported in masses smaller than 2.5 cm.[30] Logic would suggest that all malignant tumours must at some stage have been small. Evidence of malignancy in small adrenal masses should therefore be carefully sought for. This may be provided by CT appearances: non-homogeneous tumours, those with irregular edges and marked enhancement after the administration of intravenous contrast all support the diagnosis of malignancy. MRI can be helpful as adrenal carcinomas have a low fat content when compared with adrenal adenomas and, with gadolinium contrast, malignant tumours have a high rate of enhancement with a long wash-out phase (**Figs 3.8**

Standard cytotoxic chemotherapy and radiotherapy have a very limited role. Single-agent use is disappointing and multiple-agent chemotherapy only has a response rate in the region of 30%.[32]

Prognosis

The overall outcome of treatment for adrenocortical carcinoma is poor. Most series report 5-year survival rates between 20 and 35% for those who have undergone potentially curative surgery.[15] Median survival is 20–25 months but depends upon the stage at diagnosis. Non-curative surgery has a median survival of 9 months.[33] Endocrine function of the tumour makes no difference to the survival,[34] although those presenting as an acute Cushing's syndrome have an even poorer mean survival of 3 months.

PHAEOCHROMOCYTOMA

Phaeochromocytoma is the term given to a functioning tumour of the adrenal medulla producing excessive amounts of catecholamines or their derivatives. Most commonly these tumours are benign; they arise within the adrenal gland and are unilateral. However, approximately 10% can be malignant, some occur in both adrenal glands (10%), and they can occur in ectopic sites where there is any embryological chromaffin tissue derived from the neural crest (10%). A diagram of the extra-adrenal chromaffin tissue is shown in **Fig. 3.11.** Phaeochromocytomas are most commonly sporadic, but rarely they can be associated with multiple endocrine neoplasia syndrome or in association with von Recklinghausen's disease (**Fig. 3.12**), von Hippel–Lindau syndrome and occasionally as familial inherited autosomal dominant tumours. Of the extra-adrenal tumours approximately 2% are situated in the neck and the thorax, and they can even be in the myocardium (**Figs 3.13 and 3.14**). Multiple, bilateral and extra-adrenal tumours are more common in children, and malignancy is also more common in extra-adrenal tumours.[35] Phaeochromocytomas can also occur in association with Sturge–Weber syndrome and tuberosclerosis. Autopsy studies suggest 0.3% of all autopsies have an undiagnosed phaeochromocytoma, and the

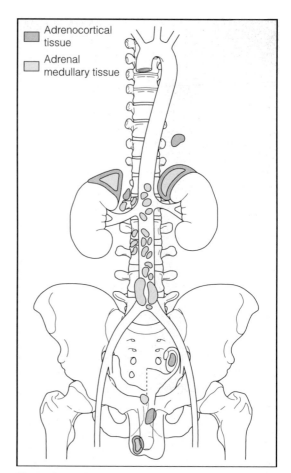

Adrenocortical tissue

Adrenal medullary tissue

Figure 3.11 • Sites of chromaffin tissue.

estimated incidence of phaeochromocytoma is 1–2 per 100 000 adults per year.[36] It is probable that this rare condition is underdiagnosed and underrecognised in life.

Clinical presentation

The diverse hormones produced by these tumours and their widespread effects produce a wide spectrum of clinical presentations. Hypertension and its associated complications is the commonest presentation. The patient may have headaches, dizziness or visual problems secondary to hypertensive retinopathy or, rarely, papilloedema. Secondary effects on the cardiovascular system include palpitations, heart failure, myocardial ischaemia and arrhythmia. The characteristic feature of all presenting symptoms is that they are

Figure 3.12 • von Recklinghausen's disease.

(a)

(b)

Figure 3.13 • MRI and CT scan of cervical phaeochromocytoma.

Figure 3.14 • MIBG and MRV scan of right atrial phaeochromocytoma.

intermittent or paroxysmal. This reflects the intermittent secretion of catecholamines into the circulation and further makes the diagnosis difficult as the patient may be perfectly well for reasonable periods of time and then have paroxysmal attacks of symptoms that may or may not be witnessed by anybody else. Typically during one of these paroxysms the patient will appear pale, sweaty and tremulous and relatives will describe them as looking 'ghostlike'. During such a paroxysm patients will commonly complain of a desperate and unpleasant sense of doom.

Direct trauma to the tumour or any stress (including anaesthesia and surgery) may precipitate symptoms. Attacks and symptoms may last for minutes or hours. Symptoms in virtually all of the major systems of the body can be caused by phaeochromocytoma, and the diagnosis will only be made if the clinician is alert to the possibility of the disease.

Conditions associated with phaeochromocytoma

MULTIPLE ENDOCRINE NEOPLASIA (MEN)

Phaeochromocytoma is a component of multiple endocrine neoplasia (MEN) types 2A and 2B (see Chapter 4). In these patients screening for the disease annually will often identify the condition before it is clinically evident. Phaeochromocytoma may be the presenting feature of MEN 2A or 2B and therefore a careful family history and history of other endocrine disease within the patient should be sought in everyone presenting with a phaeochromocytoma. In MEN 2B there are other clues to the syndrome, namely multiple mucosal neuromas, a megacolon and a typical marfanoid habitus. Screening for MEN 2A using RET mutation analysis now allows individuals susceptible to developing phaeochromocytoma and other components of the syndrome to be identified and to be monitored on an annual basis with early detection of the disease.[37]

NEUROFIBROMATOSIS

Phaeochromocytoma is associated with neurofibromatosis (Fig. 3.12). The features of the disease may not be as prominent as those shown in Fig. 3.12, but nevertheless neurofibromas, axillary freckling and a family history of this syndrome should raise the clinician's level of alertness to the diagnosis of phaeochromocytoma.

VON HIPPEL–LINDAU SYNDROME

This syndrome, which consists of cerebellar haemangiomas, renal tumours and phaeochromocytomas, is rare and can be tested for by analysis of the VHL gene.[38,39]

Very rarely the phaeochromocytoma can appear as a familial autosomal dominant condition in young individuals due to a mitochondrial enzyme defect,[40] caused by a mutation in the gene encoding succinate dehydrogenase complex subunit D (SDHD).

Diagnosis and preoperative management

Diagnosis is made on clinical suspicion first and then confirmatory biochemical tests. These will include measurement of excessive catecholamine excretion in the urine. Traditionally this is performed with 24-hour urinary collections, but overnight excretion of urinary catecholamines and their metabolites can be helpful in the detection of phaeochromocytoma and is often more socially acceptable.[41] In addition to confirmation of excess levels of urinary catecholamines, it is traditional also to measure plasma catecholamines, but these are difficult and costly to measure. The patient should be at rest when the blood is drawn, the blood rapidly centrifuged in a chilled centrifuge and then frozen pending batch analysis. Phaeochromocytoma should be actively excluded before operating on the thyroid of any patients with MEN 2 or medullary thyroid carcinoma to ensure that there is not a silent tumour awaiting activation by the anaesthetic and thyroidectomy. Once the biochemical diagnosis is made immediate blockade with α-adrenergic drugs should be instituted prior to scanning. Uncontrollable hypertension and uncontrollable paroxysmal hypertension are dangerous and take priority over localisation studies. Phenoxybenzamine is the agent most frequently used, in a dose initially of 20 mg twice daily, escalating the dose until postural hypotension occurs and the patient is maximally vasodilated. A safe and satisfactory alternative to phenoxybenzamine is doxazosin.[42] Once alpha blockade has been instituted localisation studies can begin; these will include CT scan, which is probably the most sensitive, but should be from at least the diaphragm down to the symphysis with small cuts through the adrenal gland. Ultrasound rarely may add to the value of the CT, as may MRI. Additional localisation with radioisotopes, including ^{131}I-MIBG, is helpful (Fig. 3.15). Meta-iodo benzylguanidine (MIBG) is taken up in areas of catecholamine production within chromaffin tissue and can subsequently identify not only the primary lesion but also secondary deposits in cases of malignancy. When labelled with an appropriate radiopharmaceutical it can be used as a therapeutic method of ablating irremovable metastases or recurrences.[43]

Further preoperative preparation will need to take place once localisation has been achieved, and this will include escalation of the dose of alpha-blocking agents being used, and the possible introduction of a beta-blocker if the patient is tachycardic (a beta-blocker should never be used unopposed to block a

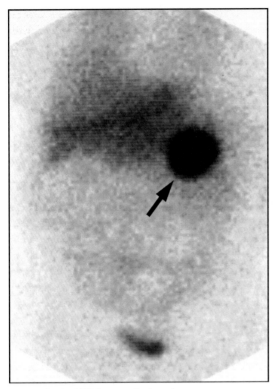

Figure 3.15 • MIBG scan of adrenal phaeochromocytoma.

may be more easily managed by open operation. Careful liaison between surgeon and anaesthetist during the operation is essential. Undue handling of the tumour can result in secretion of catecholamines and wide dispersions in blood pressure. Once the tumour is devascularised a significant fall in catecholamines will occur and the patient's blood pressure may subsequently fall requiring significant volume replacement and/or inotropes. Phaeochromocytomas can be diagnosed during a coincidental operation when, in the unblocked patient, characteristic rises in blood pressure and pulse and arrythmias may occur during induction of anaesthesia and in surgery (**Fig. 3.16**). If a surgeon encounters an undiagnosed phaeochromocytoma at laparotomy no attempt should be made to remove this. The tumour should be handled as little as possible. The primary disease for which the laparotomy was indicated should be treated providing the patient is stable, and immediate blockade, work-up, and subsequent elective removal of the phaeochromocytoma should be planned in the postoperative period. Surges in blood pressure during the operation can be controlled by the anaesthetist with agents such as nitroprusside. Full cardiac monitoring including the use of a Swan–Ganz catheter to measure cardiac output and epidural anaesthesia is advised, if an open approach to the phaeochromocytoma has been employed.

In the postoperative period the patient should be returned to a high-dependency or intensive care unit for regular monitoring of blood pressure and cardiovascular status. In addition, regular monitoring of the blood sugar is advised as the metabolic consequences of removing a phaeochromocytoma and a sudden reduction in circulating catecholamines include hypoglycaemia, which can on occasions be severe and profound. This is due to the sudden removal of the lipolytic, glycolytic and glycogenolytic effects of catecholamines that were produced by the phaeochromocytoma.

phaeochromocytoma because this can result in a severe hypertensive crisis). The period of blockade will depend upon the activity of the tumour and the patient's general cardiovascular condition. During blockade regression of cardiomyopathy is to the advantage of the patient and a sustained improvement in blood pressure allows the heart to recover and the patient to be fitter for surgery. There is no need to rush into surgery for phaeochromocytoma, and although various crash blockade and rapid blockade programmes have been advocated, a cautious approach to getting the patient into the optimal condition for surgery is advised. Typically this is going to take around 2–4 weeks, but in cases of severe cardiomyopathy may take longer.

Surgical removal

The treatment of choice for phaeochromocytoma in the 21st century is laparoscopic adrenalectomy. Most tumours will be amenable to this, but extremely large tumours and malignant tumours

Phaeochromocytoma in pregnancy and in special circumstances

As mentioned above the removal of an adrenal tumour found coincidentally at laparotomy for

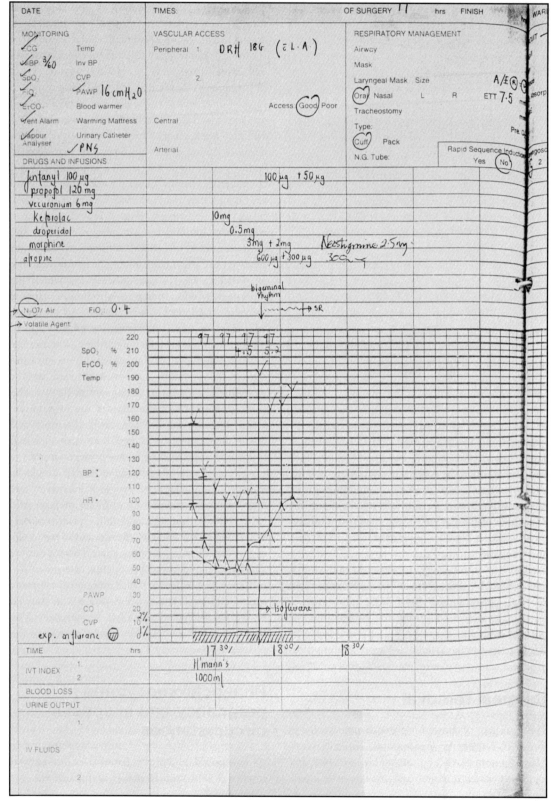

Figure 3.16 • Anaesthetic chart of patient undergoing general anaesthesia and surgery for melanoma, with an undiagnosed phaeochromocytoma.

some other reason is ill-advised in case it is a phaeochromocytoma. A profound fall in blood pressure and cardiovascular instability can occur in this setting, and it would be advisable to leave the tumour alone, investigate, block and remove it at a later date. Phaeochromocytoma in pregnancy is rare, but dangerous. There is a significant mortality both for the infant and the mother.[44] When the diagnosis is made during pregnancy it is customary to block the tumour with alpha blockade and then in the third trimester carry out a Caesarean section with or without a synchronous adrenalectomy. Vaginal delivery is contraindicated, and early operation after Caesarean section to deal with the phaeochromocytoma once the haemodynamics and raw area of the uterus has healed is controversial.

In children the treatment and diagnosis are similar to the approach in adults, but awareness of inherited syndromes will be higher.[45]

Malignant phaeochromocytomas are difficult to diagnose on the basis of histopathology. All phaeochromocytomas show bizarre cellular arrangements within the tumour. They are highly vascular, and there are multiple mitotic figures – this applies equally to benign and subsequently proven malignant tumours. Frank invasion of local structures will of course increase the likelihood of a tumour being malignant (**Fig. 3.10**) as will demonstrable metastases. The treatment of metastases is best dealt with by using radiolabelled MIBG.[43] External beam radiotherapy is unproven, but a variety of chemotherapeutic regimens can be tried, though no randomised control trials exist to inform the best choice of medication.

PRIMARY ALDOSTERONISM (CONN'S SYNDROME)

Primary aldosteronism is due to autonomous adrenal cortical tissue secreting excessive amounts of aldosterone. It presents as a result of investigations for hypertension or hypokalaemia.

Whilst a single benign adenoma of the adrenal cortex is the most common cause of primary hyperaldosteronism (**Fig. 3.17**), rarely the disease can be due to bilateral micronodular or macronodular hyperplasia of the zona glomerulosa of the adrenal gland. Exceptionally rare are aldosterone-secreting carcinomas of the adrenal and the so-called familial

Figure 3.17 • Typical Conn's tumour.

glucocorticoid-suppressible hyperaldosteronism syndrome, which is dominantly inherited. The anatomy and physiology of the adrenal cortex was reviewed at the beginning of the Chapter and it can be seen that aldosterone is the final common product of the pathway of hydroxylase enzymes converting pregnenolone into progesterone, corticosterone and ultimately aldosterone. Aldosterone produced by the zona glomerulosa controls the resorption of sodium by the distal renal tubules through the Na^+/K^+ and H^+ pumps. Along with the resorption of sodium (an active transport mechanism) water will follow, thus aldosterone will cause retention of water and an increase in the circulatory volume. The secretion of aldosterone is controlled primarily by angiotensin II, which in turn is generated through the activity of renin and angiotensin-converting enzyme on angiotensinogen. Renin, secreted from the juxtaglomerular apparatus of the kidney, is traditionally measured as well as aldosterone in reaching a diagnosis.[46] Aldosterone will also be increased by an increase in serum potassium concentration, and secondary hyperaldosteronism occurs in the presence of liver disease, cardiac failure and nephrotic syndrome. The feedback loop controlling renin and aldosterone secretion exists to regulate intravascular volume and electrolyte balance. Disturbance in the renin–aldosterone loop can be complex and the factors leading up to the onset of autonomous aldosterone production are varied.[47] In early disease more than half the patients with primary aldosteronism will have a normal circulating potassium level, and hence if this alone is used to diagnose the disease or lead to its investigation, a significant number of cases will be missed. Indeed Jerome Conn, who first described hypertension caused by a benign adrenal cortical tumour in 1954, recognised that hypokalaemia was not present in all cases.[48] Selective venous sampling is the most accurate way of diagnosing the syndrome, by measuring aldosterone, cortisol and renin from the adrenal gland via a catheter in the inferior vena cava.[49] In cases of bilateral adrenal hyperplasia this will also allow the dominant side to be identified in case unilateral adrenalectomy is indicated. Using these more sensitive, but invasive investigative tests the incidence of Conn's syndrome in the population is approximately 5%. In addition the use of the fludrocortisone suppression test may also be helpful in confirming the diagnosis. In the experimental setting, there is a correlation between the in vitro release of aldosterone and cortisol and the expression of genes responsible for steroid-synthesising enzymes (hydroxylases). This enables confirmation that these tumours not only have the **potential** to secrete aldosterone but do so.[50]

All the hormonal assays described above must be performed without the influence of drugs that may affect the renin–angiotensin–aldosterone axis. Therefore spironolactone, ACE inhibitors and diuretics must be stopped several weeks before the assays are performed. Once the biochemistry is confirmed then localisation with CT scan and/or MRI can be performed. In cases where imaging is inconclusive or confusing selective venous sampling (see above) may be helpful. Iodocholesterol scanning may be a further imaging modality if there remains doubt, and it has been estimated that this has an 83% positive predictive value for the diagnosis of adenoma.[51] Once the diagnosis is confirmed and the disease localised, blood pressure and potassium where abnormal must be corrected prior to operative intervention. Single adenomas are eminently treated by surgery, nowadays most typically this will be laparoscopic (see below). In bilateral disease selective venous sampling may identify the dominant side, removal of which can significantly reduce medications. Patients with glucocorticoid-remediable hyperaldosteronism should be treated with steroids. A typical postoperative stay after laparoscopic surgery will be 3 days.[52] At best two-thirds of patients will be cured of their hypertension, and of those continuing with antihypertensives the vast majority will benefit from reduced medication requirement. The typical appearance of an adenoma is shown in **Fig. 3.17**.

NEUROBLASTOMA

Neuroblastoma is a malignant tumour of childhood arising in the developing neuroendocrine system. Most (80%) produce abnormal levels of sympathetic amines. The incidence is 8–10/million/year in children up to 15 years of age. It is the most common solid tumour in childhood and accounts for 10% of all paediatric malignancies, although it is the most frequent malignancy in children aged under 5 and has a median age at diagnosis of 2 years. Generally speaking, the younger the child at presentation, the better the prognosis.[53]

Presentation

Most neuroblastomas present as an asymptomatic abdominal mass and may be very large, with any symptoms attributable to the organ that is being compressed. Twenty percent are in the posterior mediastinum rather than the abdomen, and rarely the tumour may present in the neck or pelvis. The tumour has usually metastasised by the time it is discovered, with the bone and bone marrow being the most commonly affected secondary sites.

Diagnosis

The primary tumour is usually confirmed by imaging – most commonly CT scan and/or MRI. The diagnosis requires histological confirmation, as the differential diagnosis includes other small-cell tumours including lymphoma and Ewing's sarcoma. Urinary catecholamines may be raised and urinary levels of VMA, HVA and dopamine will be elevated in 90% of patients. Infiltration of bone marrow produces classical pseudorosettes in the aspirate, and this may also be diagnostic. Skeletal metastases are detected with MIBG scans or a technetium scan. Various gene abnormalities have been identified with neuroblastomas. Amplification of the *MTCN* oncogene is associated with a poor prognosis. DDX1, NAG and N-cym have also been demonstrated to be co-amplified.[54]

Treatment

Neuroblastoma exists in three clinical patterns: non-metastatic loco-regional disease, metastatic disease, and the spontaneously regressing widespread disease (stage IVs). Treatment must be tailored to the type and stage of the tumour as well as the age of the patient. Surgical resection is most effective in low-stage tumours, but localised, operable tumours account for only 20% of neuroblastomas. In 20–25% the presentation is with disease that has spread beyond the midline, and is therefore inoperable.[55,56] Chemotherapy is the mainstay of treatment for these children, followed by surgery if the tumour has regressed sufficiently. For those children with disseminated disease at presentation, the outcome is poor if they are over 1 year old. Chemotherapy response rates have improved recently with the intensification of doses used. Multifocal disease (stage IVs) is most commonly found in children aged under 1 year and accounts for 5–10% of patients. Bizarrely, this small group of patients have a good long-term survival rate as spontaneous remission of the disease may occur after resection of the primary tumour.[57] Increased understanding of tumour biology should in future allow appropriate selection of therapies.[58]

INCIDENTALOMA

Adrenal masses are found in approximately 1% of patients having cross-sectional imaging of the abdomen for a variety of indications. The incidence of adrenal tumours presenting as clinical problems is approximately 10 per million of the population so it is self-evident that more masses are found in the adrenal gland than produce symptoms, and thus a careful strategy is required to identify those that need intervention and investigation and those that can be safely ignored. Investigation and management of an incidental finding of an adrenal mass requires a thorough understanding of adrenal pathophysiology. Only a small percentage of such incidentally found tumours are found to be malignant (5%) and a further small percent are metastases from an otherwise occult primary tumour.[59] Nevertheless a significant number will be metastases from a known primary tumour, roughly a third will be benign cortical adenomas (either functioning or non-functioning), and a further 5% will be phaeochromocytomas. **Box 3.1** summarises the differential diagnosis of adrenal masses incidentally noted while imaging the abdomen. Initial assessment of a patient with an incidentaloma should

Box 3.1 • Differential diagnosis of adrenal masses incidentally noted while imaging the abdomen

FUNCTIONAL

Adrenal cortex

- Adenoma
- Nodular hyperplasia
- Carcinoma

Adrenal medulla

- Phaeochromocytoma
- Ganglioneuroma
- Ganglioneuroblastoma

NON-FUNCTIONAL

Adrenal masses

- Myelolipoma
- Cyst
- Haematoma
- Hamartoma
- Amyloidosis
- Xanthomatosis
- Neurofibroma
- Teratoma
- Granulomatosis

Metastases

- Breast
- Lung
- Lymphoma
- Leukaemia

Pseudo-adrenal masses

- Lymph nodes
- Renal
- Splenic
- Pancreas
- Vessels

Imaging artefacts

start with the patient and not by focusing on the X-ray. Reflex biopsy and unconsidered investigation of coincidentally found adrenal masses can lead to disasters, and a careful strategy must be employed to elucidate the cause of the problem. Clinical examination should be carefully undertaken looking for evidence of Cushing's disease, hypertension, diabetes or any other symptoms that could be associated with pituitary–adrenal axis imbalance. A past medical history of malignant disease or a family history of endocrine disease should also be sought. Simple investigations, including a chest X-ray, urea and electrolyte estimation and a full blood count, may lead to a diagnosis, but if there is still no obvious cause for the abnormality then specialist endocrine investigations will be required.[60] These may include exclusion of a phaeochromocytoma by measuring urinary catecholamine excretion,[41] urinary cortisol levels, plasma cortisol levels and ACTH levels. These can, however, be insensitive tests in the setting of preclinical Cushing's syndrome. The gold standard for a diagnosis of autonomous cortisol production is the overnight dexamethasone suppression test (2 mg). Conn's syndrome may need to be considered (see above) and evidence of androgen secretion by the adrenal gland should be investigated by measuring serum testosterone levels and dehydroepiandrosterone sulphate (DHEA-S). If any of these investigations prove positive then appropriate treatment can be instituted. In a significant number of individuals, however, there will be no endocrine function of the adrenal mass and further investigation is required to elucidate the cause of the enlarged adrenal gland. In a patient with a history of malignant disease in the recent past, guided fine-needle aspiration biopsy may be helpful. Cells retrieved that resemble those of the original primary tumour can be diagnostic and save unnecessary surgery on occasions. In the absence of a history of previous malignant disease then fine-needle aspiration biopsy or core biopsy is generally unhelpful as the interpretation of primary adrenal pathology is difficult if not impossible in such small samples. Dynamic gadolinium-enhanced MRI may be helpful in predicting the status of adrenal masses,[61] but it is likely that a combination of CT scan, MRI and, where appropriate, fine-needle aspiration biopsy will identify the cause of the adrenal mass in the majority of cases[62] (**Figs 3.6–3.9**). In small (<3 cm) apparently benign adrenal tumours a watch policy with serial CT scanning on a yearly basis seems safe.[63] In tumours over 3.5 cm the threshold for surgical removal is less because there appears to be a significant risk of malignancy in larger tumours.[64] Incidentalomas that are growing on serial scanning or in which there is any suspicion of malignancy should be removed surgically and the laparoscopic approach will usually be the preferred option.

The management of incidentalomas should be conducted in the context of a full endocrine work-up and should not be handled by surgeons, anaesthetists or physicians unfamiliar with the routine management of such patients. In this way the inadvertent operation on an unsuspected phaeochromocytoma or removal of an adrenal containing autonomous cortisol-secreting tissue resulting in postoperative Addison's disease can be avoided.

ADDISON'S DISEASE (ADRENAL INSUFFICIENCY)

Adrenal insufficiency is most commonly caused by autoimmune adrenalitis or more rarely by pituitary disease resulting in failure of the hypothalamic–pituitary–corticotropic axis. In addition adrenal insufficiency can be caused by removal of overactive adrenal tissue and a failure to recognise hypofunction in a suppressed normal adrenal gland remaining on the contralateral side. The main presenting features of adrenal insufficiency include fatigue, anorexia and weight loss, and in the acute postoperative phase failure to wean off the ventilator, poor healing and hypotension.[65]

Glucocorticoid replacement therapy and mineralocorticoid replacement therapy are life saving, but clearly the disease must be recognised first. In addition to the above causes of adrenal insufficiency, therapeutic glucocorticoid administration will cause secondary adrenal insufficiency if steroid replacement therapy is withdrawn or not increased at times of stress. Adrenal infiltration by a secondary tumour or haemorrhage into the adrenal gland are rare causes of primary adrenal insufficiency, but in the context of disseminated malignancy, shock or other surgical interventions these must be borne in mind. The natural history, evolution and development of primary Addison's disease is a lengthy one and patients who are stressed by, for example, surgery can be tipped into full acute adrenal insufficiency.

Diagnosis

Concentrations of ACTH and cortisol vary throughout the day due to the diurnal rhythm. Random samples are therefore not generally helpful. Hence, the combined measurement of an early morning serum cortisol and plasma ACTH level is helpful. The short Synacthen test will expose an inability of the adrenal cortex to respond to ACTH. Serum cortisol levels are measured before and 30 or 60 minutes after intravenous or intramuscular injections of ACTH. In healthy individuals this will lead to an increase in serum cortisol to a level of >500 nmol/L. In patients who have primary adrenal failure the exogenous administration of extra ACTH will not normally produce any further increase in serum cortisol. Caution must be taken in interpreting these investigations in critically ill patients in whom the corticotropic axis is greatly activated. In this setting there is reduced sensitivity to dexamethasone and enhanced responses to ACTH and cortisol concentrations after the administration of corticotropin-releasing hormone. In settings where there is doubt about whether or not there has been acute adrenal failure, blood samples should be drawn to estimate ACTH and serum cortisol levels followed by the administration of exogenous glucocorticoid, pending the results of the blood work.

ADRENALECTOMY

The operation of adrenalectomy should never be commenced without a working diagnosis of the lesion, and in particular an assessment of its function. If an adrenalectomy is performed for an unrecognised phaeochromocytoma, then there is a high mortality rate. If an undiagnosed adenoma producing cortisol is excised, then a postoperative Addisonian crisis may ensue (see above). Preparation of patients prior to adrenalectomy is discussed in each section of this chapter. The operation should nearly always aim for total excision of the affected adrenal gland. Laparoscopic adrenalectomy has become widely accepted as the procedure of choice, and should be regarded as the norm for benign adrenal surgery. Benefits for patients from this approach have been widely reported, although a truly randomised trial has not been published. Most

surgeons would choose to perform an open adrenalectomy for tumours with a high degree of suspicion for malignancy as open access to the major blood vessels may be essential but difficult if not impossible laparoscopically. The basic principles of adrenalectomy are the same for both the open and laparoscopic approaches to the glands; in each case the procedure is essentially the same, but with different access.

Open adrenalectomy

Open adrenalectomy has been the main means of access to the adrenal gland for many years. The first reported adrenalectomy was performed in 1889 by Thornton, who utilised a transabdominal approach. The first description of a phaeochromocytoma was in 1886, and the first successful adrenalectomy for phaeochromocytoma was performed in 1927 by Charles Mayo. Traditionally, three approaches have been used – transperitoneal, loin or posterolateral, and posterior. In addition a thoraco-abdominal approach may be needed for large tumours. The approach employed by the surgeon depends upon the size of the tumour, any invasion of surrounding tissues, bilateral disease, previous surgery and coexisting disease.

ANTERIOR APPROACH

This may be achieved with either a subcostal or midline incision – the advantage of the latter being that both glands can be more easily explored. Traditionally, phaeochromocytomas have been approached anteriorly, so that extra-adrenal or bilateral lesions can be excised. This has rather fallen into obsolescence as MIBG scans and better imaging with CT and MRI have improved pre-operative detection and rendered this approach unnecessary. The main disadvantage of this approach is the morbidity associated with a major laparotomy. The blood loss, postoperative stay and operative time have all been shown to be higher with an anterior approach when compared with other open approaches (and especially when compared with laparoscopic approaches).

LOIN APPROACH

This is generally the most popular open approach to the adrenal gland and is widely accepted as the normal approach to the kidney. The patient is positioned in the lateral decubitus position with the table broken to open the space between the 12th rib and the iliac crest. An incision is made along the line of the 11th rib, which is then excised. The adrenal is exposed taking care to injure neither the pleura nor the peritoneum. This gives more limited exposure than an anterior approach, but better exposure than the posterior approach to the glands. Only one side can be operated upon, and if bilateral surgery is required the patient needs to be moved after completion of one side and repositioned.

POSTERIOR APPROACH

This gives the most direct access to the adrenals and both are able to be operated upon without moving the patient. This approach was initially described in 1936 by Hugh Young. It involves positioning the patient prone and flexing the back by jack-knifing the table. A near-vertical incision (moving slightly towards the iliac crest) is then made and the neck of the 12th rib divided (or completely excised) to expose the gland. The advantage of the posterior approach is that a bilateral adrenalectomy may be performed without moving the patient by the use of bilateral parallel incisions. Access is limited, however, particularly in the obese, and excision of tumours larger than 5 cm should not be attempted by this approach. This is frustrating as bilateral adrenalectomy is most commonly indicated in Cushing's syndrome, and these are the most obese patients and technically most difficult to approach in this way.

THORACO-ABDOMINAL APPROACH

This is indicated only for large malignant adrenal tumours as it provides the widest exposure to the adrenal and in particular its vessels and adjacent organs.[66]

Laparoscopic adrenalectomy

Laparoscopic adrenalectomy was initially described by Michel Gagner in 1992.[67] It has rapidly become widely accepted by surgeons, anaesthetists and patients, and should now be considered the standard technique for adrenalectomy.[68] It has been demonstrated to have lower blood loss, shorter hospital stay, faster return to normal daily activities and lower postoperative pain than open adrenalectomy, but a slightly longer operative time.[69–71] The intra-abdominal procedure is the same as in the open operation and there are three approaches in laparoscopic surgery as in open surgery: transperitoneal, lateral retroperitoneal and posterior retroperitoneal.

The choice of approach chosen by the surgeon will depend upon his or her experience but certain factors should be taken into account when contemplating surgery. Any surgeon who is going to attempt a laparoscopic adrenalectomy should also be comfortable with the open procedure. The size of the tumour is important both for access by laparoscopic surgery[69] and for the risk of malignancy, which should be regarded as a relative contraindication to laparoscopic surgery.[72] Most surgeons would regard a tumour size of 6–10 cm as the upper limit for laparoscopic surgery, although Gagner will operate laparoscopically on tumours up to 15 cm in diameter.[73] Bear in mind that the duration of surgery is relative to the size of the tumour, and large tumours will require more surgical time and are more difficult dissections. Phaeochromocytoma is not a contraindication to laparoscopic surgery assuming the patient has been adequately prepared preoperatively.[74] Relative contraindications to laparoscopic adrenalectomy include a coagulopathy, and previous surgery in the area (particularly nephrectomy and splenectomy). Conversion rates to the open approach are usually quoted as 5–10%.

TRANSPERITONEAL APPROACH

This is the most commonly used approach to the adrenal glands laparoscopically. The patient is placed in the lateral decubitus position with the table jack-knifed to open the lumbar space between the ribs and the iliac crest (similar to the open loin approach). The patient is placed slightly head-up so irrigation fluid, the omentum and intra-abdominal contents will tend to fall away from the site of dissection. The operation can also be performed with the patient supine although access to the adrenal will be more difficult. The advantage of the flank approach is that the organs act as their own retractors and gravity is used to facilitate access to retroperitoneal structures.

Left adrenalectomy

Once the patient has been correctly positioned, a 10 or 12-mm trocar is introduced into the peritoneal cavity under direct vision in the left subcostal space and the pneumoperitoneum is created. Two further subcostal ports are then placed under direct vision (**Fig. 3.18**). The splenic flexure is mobilised and the lienorenal ligament is divided. The spleen retracts forwards under gravity to allow entry into the retroperitoneum behind the lesser sac. The adrenal will be recognised superomedial to the kidney in the perinephric fat by its characteristic colour. The ease with which the adrenal gland is then dissected out of the fat depends upon the vascularity of the gland and density of the periadrenal fat. The dissection can be performed by diathermy or the use of a harmonic scalpel (preferred by the authors). Care must be taken to ensure that the adrenal vein is identified and is controlled by Ligaclip (Ethicon, Cornelia, GA). Adjacent organs must be protected from injury, particularly the spleen and the tail of the pancreas as it lies just in front of the adrenal gland. When freed from blood vessels and surrounding structures the adrenal gland is placed in a bag prior to removal from the abdomen.

Right adrenalectomy

Once the patient has been placed in the correct position, the trocars are introduced in a similar fashion as on the left side. A fourth trocar is more often required on the right to retract the liver. The right triangular ligament of the liver is divided to mobilise the liver, which allows retraction of the liver medially and good exposure of the space between the right adrenal and the inferior vena cava. The peritoneum below the liver and overlying the adrenal gland is then divided above and medial to the right kidney. Once the gland has been identified by its characteristic colour, it is dissected from the surrounding tissue. It is advisable to dissect the superior pole of the adrenal first, so that the gland remains attached to the kidney and does not migrate further away from the dissection point and upwards. Again, great care must be taken to ensure that the adrenal vein is identified and controlled prior to division from the vena cava.

RETROPERITONEAL APPROACH

The retroperitoneal approach is similar to the traditional open loin approach to the adrenal gland. It is less widely used than the transperitoneal approach in the UK. The surgeon positions the patient in the same lateral decubitus position as for an open or transperitoneal approach. A port is placed under direct vision through the muscles in the subcostal plane and into the retroperitoneal tissue. A balloon is then inflated to create a space. This balloon may be either passed down the port and then inflated, or some ports are produced with the balloon attached as an integral part of the port itself. This approach is limited as the space provided is smaller, and thus the size of the adrenal that can be removed may be more restricted. Bleeding may be more difficult to control and hypercapnoea and surgical emphysema are more likely to occur. However, it has been claimed that postoperative pain control is better and the duration of hospital stay is shorter.

POSTERIOR RETROPERITONEAL APPROACH

Again, the patient is positioned in the same position as for the open posterior approach; i.e. prone with the table jack-knifed. Three ports are used for each side, in a line in the subcostal plane. This has the same advantages and disadvantages in comparison with the open posterior approach as the laparoscopic loin approach has compared with the open loin approach.

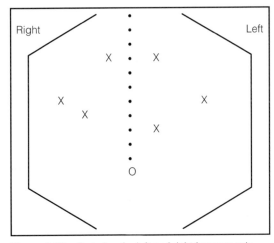

Figure 3.18 • Port sites for left and right laparoscopic adrenalectomy.

In conclusion, the different techniques that are available all have their supporters.[75] The laparoscopic approach to the adrenal gland is now considered the 'gold standard' technique for benign tumours. Different surgeons use different techniques, but no approach has been demonstrated as yet to have significantly better results in all hands.

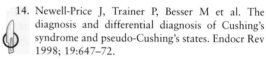

Key points

- Adrenal function is essential to sustain normal healthy life.
- Adrenal malfunction is rare.
- Tumours of the adrenal can be functioning or non-functioning, benign or malignant.
- Via the negative-feedback loop cortisol over-production by one adrenal will suppress the contralateral gland.
- Functioning or familial syndromes must be excluded before removing any adrenal gland.
- Most adrenal pathology can be safely and optimally removed by the laparoscopic route.

REFERENCES

1. Young MB, Hughes IA. The response to treatment of congenital adrenal hyperplasia in infancy. Arch Dis Child 1990; 65:441–4.

2. Merke DP, Bornstein SR, Avila NA et al. NIH conference. Future directions in the study and management of congenital adrenal hyperplasia due to 21-hydroxylase deficiency. Ann Int Med 2002; 136:320–4.

3. Van Wyk JJ, Ritzen EM. The role of bilateral adrenalectomy in the treatment of congenital adrenal hyperplasia. J Clin Endocrinol Metab 2003; 88:2993–8.

4. Clutter WE. Cushing's syndrome; hypercortisolism. In: Doherty GM, Skogseid B (eds) Surgical endocrinology. Philadelphia: Lippincott Williams & Wilkins, 2001; p. 237.

5. Ross EJ, Lynch CD. Cushing's syndrome: killing disease. Lancet 1982; ii:64–9.

6. Cushing H. The basophil adenomas of the pituitary body and their clinical manifestations (pituitary basophilism). Bull Johns Hopkins Hosp 1932; 50:137–95.

7. Wajchenberg BL, Mendonca BB, Liberman B et al. Ectopic ACTH syndrome. Endocr Rev 1994, 15:752–87.

8. Delisle L, Boyer MJ, Warr D et al. Ectopic corticotropin syndrome and small-cell carcinoma of the lung: clinical features, outcome and complications. Arch Intern Medicine 1993; 153:746–52.

9. Limper AH, Carpenter PC, Scheithauer B et al. The Cushing syndrome induced by bronchial carcinoid tumours. Ann Intern Medicine 1992; 117:209–14.

10. Young WF, Carney JA, Musa BU et al. Familial Cushing's syndrome due to primary pigmented nodular adrenocortical disease. N Engl J Med 1989; 321:1659–64.

11. Samuels MH, Loriaux DL. Cushing's syndrome and the macronodular adrenal gland. Endocrinol Metab Clin North Am 1994; 23:555–69.

12. Crapo L. Cushing's syndrome: a review of diagnostic tests. Metab Clin Exp 1979; 28:955–77.

13. Orth DN. Cushing's syndrome. N Engl J Med 1995; 332:791–803.

14. Newell-Price J, Trainer P, Besser M et al. The diagnosis and differential diagnosis of Cushing's syndrome and pseudo-Cushing's states. Endocr Rev 1998; 19:647–72.

15. Icard P, Goudet P, Charpenay C et al. Adrenocortical carcinomas: surgical trends and results of a 253-patient series from the French Association of Endocrine Surgeons Study Group. World J Surg 2001; 25:891–7.

16. Copeland PM. The incidentally discovered adrenal mass. Ann Intern Med 1983; 98:940.

17. Prager G, Heinz-Peer G, Passler C et al. Can dynamic gadolinium-enhanced magnetic resonance imaging with chemical shift studies predict the status of adrenal masses? World J Surg 2002; 26:958–64.

18. Katznelson L, Bogan JS, Trob JR et al. Biochemical assessment of Cushing's disease in patients with corticotroph macroadenomas. J Clin Endocrinol Metab 1998; 83:1619–23.

19. Dichek HL, Nieman LK, Oldfield EH et al. A comparison of the standard high-dose dexamethasone suppression test and the overnight 8 mg dexamethasone suppression test for the differential diagnosis of ACTH-dependent Cushing's syndrome. J Clin Endocrinol Metab 1994; 78:418–22.

20. Zovickian J, Oldfield EH, Doppman JL et al. Usefulness of inferior petrosal sinus venous endocrine markers in Cushing's disease. J Neurosurg 1988; 68:205–10.

21. Oldfield EH, Doppman JL, Nieman LK, et al. Petrosal sinus sampling with and without corticotropin-releasing hormone for the differential diagnosis of Cushing's syndrome. N Engl J Med 1991; 325:897–905.

22. Findling JW, Doppman JL. Biochemical and radiological diagnosis of Cushing's syndrome. Endocrinol Metab Clin North Am 1994; 23:511–37.

23. Nagesser SK, van Seters AP, Kievit J et al. Long-term results of total adrenalectomy for Cushing's disease. World J Surg 2000; 24:108–13.

24. Sarkar R, Thompson W, McLeod MK. The role of adrenalectomy in Cushing's syndrome. Surgery 1990; 108:1079–84.

25. Moore TJ, Dluhy RG, Williams GH et al. Nelson's syndrome: frequency and effect of prior pituitary irradiation. Ann Int Med 1976; 85:731.

26. Nagesser SK, Kievit J, Derksen J et al. Autologous adrenal transplantation for Cushing's disease. In: Clark OH, Duh QY (eds) Textbook of endocrine surgery. Philadelphia: WB Saunders, 1997; pp. 506–11.

27. Aniszewski JP, Young WF, Thompson GB et al. Cushings syndrome due to ectopic adrenocorticotropic hormone secretion. World J Surg 2001; 25:934–40.

28. Wooten MD, King DK. Adrenal cortical carcinoma. Epidemiology and treatment with mitotane and a review of the literature. Cancer 1993; 72:3145–55.

29. Mighell AJ, High AS. Histological identification of carcinoma in 21-guage needle tracks after fine-needle aspiration biopsy of head and neck carcinoma. J Clin Pathol 1998; 5:241–3.

30. Lee MJ, Hahn PF, Papanicolau N et al. Benign and malignant adrenal masses: CT distinction with attenuation coefficients, size and observer analysis. Radiology 1991; 179:415–18.

31. Gross MD, Wilton GP, Shapiro B et al. Functional and scintigraphic evaluation of the silent adrenal mass. J Nucl Med 1987; 28:1401–7.

32. Ahlman H, Khorram-Manesh A, Jansson S et al. Cytotoxic treatment of adrenocortical carcinoma. World J Surg 2001; 25:927–33.

33. Pommier RF, Brennan MF. An eleven-year experience with adrenocortical carcinoma. Surgery 1992; 112:963–71.

34. Venkatesh S, Hickey RC, Sellin RV et al. Adrenal cortical carcinoma. Cancer 1989; 64:765–9.

35. Kebebew E, Duh Q-Y. Benign and malignant phaeochromocytoma. Diagnosis, treatment and follow up. Surg Oncol Clin N Am 1998; 7:765–89.

36. St John Sutton MG, Sheps SG, Lie TJ. Prevalence of clinically unsuspected phaeochromocytoma: review of a 50 year autopsy series. Mayo Clin Proc 1981; 56:354–60.

37. Williams DT, Dann S, Wheeler MH. Phaeochromocytoma – views on current management. Eur J Surg Oncol 2003; 29:483–90.

38. Richard D, Beigelman C, Dudas J-M et al. Phaeochromocytoma as the first manifestation of Von Hippel–Lindau disease. Surgery 1994; 116:1076–108.

39. Woodward ER, Eng C, McMahon R et al. Genetic predisposition to phaeochromocytoma: analysis of candidate genes GDNF, RET, and VHL. Hum Mol Genet 1997; 6:1051–6.

40. Astuti D, Douglas F, Lennard TWJ et al. Germline SDHD mutation in familial phaeochromocytoma. Lancet 2001; 357:1181–2.

41. Peaston RT, Lennard TWJ, Lai LC. Overnight excretion of urinary catecholamines and metabolites in the detection of phaeochromocytoma. J Clin Endocrinol Metab 1996; 81:1378–84.

42. Prys-Roberts C, Farndon JR. Efficacy and safety of doxazocin for perioperative management of patients with phaeochromocytoma. World J Surg 2002; 26:1037–42.

43. Bouloux PG, Fakeeh M. Phaeochromocytoma. In: Sheaves R, Jenkins PJ, Wass JH (eds) Clinical endocrine oncology. Blackwell Science, 1988; pp. 299–305.

44. Dreier DT, Thompson NW. Phaeochromocytoma and pregnancy: the epitome of high risk. Surgery 1993; 114:1148–52.

45. Hume DM. Phaeochromocytoma in the adult and in the child. Am J Surg 1960; 99:458.

46. Hiramatsu K, Yamada T, Yukimura Y et al. A screening test to identify aldosterone producing adenoma by measuring plasma renin activity. Arch Intern Med 1981; 141:1589.

47. Gordon RD, Stowasser M, Rutherford JC. Primary aldosteronism: Are we diagnosing and operating on too few patients? World J Surg 2001; 25:941–7.

48. Conn JW. Plasma renin activity in primary aldosteronism: importance in differential diagnosis and in research of essential hypertension. JAMA 1964; 190:222.

49. Melby JL, Spark RF, Dale S et al. Diagnosis and localization of aldosterone producing adenomas by adrenal vein catheterization. N Engl J Med 1967; 277:1050.

50. Enberg U, Farnebo LO, Wedell A et al. In vitro release of aldosterone and cortisol in human adrenal adenomas correlates to mRNA expression of steroidogenic enzymes for genes CYP 11 B2 and CYP 17. World J Surg 2001; 25:957–66.

51. Wheeler MH, Harris DA. Diagnosis and management of primary aldosteronism. World J Surg 2003; 27:627–31.

52. Harris DA, Au-Yong I, Basnyat PS et al. Review of surgical management of aldosterone secreting tumours of the adrenal cortex. Eur J Surg Oncol 2003; 29:467–74.

53. Hayes FA, Smith EI. Neuroblastoma. In: Pizzo PA, Poplack DG (eds) Pediatric oncology, principles and practice. Philadelphia: JB Lippincott, 1989; pp. 607–22.

54. Scott D, Elsden J, Pearson A et al. Genes co-amplified with MYCN in neuroblastoma: silent passengers or co-determinants of phenotype? Cancer Letters 2003; 197:81–6.

55. De Bernardi B, Conte M, Mancini A et al. Localised resectable neuroblastoma: results of the second study on the Italian Co-operative Group for neuroblastoma. J Clin Oncol 1995; 13:884–93.

56. Garaventa A, De Bernardi B, Pianca C et al. Localised but unresectable neuroblastoma: treatment and outcome of 145 cases. J Clin Oncol 1993; 11:1770–9.

57. De Bernardi B, Milanaccio C, Occhi M. Neuroblastoma. In: Sheaves R, Jenkins PJ, Wass JAH et al. (eds) Clinical endocrine oncology. Oxford: Blackwell Scientific Publications, 1997; pp. 306–11.

58. Brodeur GM. Neuroblastoma: biological insights into a clinical enigma. Nature Reviews 2003; 3:203–16.

59. Lumachi F, Borsato S, Tregnaghi A et al. CT scan, MRI and image guided FNA cytology of incidental adrenal masses. Eur J Surg Oncol 2003; 29:689–92.

60. Ross NS, Aron OC. Hormonal evaluation of the patient with an incidentally discovered adrenal mass. N Engl J Med 1990; 323:1401–5.

61. Prager G, Heinz-Peer G, Passler C et al. Can dynamic gadolinium-enhanced magnetic resonance imaging with chemical shift studies predict the status of adrenal masses? World J Surg 2002; 26:958–64.

62. Patel HRH, Harris AM, Lennard TWJ. Adrenal masses: the investigation and management of adrenal incidentalomas. Ann R Coll Surg Engl 2001; 83:250–252.

63. Siren J, Tervahartiola P, Sirula A et al. Natural course of adrenal incidentalomas: seven year follow up study. World J Surg 2000; 24:579–82.

64. Kjellman M, Larsson C, Backdahl M. Genetic background of adrenocortical tumour development. World J Surg 2001; 25:948–56.

65. Arlt W, Allolio B. Adrenal insufficiency. Lancet 2003; 361:1881–93.

66. Prinz RA, Falimirski. Operative approaches to the adrenal glands. In: Clark OH, Duh QY (eds) Textbook of endocrine surgery. Philadelphia: WB Saunders, 1997; pp. 529–34.

67. Gagner M, Lacroix A, Bolte E. Laparoscopic adrenalectomy in Cushing's syndrome and phaeochromocytoma. N Engl J Med 1992; 327:1003.

68. Gagner M. Laparoscopic adrenalectomy. Surg Clin North Am 1996; 76:523–37.

69. Prinz RA. A comparison of laparoscopic and open adrenalectomies. Arch Surg 1995; 130:489–94.

70. Dudley NE, Harrison BJ. Comparison of open posterior versus transperitoneal laparoscopic adrenalectomy. Br J Surg 1999; 86:656–60.

71. Duh QY, Siperstein AE, Clark OH et al. Laparoscopic adrenalectomy: comparison of the lateral and posterior approaches. Arch Surgery 1996; 131:870–5.

72. Henry JF, Sebag F, Iacobone M et al. Result of laparoscopic adrenalectomy for large and potentially malignant tumours. World J Surg 2002; 26:1043–7.

73. Gagner M, Pomp A, Heniford BT et al, Laparoscopic adrenalectomy: lessons learned from 100 consecutive procedures. Ann Surg 1997; 226:238–46.

74. Gagner M, Breton G, Pharand D et al. Is laparoscopic adrenalectomy indicated for phaeochromocytomas? Surgery 1996; 120:1076–80.

75. Lezoche E, Guerrieri M, Feliciotti AM et al. Anterior, lateral and posterior retroperitoneal approaches in endoscopic adrenalectomy. Surg Endosc 2002; 16:96–9.

Four

Familial endocrine disease: genetics, clinical presentation and management

Stephen G. Ball, Fiona S. Douglas and T.W.J. Lennard

INTRODUCTION

The role of clinical genetics for all specialities has grown over recent years. This is true for endocrine disease. While inherited disorders of the endocrine system remain relatively uncommon it is becoming important for all clinicians involved in the care of such patients to recognise and ensure that they enter appropriate care pathways. For the individual patients affected by an inherited predisposition to endocrine disease it is of great importance that their condition is recognised such that not only are they offered screening and care but that risks for other family members can be addressed. A multidisciplinary team-based approach is recommended to ensure high quality of care for these patients.[1]

Another important aspect of care covers issues of consent and confidentiality. Inherited disease is by its nature rarely of significance to one person only. One of the challenges facing clinical genetics is that the shared or familial nature of genetic information must be addressed in the process of consent thereby avoiding the problem of breach of confidentiality.

The issue of **when** to test for a genetic predisposition to disease must also be carefully considered. In the UK it is generally recommended that testing for an adult-onset disorder should not be undertaken in childhood.[2] However, if the disease is likely to manifest in childhood or adolescence, then testing in childhood is appropriate because it can inform management.

For each of the conditions described in this chapter there are certain symptoms and signs, both at an individual and familial level, that in most cases enable the diagnosis of a hereditary disorder to be made.

This chapter will cover:

- Multiple endocrine neoplasia type 1 (MEN 1)
- Multiple endocrine neoplasia type 2 (MEN 2) and familial medullary carcinoma of the thyroid (FMTC).
- Familial non-medullary carcinoma of the thyroid: Cowden's/Bannayan–Zonana syndrome, papillary carcinoma of the thyroid, familial adenomatous polyposis.
- Familial parathyroid syndromes.
- Phaeochromocytomas: von Hippel–Lindau syndrome (VHL), neurofibromatosis type 1 (NF1) and hereditary paragangliomatosis.
- Other adrenal syndromes: Carney's syndrome, familial primary hyperaldosteronism, adrenocortical carcinoma.

Genetic aspects of the conditions are considered first, followed by the clinical manifestations.

MULTIPLE ENDOCRINE NEOPLASIA TYPE 1 (MEN 1)

This is an autosomal dominant disorder: in approximately 10% of cases it is due to a new mutation. Its exact prevalence is unknown and this probably reflects the variability in expression of the gene even though penetrance is high. Penetrance refers to the likelihood of the syndrome manifesting itself in any form, whereas expression refers to the particular manifestations of a syndrome. The principal clinical features of MEN 1 are tumours of the parathyroid glands, anterior pituitary and gastrointestinal endocrine cells. MEN 1 should be suspected when either two close relatives share a characteristic feature or one individual has relevant tumours at two or more sites.

In 1995 familial cases of MEN 1 were shown to be associated with chromosome 11q13, and subsequently the *MEN 1* gene was cloned.[3] However, some families with an apparent diagnosis of MEN 1 have not been demonstrated to have mutations in this gene. There are a number of explanations: chance will occasionally generate an apparent family history of MEN 1 such that more than one member of a family has a sporadic tumour that could be in keeping with MEN 1. Some families appear only to manifest hyperparathyroidism; this could be due to mutations in another gene. Other families have some features of MEN 1 but others that would not be expected; again this could represent a different inherited predisposition syndrome. Finally, in some families there may be a mutation affecting the *MEN1* gene that is hard to identify: for example, a mutation in a promoter region, a missense mutation or an in-frame deletion.

The majority of mutations identified in the *MEN1* gene result in loss of function of the menin protein for which this gene encodes.

What are the functions of menin?

Loss of heterozygosity of the *MEN1* gene has been demonstrated in tumours from individuals with MEN 1 implying that it functions as a tumour suppressor. Menin is known to bind the signalling proteins JunD and Smad3. Smad3 affects transforming growth factor β (TGF-β) signalling and hence cell proliferation.[4]

It is recognised that not all of the features of MEN 1 will occur in one person nor indeed in one family. This could imply that particular mutations are more likely to predispose to a particular set of features; however, such genotype-phenotype correlation has not been demonstrated.

There is some evidence of a founder effect; mutations at 512delC and 416delC in different families have identical haplotypes around the *MEN1* gene locus. Having said that there is also evidence of mutations arising as a new event; one study found *MEN1* mutations in 8/11 sporadic cases of MEN 1.[5]

Genetic counselling in MEN 1 needs to address the pattern of inheritance and information about penetrance and expression. As some of the features can manifest in childhood it is appropriate to consider predictive testing in childhood.

MULTIPLE ENDOCRINE NEOPLASIA TYPE 2 AND FAMILIAL MEDULLARY CARCINOMA OF THE THYROID GLAND

On clinical grounds multiple endocrine neoplasia type 2 (MEN 2) can be divided into MEN 2A and MEN 2B (see below). Familial medullary carcinoma (FMTC) of the thyroid alone is a separate clinical entity. All three conditions are now known to be allelic, being caused by mutations in the *RET* gene; all are inherited as autosomal dominant traits. MEN 2A is the most common. It is important to realise that not all cases of medullary carcinoma of the thyroid (MTC) represent an inherited tendency. In cases of apparently sporadic MTC an underlying germ-line mutation can be expected in approximately 25%.

MEN 2A

The clinical features of MEN 2A are the combination of medullary thyroid carcinoma, phaeochromocytoma and hyperparathyroidism. (Hyperplasia or an adenoma of the parathyroid glands may be present.) C-cell hyperplasia is regarded as the premalignant lesion for medullary thyroid carcinoma.

MEN 2A shows variable penetrance, thus approximately 40% of gene carriers develop clinical manifestations by age 50 and 60% by age 70. Biochemical screening can lead to earlier identification of gene carriers: approximately 90% of individuals with MEN 2A have biochemical abnormality by age 30 even if there are no overt signs of MEN 2A, emphasising the silent nature of the condition. Some patients with MEN 2A also have Hirschsprung's disease.

MEN 2B

Individuals with MEN 2B have the thyroid and adrenal features of MEN 2A but without hyperparathyroidism. They manifest additional features of multiple mucosal neuromas and intestinal ganglioneuromatosis. They also have a marfanoid habitus with joint laxity, neurological abnormalities (and possibly muscle weakness), café-au-lait patches and facial lentigines. The café-au-lait patches make MEN 2B a differential diagnosis to be considered in the diagnosis of neurofibromatosis type 1.

Familial medullary carcinoma of the thyroid gland (FMTC)

This is a condition in which affected individuals only develop medullary thyroid carcinoma. In order to be certain of the diagnosis of FMTC it is necessary for the family concerned to be large with no affected individuals suffering from any of the other features of MEN 2A. Although there is some phenotype-genotype correlation this is not sufficient to make a certain diagnosis of FMTC as opposed to MEN 2A.

The *RET* gene

The *RET* gene codes for a protein that is part of a family of tyrosine kinase receptors. Most cancer predisposition syndromes are caused by mutations in tumour suppressor genes. *RET* is one of the few identified exceptions to this rule; it is a proto-oncogene, mutations thus converting it to an oncogene.

The RET protein has three domains: extracellular; transmembrane; and intracellular. The intracellular domain contains two, discrete tyrosine kinase sub-domains. Activation of these sub-domains through phosphorylation initiates a downstream signal transduction cascade.[6]

For the majority of families with MEN 2A and FMTC the mutations in *RET* affect cysteine residues in the extracellular domain of the tyrosine kinase receptor. The exact position of the cysteine residue involved by any particular mutation affects the likelihood of the phenotype being either MEN 2A or FMTC. Virtually all mutations in MEN 2A are found in exons 10 and 11 of the *RET* gene but there is a strong case for looking at other exons if 10 and 11 are negative. For FMTC, mutations may be found in exons 13–15 as well as some in exons 10 and 11. For MEN 2B, 95% have a mutation in exon 16 (codon 918), at a site that is prone to somatic mutation.[7] This leads to a methionine amino acid being replaced by threonine and affects the process of catalysis of the tyrosine residues.

The mutations identified in MEN 2A, FMTC and MEN 2B all result in constitutive activation of the RET protein and aberrant cell growth and proliferation. This has been neatly demonstrated by transfection experiments leading to transformation in cell lines.[8]

Loss of function mutations in *RET* have been demonstrated in some kindreds with familial Hirschsprung's disease. In contrast to the mutation hot-spots noted in MEN 2, these mutations are distributed throughout the gene.

Genetic counselling for these conditions should cover the pattern of inheritance, penetrance and both common and rare manifestations. Because all may present in childhood it is reasonable to undertake predictive testing at a early age to help management decisions. Consideration needs to be given to whether or not genetic testing should be offered to patients presenting with a medullary carcinoma of thyroid as an apparently sporadic event. This is particularly relevant for those presenting in early adulthood. It is possible to test for specific *RET* mutations in the tumour itself. Somatic *RET* codon 918 mutations are found at moderate frequency in sporadic tumours. Confirmation of this mutation in tumour tissue and its absence in germ-line DNA (consistent with a somatic event) may help in establishing a case of MTC as sporadic. If DNA testing is to be offered, it is important that issues of consent are addressed carefully in view of the potential consequences of identifying germ-line *RET* mutations for both the inidividual and other family members.

Consent must therefore cover both the implications of such a test and further illness in the future, and also information sharing with relevant family members.

NON-MEDULLARY CARCINOMA OF THE THYROID GLAND

The main types of non-medullary thyroid carcinoma are:

- Cowden's/Bannayan Zonana syndrome
- papillary carcinoma of the thyroid
- familial adenomatous polyposis

Cowden's syndrome

This is a dominantly inherited disorder, but penetrance may be variable. The clinical features are hamartomatous lesions of the skin, thyroid gland and breast tissue. Other features are macrocephaly, mild to moderate learning difficulties and occasionally Lhermitte–Duclos disease (LDD), which is an unusual condition of cerebellar ganglion cell hypertrophy, causing ataxia and seizures. It is also unusual in that gene carriers may suffer from a variety of thyroid disorders: adenomatous goitre, hypothyroidism or hyperthyroidism and thyroid cancer.[9] Females with Cowden Syndrome can also suffer from benign breast disease, and the incidence of breast cancer is also high – approximately 25–30%. The average age of onset is 38 but it has been reported in adolescence.[10]

Bannayan–Zonana syndrome

This autosomal dominant condition has more names than most, and may also be called Ruvalcaba–Mhyre–Smith or Bannayan–Riley–Ruvalcaba syndrome. Like Cowden's syndrome this is a condition manifested by multiple hamartomas. It is characterised particularly by intestinal polyps, haemangiomas and lipomas, café-au-lait patches on the penis and macrocephaly.[11] Other features are breast cancer, lipid storage disorder, protein-losing enteropathy and thyroid disease including thyroid cancer.

Cowden's syndrome and Bannayan–Zonana syndrome have both been shown to be caused by mutations in *PTEN*. There are some reports of both occurring in the same family and presumably due to the same mutation.[12] It is not understood why penetrance and expression of mutations in *PTEN* can be so variable.

FUNCTION OF *PTEN*

The *PTEN* gene codes for a protein tyrosine phosphatase. *PTEN* expression blocks cell cycle progression in the G1 phase.[13] *PTEN* mutation testing remains an area of research and the usefulness of testing in the clinical setting remains uncertain. Currently, for the vast majority of families, diagnosis of both Cowden's and Bannayan–Zonana syndrome is based on clinical findings.

Papillary carcinoma of the thyroid gland

A small number of families have been reported in which there appears to be an autosomal dominant trait of papillary thyroid cancers. The underlying genetic aetiology remains unknown. There may be a separate syndrome of breast and thyroid cancer being inherited, again as an autosomal dominant trait that is distinct from those syndromes caused by *PTEN* mutations.

Familial adenomatous polyposis (FAP)

FAP is an autosomal dominant condition whose primary feature is polyp formation in the gastrointestinal tract. If left untreated these individuals have a very high risk of large bowel cancer, which usually occurs in the fourth decade. There is also, particularly for women, an increased risk of papillary thyroid cancer. However, the frequency of this in FAP is sufficiently low (affecting approximately 1% of those with FAP) that apart from an awareness of this as a risk it is unnecessary to organise a screening programme of the thyroid gland.[14] There is some evidence, however, of familial aggregation of this thyroid cancer in FAP, so for rare families who demonstrate such aggregation it is important to raise it with the at-risk family members and perhaps in this group consider screening. FAP is caused by mutations in the *APC* gene.

FAMILIAL PARATHYROID SYNDROMES

Apart from their occurrence as part of MEN 1 and MEN 2A, familial parathyroid syndromes are rare. There are occasional reports of families with hyperparathyroidism only and no other features of multiple endocrine neoplasia. These families are likely to have mutation in genes other than *MEN1* or *RET*.[15,16]

Hyperparathyroidism jaw tumour syndrome

This is an autosomal dominant condition. The gene has been identified as *HRPT2*, so it is now possible to offer genetic testing to these rare families. As the jaw tumours may be occult, this condition should be borne in mind in families thought to have familial primary hyperparathyroidism alone.

McCune–Albright syndrome

This condition features polyostotic fibrous dysplasia of bone, café-au-lait patches, and endocrinopathies – precocious puberty, hyperparathyroidism, acromegaly, Cushing's syndrome and hyperprolactinaemia.[17] It occurs as a sporadic mutation. It is due to mosaicism involving the gene encoding the α subunit of the G protein G_s. If mutations in this gene were present in all cells of the body it is thought this would cause early lethality.[18] Mosaicism is the name given to a somatic mutation occurring at some point in embryogenesis. The earlier it occurs the more cells are affected and the worse the phenotype that is seen.

PHAEOCHROMOCYTOMAS

von Hippel–Lindau syndrome (VHL)

This is an autosomal dominant syndrome with an incidence of the order of 1 in 40 000.[19] It demonstrates variable penetrance and expression, this variability being both intra- and interfamilial. It may also occur in an individual as the result of a new mutation. The main features of VHL are ocular angioma, cerebellar and spinal haemangioblastoma, phaeochromocytoma and renal cancer. Other features that are less serious are renal, hepatic, pancreatic and epididymal cysts. A rare but serious complication is pancreatic neuroendocrine tumour. These can secrete peptides and may be benign or malignant.

THE *VHL* GENE

The gene responsible for this syndrome (*VHL*) was identified in 1993. It is a tumour suppressor gene, and this was demonstrated by showing loss of the wild-type allele in tumours from individuals known to have VHL. *VHL* has three exons: exon 2 is alternatively spliced giving two products of different sizes. Expression of both occurs in adult tissues. In fetal tissue expression varies in different tissues; it may be that the longer transcript that is expressed in fetal kidney has a specific developmental role here. It is now known that the gene product interacts with the elongin complex and is thus involved in the detection and response to hypoxia. The tumours seen in VHL are all very vascular with pronounced angiogenesis. Their cells exhibit overexpression of vascular endothelial growth factor (VEGF). Production of VEGF is mediated by a pathway of hypoxia detection involving the VHL protein and the elongin complex. Many hypoxia-inducible genes are controlled by hypoxia-inducible factor (HIF). HIF is composed of an α subunit and a β subunit. The HIF α subunit is degraded if oxygen is present; this requires functioning VHL protein. Why mutations in *VHL* lead to pathologies at characteristic sites is not known.

In VHL there is evidence of genotype–phenotype correlation. Type 1 VHL refers to those families without phaeochromocytoma. These families are most likely to have deletions or premature termination mutations. Type 2 families do have phaeochromocytomas and are more likely to have missense mutations.[17] Mutations should be found in the majority of families with VHL.

The mean age of diagnosis in VHL is 26 years but some of the complications can present at a much younger age, hence recommended clinical screening in the UK starts at the age of 5 with annual eye examinations.[19] It could be argued that this means predictive genetic testing for this condition should be undertaken at this young age. However, genetic screening for VHL usually starts at age 15, so it is thus unusual for predictive testing to be requested in children before they can be involved in the decision-making process. It is not advisable to recommend a fixed policy with regard to age of testing for VHL, and each case should be judged on its merits.

Neurofibromatosis type 1 (NF1)

This is also an autosomal dominant disorder, previously referred to as von Recklinghausen's disease. It is relatively common, with a birth incidence of approximately 1 in 3000 and a prevalence of approximately 1 in 4000. However, 50% of those affected have NF1 due to a new mutation, hence such individuals do not have a family history of NF1. It is also possible for a person to have segmental NF1 due to a mutation developing at some point during embryogenesis and causing mosaicism. For those with a germ-line mutation penetrance is essentially 100%. Expression of NF1 can be very variable notwithstanding well-established diagnostic criteria:

- six or more café-au-lait patches;
- two or more neurofibromas;
- one plexiform neurofibroma;
- axillary or inguinal freckles;
- two or more Lisch nodules;
- optic glioma;
- bone lesions;
- sphenoid dysplasia;
- cortical thinning of long bones;
- pseudoarthrosis;
- first-degree relative with NF1.

It is a diagnosis that can be made in childhood: all gene carriers have six or more café-au-lait patches by age 5. It is important to emphasise that café-au-lait patches are not pathognomonic of NF1 and are seen in other inherited predisposition syndromes.

Phaeochromocytomas are a feature of NF1, although not common, affecting 0.7% of NF1 gene carriers. The most likely age of presentation is in the fifth decade. Phaeochromocytoma is rare in adolescence and extremely rare in children with NF1; they may be bilateral.

People with NF1 also have a risk of duodenal carcinoid:[20] a somatostatinoma with a particular histology, namely psammoma bodies and somatostatin immunoreactivity. The frequency of this complication is 1.5% in NF1 gene carriers. There is some evidence of an association between these two tumours.

The *NF1* gene is located on the long arm of chromosome 17 (17q11.2). It is a large gene that unfortunately has no mutation hotspots. This means that genetic analysis is not guaranteed to be clinically useful given the difficulties of identifying a mutation. Mutations in *NF1* result in loss of the protein product, in keeping with *NF1* being a tumour suppressor gene. This is supported by loss of heterozygosity that has been described in NF1-typical tumours. There is some evidence of a more severe phenotype for those with an intragenic deletion, and in this group it may be useful to identify the mutation as it could influence management. The *NF1* gene codes for a protein called neurofibromin. It acts like a GTPase-activating protein (GAP). These proteins interact with RAS protein thus downregulating it. Loss of neurofibromin leads to unopposed RAS activity and hence cell proliferation.

Hereditary paragangliomatosis (HP)

Although it has been recognised for some time that there are rare families with an inherited predisposition to phaeochromocytomas and carotid body tumours, it is only recently that the underlying genetic mechanisms have been elucidated. In some families hereditary paragangliomatosis (HP) follows an autosomal dominant inherited pattern, but in others the pattern is more complex, following an autosomal dominant pattern with imprinting. This is the name given to the switching off of one of a pair of genes depending on which parent it has been inherited from. For some conditions the maternally derived gene is switched off, as is the case in hereditary paragangliomatosis; in others it is the paternally derived gene that is switched off.[21]

The clinical picture is of tumours of the sympathetic chain; phaeochromocytomas, both adrenal and extra-adrenal; carotid body tumours and glomus jugulare tumours. Age at presentation varies from childhood to old age. There is apparent anticipation – the age at presentation seems to be younger in successive generations. Anticipation is a recognised genetic phenomenon and in all other situations is due to an unstable type of mutation called an expansion, which may change in size from one generation to the next. However, this is not the case for the mutations responsible for HP.

HP is caused by mutations in succinate dehydrogenase genes; *SDHB*, *SDHC* and *SDHD*.[22] Mutations in the fourth gene of the succinate dehydrogenase gene family, *SDHA*, cause Leigh's syndrome, a rare autosomal recessive disorder characterised by encephalopathy, lactic acidosis, respiratory failure and retinopathy. The protein products of these four genes form a complex that is involved in the respiratory cycle of mitochondria. It remains to be explained why mutations in these genes cause hereditary paragangliomatosis.

SDHB AND *SDHC*

Mutations in either of these genes cause an autosomal dominant condition, and expression, particularly age at presentation, is variable.[23]

SDHD

Mutations in *SDHD* demonstrate imprinting; if a person inherits the mutated *SDHD* gene from their mother he or she will remain clinically unaffected as the maternal gene is switched off. But if a person inherits the mutation paternally then that person will develop features of HP.[24]

ADRENOCORTICAL CARCINOMA

When this occurs in childhood it is likely to be due to a germ-line TP53 mutation. In a series of 14 such cases, 9/14 were shown to be due to TP53 and 2/14 were likely to have TP53 mutations that could not be identified. The one case not due to a TP53 mutation occurred in a child with hemihypertrophy due to Beckwith–Wiedemann syndrome.

Carcinoid tumours

As already described, carcinoid may be a feature of MEN, NF1 and, very rarely, VHL syndrome. There have been occasional reports of carcinoid tumours being inherited in an autosomal dominant fashion.[25]

FAMILIAL ENDOCRINE DISEASE: GENETICS AND EARLY TREATMENT

The diagnosis and management of familial endocrine syndromes epitomises the complex and changing interface between surgery, medicine and molecular genetics. The last decade has seen an explosion in our understanding of the molecular basis of these rare syndromes, and the rapid translation of research-based findings into clinical practice. As a result, we are already witnessing genetic testing leading to highly effective, targeted intervention. The next decade is likely to see continued progress, with expansion and refinement of molecular diagnostics and further integration of these developments into clinical practice.

Multiple endocrine neoplasia type 1 (MEN 1)

PRESENTATION

MEN 1 is an autosomal dominant familial syndrome characterised by the development of multiple and metachronous endocrine and non-endocrine tumours (**Table 4.1**). Approximately 10% of cases arise de novo, without a prior family history of the syndrome. The hallmark features of MEN 1 are endocrine tumours of the pituitary, pancreas and parathyroid. Presentation is dependent upon the herald lesion. More than one component may be apparent at presentation.

Primary hyperparathyroidism

Primary hyperparathyroidism (PHP) is the most common endocrinopathy in MEN 1, and is thought to be present in at least 90% of cases aged 50 years or over. It is also the most common initial clinical expression of MEN 1, with typical detection or

Table 4.1 • Clinical features of multiple endocrine neoplasia type 1 (MEN 1)

Tumour/site*	Hormonal/ other characteristics*
Parathyroid adenoma (90%)	
Enteropancreatic islet tumour (30–80%)	NF (80%) Gastrinoma (40%) Pancreatic polypeptidoma (20%) Insulinoma (10%) Glucagonoma VIPoma Somatostatinoma ACTHoma (rare) GRFoma (rare)
Anterior pituitary tumour (10–60%)	Prolactinoma (20%) NF (6%) GHoma (5%) ACTHoma (2%)
Foregut carcinoid	Gastric ECL tumour (10%) Thymic carcinoid (2–8%) Bronchial carcinoid (2%)
Adrenocortical tumour	Non-functioning adenoma (25%) Adrenocortical carcinoma (rare) Hyperaldosteronism (rare)
Cutaneous manifestations	Lipoma (30%) Angiofibroma (85%) Collagenoma (70%)

*Values in brackets are estimates of penetrance of given characteristic at age 40.
NF, non-functioning; ACTH, adrenocorticotropin; ECL, enterochromaffin-like; GH, growth hormone; GRF, growth hormone releasing factor; VIP, vasoactive intestinal peptide.

presentation in the third decade of life, significantly earlier than that found in sporadic PHP. Patients with MEN 1 generally have asymmetric, independent parathyroid adenomas in 3–4 glands. PHP often recurs following subtotal parathyroidectomy. PHP can exacerbate coexistent hypergastrinaemia from gastrinoma.

Enteropancreatic islet tumours

The prevalence of enteropancreatic islet tumours in patients with MEN 1 may be as high as 80%, although the majority of such tumours are clinically silent and non-functional. Functional tumours can present in the second decade of life. Many

asymptomatic patients have radiologically detectable tumours by the third decade. Tumours can arise throughout the pancreas and the duodenal submucosa. They are commonly multicentric, metachronous and range in size and characteristics from micro- and macroadenomas to invasive and metastatic carcinoma. The prognosis of these tumours may relate to their specific molecular mutations.[26]

Up to 40% of patients with MEN 1 develop gastrinoma, and current data suggest that up to 25% of all patients with gastrinoma have MEN 1. Though presentation with invasive or metastatic disease is unusual before 30 years of age, metastatic disease (possibly occult) can be present in up to 50% of MEN 1-associated gastrinoma at diagnosis. Tumours secreting pancreatic polypeptide are manifest biochemically and radiologically, but are generally clinically silent.[27]

Pituitary tumours

The prevalence of pituitary tumours in MEN 1 is uncertain, due to the range of patients and methods employed in the majority of studies to date. A large European multicentre study of 324 patients with MEN 1 found pituitary tumours in 42% of cases.[28] The most common pituitary lesion is prolactinoma. There are few prospective data on age-related penetrance of pituitary disease. However, MEN 1-associated pituitary macroadenoma has occurred as early as 5 years of age.[29]

Foregut carcinoids

MEN 1-associated foregut carcinoid tumours are found in the thymus, stomach and bronchi. They are not generally hormonally active, and do not present with carcinoid syndrome. Their true prevalence is unclear. Gastric enterochromaffin-like (ECL) tumours are generally discovered at endoscopy. They are promoted by hypergastrinaemia and thus generally arise in MEN 1 patients with gastrinoma. Thymic carcinoid disease has been highlighted as a major cause of mortality in MEN 1. However, relatively little is known about its natural history. A recent prospective study of 85 patients with MEN 1 found an incidence of 8% over a mean follow-up period of 8 years.[30] Patients were all male, and most had no symptoms of the tumour at the time of detection. Interestingly, 4/7 of the tumours did not show somatic loss of heterozygosity at the *MEN1* locus, raising questions as to the mechanism of tumour development. Serum chromogranin A was elevated in 6/7 tumours. Mean time interval between diagnosis of MEN 1 and development of thymic carcinoid was 19 years. It may be that as early mortality reduces in MEN 1 due to improved surgical and medical treatment, this relatively late expression of the disease increases in prevalence and impact.

Adrenocortical tumours

Adrenocortical disease occurs in 20–40% of patients with MEN 1. It is unusual in patients who do not have pancreatic disease. Pathology may include diffuse hyperplasia, solitary adenoma and carcinoma.[31] Disease can be bilateral. Excess hormone secretion is rare, and the majority of lesions are detected on routine radiological monitoring.[32]

Cutaneous manifestations

A variety of cutaneous pathologies are now firmly established as components of MEN 1. Cutaneous lipomas are often nodular and multicentric. Visceral lipomas have also been described. Cutaneous manifestations of MEN 1 are useful clinically in the presymptomatic diagnosis of MEN 1 in affected kindreds.[33]

DIAGNOSIS

Diagnosis of MEN 1 is considered in any patient presenting with two synchronous or metachronous tumours in the three characteristic sites (pituitary, pancreas and parathyroid). If there is a first-degree relative with a lesion typical of MEN 1, the diagnosis should be considered in the presence of a single lesion. Patients with recurrent PHP, especially multiglandular disease, should have the diagnosis excluded.

The application of molecular diagnostics is altering the spectrum of presentation of MEN 1, highlighting both asymptomatic individuals and those with atypical presentations. Furthermore, it is likely to refine diagnostic criteria in the light of discrepancies between phenotype and genotype. The association of an endocrine tumour that has a low population prevalence – such as growth hormone(GH)-secreting pituitary tumour – with PHP may represent *MEN 1* or *MEN 1* phenocopy.

Recent data suggest that mutations in the menin coding region are infrequent in those patients without a family history of MEN 1 who develop a combination of PHP and acromegaly due to GH-secreting pituitary tumour.[34]

MANAGEMENT

MEN 1 is associated with premature death, most commonly (30%) through metastatic islet cell tumours.[35] Advances in the medical management of gastrinoma and hyperparathyroidism may result in a paradoxical increase in cumulative morbidity from other facets of the condition in the coming decade. The principal organs involved in MEN 1 are difficult to screen for early tumours, and prophylactic surgery is either not appropriate or has not been shown to prevent the development of tumour (cervical thymectomy).[30] The challenge is therefore to improve morbidity and mortality through targeted surgical and medical interventions as directed by surveillance and molecular screening programmes that aim to detect disease expression at an early stage in an inclusive manner.[36]

Primary hyperparathyroidism

PHP in MEN 1 is characterised by asynchronous involvement of all parathyroid glands. However, there remains debate as to the optimum type and timing of parathyroid surgery. Subtotal parathyroidectomy for PHP in MEN 1 is associated with a surgical cure rate (as defined by the number of patients not hypercalcaemic) of 60% at 10 years and 51% at 15 years.[37] The alternative, total parathyroidectomy with or without autograft, is associated with postoperative hypoparathyroidism and lifelong treatment with vitamin D analogues. Preoperative imaging and minimally invasive approaches may be difficult because of the need to examine all four glands. Transcervical thymectomy is recommended at the time of parathyroidectomy.

Enteropancreatic islet tumours

Enteropancreatic tumours in MEN 1 are often multiple, recurrent and heterogeneous in behaviour. Correct management requires the correlation of symptoms, hormonal and imaging studies (which may be discordant) and experience in the natural history of the pathology. This can pose a significant challenge to the clinician.

Figure 4.1 • Operative specimen of an insulinoma in the tail of the pancreas, bisected.

Figure 4.2 • Macroscopic histology of the insulinoma in **Fig. 4.1**.

Surgery is the main treatment for patients with insulinoma in MEN 1 (**Figs 4.1** and **4.2**). All other syndromes of hormone excess due to entero-pancreatic tumours respond well to medical therapy with proton-pump inhibitors (gastrinoma) or somatostatin analogues (VIPoma). The timing of surgery in the management of these conditions is debated.

Gastrinomas in MEN 1 are often multifocal and small, and can be situated in the duodenum. Extensive pancreatic-duodenal surgery can be associated with significant morbidity. Surgery for gastrinoma in MEN 1 is frequently not curative.[38] Furthermore, metastatic disease is found at surgery in a substantial number of patients in whom it is not apparent preoperatively.[39] Nevertheless, the outcome of patients treated surgically for locally advanced disease can be the same as those with limited disease. A subset of MEN 1 patients with

gastrinoma has aggressive disease and decreased survival.[40] Features associated with aggressive tumour behaviour include:

- diagnosis of MEN 1 before 35 years of age;
- onset of gastrinoma at 27 years or younger;
- markedly elevated gastrin levels at presentation;
- tumour size greater than 3 cm.

Aggressive antitumour treatment in this group needs to be considered.

Non-functioning enteropancreatic islet cell tumours and those secreting pancreatic polypeptide are generally clinically silent. There is no consensus as to best treatment in this situation. Some advocate surgical removal if the lesion is greater than 3 cm or growing on serial radiological monitoring, while others suggest excision as a preventive measure in the absence of data suggestive of aggressive behaviour.

The standard surgical approach other than for gastrinoma is spleen-preserving distal pancreatectomy (**Fig. 4.3**) and intraoperative bidigital palpation, coupled with intraoperative ultrasound and enucleation of any tumour found in the pancreatic head and duodenal submucosa. Surgery for gastrinoma should include duodenotomy.[41] A Whipple procedure may be considered for tumours at the pancreatic head. Preoperative localisation of the target lesion with corroborative intraoperative ultrasound is useful in planning the appropriate approach. This can be important in the manage-

Figure 4.3 • Spleen-preserving distal pancreatectomy specimen, showing a large neuroendocrine tumour in the body of the pancreas.

ment of functional tumours as the pancreas and duodenum may contain multiple abnormalities, leading to uncertainty as to which of several lesions is the source of excess hormone production. Surgery prompted by abnormal biochemistry but in the absence of any scan-detected lesion should be considered to prevent malignant transformation of microadenomas.

Pituitary tumours

Pituitary tumours should be managed in the same manner as in isolated pituitary disease. Prolactinomas should be treated with dopamine agonists, with biochemical and radiological confirmation of response. Normalisation of prolactin levels without tumour shrinkage suggest misdiagnosis of a non-functioning pituitary adenoma with secondary hyperprolactinaemia. Non-functioning tumours should be treated with surgery. GH-secreting adenomas are best treated with primary surgery followed by consideration of external beam radio-therapy and somatostatin analogue therapy for persistent disease.[33]

Foregut carcinoids

The optimum management of this generally late expression of MEN 1 is unclear. Resection of bronchial carcinoid is usually required to make the diagnosis. Long-term follow-up is then required to check for recurrence. The natural history and malignant potential of ECL-like gastric carcinoids is unclear. Thymic carcinoid tumours are generally asymptomatic when detected through radiological screening, and can behave aggressively. Relapse is common after surgery, and the optimum adjuvant medical and radiotherapeutic approaches are not yet established.[30]

SCREENING

The multiple and metachronous nature of endo-crine tumours associated with MEN 1 requires lifelong clinical, biochemical and radiological surveillance to detect MEN 1-associated tumour expression as soon as possible, minimising mor-bidity and optimising outcome. Genetic testing supports this process, facilitating the identification of both individuals within a kindred who will benefit from such long term surveillance, and those who do not require it.

Genetic

MEN1 gene analysis, involving sequencing of all coding exons of the MEN1 gene, should be offered to patients with MEN 1 to help in determining biochemical and radiological screening strategies for their relatives. Analysis may also be helpful in those patients with atypical presentations, but only if a MEN 1-defining mutation is found. It should not be used to exclude the disease. Identification of a MEN1 mutation in an index case should lead to a screening cascade for the same mutation within the kindred, beginning with first-degree relatives. Given that 25% of all patients with gastrinoma have MEN 1, genetic testing should be considered in patients presenting with gastrinoma, even in the absence of other features.

Absence of MEN1 coding region mutations does not exclude MEN 1, and should trigger promoter and exon dosage studies if the index of suspicion of MEN 1 is sufficient. If these prove negative in a kindred with suspected MEN 1, linkage studies may be appropriate.

Biochemical and radiological

Biochemical and radiological screening should be offered to all patients with a diagnosis of MEN 1, to asymptomatic relatives found to harbour a MEN 1-defining MEN1 mutation on genetic testing, and to those found to be at risk through haplotype and linkage studies (Table 4.2). First-degree relatives of those patients with MEN 1 in whom a MEN1 mutation has not been found should also be offered screening pending the outcome of promoter and exon dosage analyses. Biochemical and radiological screening should commence in early childhood, balancing age-dependent penetration, sensitivity of specific studies in specific age groups, and the inconvenience caused by the process. Screening should be lifelong for those patients with MEN 1, those known to harbour MEN 1-defining MEN1 mutations, and those defined as 'at risk' by haplotype and linkage studies. It should continue to the age of 50 in those kindreds in whom no genetic risk stratification is possible.

Gastrin levels are elevated in primary (atrophic) and secondary (drug-induced) achlorhydria, which can lead to false-positive screening tests for the disease. Ideally, treatment with H_2 antagonists and proton-pump inhibitors should be stopped for

Familial endocrine disease: genetics, clinical presentation and management

Chapter Four •

Table 4.2 • Outline programme for biochemical and radiological screening for MEN 1

Tumour type	Investigation	Age commencing (years)	Frequency
Parathyroid adenoma	iCa^{2+}, PTH	8	Annual
Enteropancreatic islet cell	Gastrin	20	Annual
	Glucose, insulin	5	Annual
	VIP, PP	20	Annual
	Glucagon	20	Annual
	Somatostatin	20	Annual
	MRI	20	3–5-yearly
Anterior pituitary	Prolactin	5	Annual
	IGF-1		Annual
	MRI		5-yearly
Foregut carcinoid	Chromogranin A	20	Annual
	MRI	20	3–5-yearly

Choice of radiological imaging modality may vary with local resources and expertise.
iCa^{2+}, ionised Ca^{2+}; IGF-1, insulin-like growth factor 1; PP, pancreatic polypeptide; PTH, parathyroid hormone; VIP, vasoactive intestinal polypeptide.

2 and 4 weeks, respectively, before assessment of gastrin levels. However, gastrin levels in the normal range do not exclude gastrinoma, and there should be a low threshold for complementary corroborative gastric acid studies.

Multiple endocrine neoplasia type 2 (MEN 2)

MEN 2 is an autosomal dominant familial cancer syndrome characterised by the metachronous development of medullary thyroid cancer (MTC), phaeochromocytoma and PHP. Overall penetrance of the disease is high in gene carriers although that of individual characteristics is varied. MEN 2 is subclassified into several discrete forms with clinical, pathological and molecular correlates.

- MEN 2A: MTC (90%), phaeochromocytoma (50%) and PHP (20–30%).
- MEN 2A with cutaneous lichen amyloidosis.
- MEN 2A with Hirschsprung's disease (HD).
- Familial medullary thyroid cancer (FMTC): at least 10 or more carriers or affected cases of MTC in a kindred over the age of 50 with no clinical or detectable evidence of other features of MEN 2.

- FMTC with HD.
- MEN 2B: MTC, phaeochromocytoma, decreased upper/lower body ratio, marfanoid habibtus, gastrointestinal and mucosal ganglioneuromatosis.

MEN 2B is the most aggressive form, MTC presenting at a younger age and often with more advanced disease. Historically, the majority of MEN 2B cases represent de novo mutations without a family history of the condition. Earlier diagnosis and improved management strategies may result in a change in this picture over the next 20 years.

PRESENTATION

Presentation can be with any specific feature of the condition. MEN 2B can present with signs or complications of ganglioneuromatosis (mucosal or gastrointestinal) prior to the development or recognition of an endocrinopathy.

Medullary thyroid cancer

MTC has been the first manifestation of MEN 2 in most kindreds. It can present in the first decade of life with intrathyroidal, locally advanced or disseminated disease. Historically, MTC has been the major cause of morbidity and mortality in

MEN 2. Current management approaches will alter this natural history (see later). MTC in MEN 2 is preceded by C-cell hyperplasia. Recent data have highlighted a 6.6-year window between development of MTC and progression to nodal metastases in MEN 2A patients harbouring the most common (codon 634) *RET* mutation.[42]

Phaeochromocytoma

Phaeochromocytoma can be unilateral or bilateral. Presentation can be with symptoms as in sporadic disease or as the result of positive surveillance studies. Phaeochromocytoma in MEN 2 can present in the first decade of life.

Primary hyperparathyroidism

PHP occurs in 20–30% of patients with MEN 2A, and is more common in those with RET_{634} mutations. Most patients are asymptomatic. PHP associated with MEN 2 is often less severe than that encountered in MEN 1, and synchronous involvement of all four glands is less common.

MANAGEMENT

Medullary thyroid cancer

New cases of MEN 2 presenting with MTC should be treated by thyroidectomy with central or more widespread node dissection depending on pre- and perioperative staging. Thyroidectomy for MEN 2B should include central node dissection. However, the aim of surgical management encompasses and is focused increasingly on prevention of MTC. Surgery for MTC in MEN 2 should be performed before the age at which malignant progression occurs.[43] Historically this decision was based on basal and stimulated levels of the hormone calcitonin, produced by C-cells of the thyroid and a valuable tumour marker for MTC. However, this approach has an unacceptable sensitivity and specificity. Decisions on the timing of thyroidectomy in new cases of MEN 2 without apparent MTC at presentation (such as those cases detected through genetic screening) should follow a stratified approach based on the genotype-phenotype relationships linking specific *RET* mutations with a specific natural history of MTC. Such an approach balances the earliest age at which MTC can present in association with a given *RET* genotype against the potential surgical morbidity of thyroidectomy at a

Figure 4.4 • Operative view at the conclusion of a prophylactic thyroidectomy for MEN 2B in a child aged 18 months.

young age (**Fig. 4.4**). Patients are assigned to one of three risk bands:

- **Risk level 1:** all patients with MEN 2B; patients with *RET* mutations involving codons 883, 918 and 922.
- **Risk level 2:** patients with *RET* mutations involving codons 611, 618, 620 and 634.
- **Risk level 3:** patients with *RET* mutations involving codons 609, 768, 790, 791, 804 and 891.

Patients in risk level 1 should undergo thyroidectomy in the first year of life, and preferably in the first 6 months of life. Those in risk level 2 should undergo thyroidectomy before the age of 5 years. There is no consensus on the optimum approach to patients in risk level 3. MTC presents at an older age in this group, and is commonly less aggressive. Recent data suggest that thyroidectomy need not take place before the age of 10 years, and that central node dissection is unnecessary before 20 years. However, the cumulative experience on which such recommendations are based remains limited.[42,44]

Persistence of elevated calcitonin levels following primary surgery should trigger radiological staging with CT or MRI. In-111 pentetreotide scanning can detect somatostatin receptor-positive disease. Flurodopamine PET is an additional sensitive modality for detection of occult recurrent MTC.[45] Local recurrent or residual disease is the most common cause of persistently elevated tumour markers following primary treatment. In the absence of widespread distant disease, re-operation should be considered. If more distant metastatic disease is found, repeat surgery for tumour debulking should be considered for control of local pressure symptoms or those due to humoral factors secreted by the tumour.

Standard chemotherapy regimens are not particularly effective in the management of systemic metastatic disease. External beam radiotherapy can be used for the palliative treatment of bone metastases. However, metastatic MTC can remain asymptomatic, and conservative approaches to management coupled with regular biochemical surveillance of tumour load can result in good quality of life for many years.

Phaeochromocytoma

The principles of diagnosis and intervention should be similar to those applied to sporadic disease (see Chapter 3). However, it is important to exclude active phaeochromocytoma in any patient with suspected or established disease prior to surgical intervention for a separate or linked condition, in early pregnancy and prior to labour. Analysis of both timed overnight urine metanephrines and normetanephrines, together with plasma metanephrines provides the highest degree of sensitivity and specificity in biochemical diagnostic and surveillance programmes.[46] Plasma metanephrines alone may generate significant false-positive screening data. Positive biochemistry should trigger appropriate imaging studies with MRI, supported by radionuclear imaging if necessary.

Primary hyperparathyroidism

The principles of diagnosis and indications for intervention should be similar to those in sporadic PHP; although all four glands may not be enlarged, the approaches to surgery should be similar too. If enlarged parathyroid glands are encountered at the time of thyroidectomy in a patient who is eucalcaemic, the approach should be the same as if the patient were known to have mild PHP.

BIOCHEMICAL SCREENING

All patients with MEN 2 or those identified as *RET* mutation carriers but yet to express the disease should have annual biochemical screening for endocrine components of the syndrome to detect new or recurrent disease:

- MTC: plasma calcitonin, carcinoembryonic antigen.
- Phaeochromocytoma: timed overnight urine metanephrines and normetanephrines, plasma metanephrines.
- PHP: ionised Ca^{2+}, parathyroid hormone.

In the high-risk groups (risk levels 1 and 2) biochemical screening should commence at the time of planning thyroidectomy. In remaining patients it should commence between the ages of 5 and 7 years. Catecholamine screening can be difficult in young children. Phaeochromocytoma has not been found in association with certain *RET* mutations involving codons 609, 768, $_{val}804_{met}$ and 891. It is premature to omit catecholamine screening in these groups, though reduced surveillance frequency can be considered. Positive screening data should trigger appropriate imaging studies and intervention.

GENETIC SCREENING

Germ-line *RET* mutation analysis is accurate, effective and widely available. Routine testing should include analysis of exons 10, 11, 13, 14, 15 and 16. Testing should be offered to the following groups:

- New patients presenting with two synchronous or metachronous features of MEN 2.
- Patients presenting with a single manifestation of MEN 2 who have a first-degree relative with an endocrine feature of MEN 2.
- Infants presenting with gastrointestinal or mucosal features of MEN 2B.
- Patients presenting with MTC.
- Infants presenting with HD.

First-degree relatives of those patients diagnosed with *RET* mutations should be screened for the same mutation. Failure to identify a *RET* mutation on routine screening programmes in a patient in whom the clinical suspicion of MEN 2 is high should lead to sequencing of remaining exons. In a kindred in which the clinical suspicion of MEN 2 is high and in which no *RET* mutation is identified, haplotype and linkage studies may be helpful in confirming association of the disease with the *RET* locus and in risk assessment. Such situations are unusual in MEN 2A. Absence of *RET* mutations have been described in up to 16% of families with apparent FMTC. It has also been proposed that patients presenting with apparent sporadic phaeo-chromocytoma should also undergo *RET* screening.[33,47] Failure to detect a *RET* mutation in cases of apparently sporadic MTC and phaeochromo-cytoma leaves a small possibility that the patient has MEN 2, placing their offspring at risk. This can be defined using Bayes' theorem and the prevalence of germ-line *RET* mutations in apparent sporadic isolated MTC and phaeochromocytoma found in cohort studies (taken as the prevalence of MEN 2 in such cohorts).

Familial hyperparathyroidism (FHP) syndromes

Familial hyperparathyroidism (FHP) without other features of endocrinopathy has been described extensively. However, advances in our understanding of the calcium receptor and its physiology, the recognition of additional phenotypes found in association with FHP, and the increased application of molecular diagnostics have led to the recognition that many cases may be manifestations of wider syndromes.

PRESENTATION

Familial hypocalciuric hypercalcaemia (FHH) and neonatal severe hyperparathyroidism (NSHP)

FHH is inherited as an autosomal dominant condition, and is characterised by lifelong mild to moderate hypercalcaemia that is generally asymptomatic, and normal-range values of parathyroid hormone (PTH). FHH generally presents following detection of hypercalcaemia on routine testing, or on family screening of individuals with a family history. Calcium concentrations are consistent within a kindred. Although pancreatitis has been described as a complication of FHH, most patients in whom it has occurred have had additional risk factors. Renal excretion of calcium and magnesium are characteristically reduced, and the urine calcium:creatinine ratio is less than 0.01 in 80% of cases. The diagnostic value of the urine calcium:creatinine ratio is reduced in patients taking lithium and thiazide diuretics, both of which can reduce calcium excretion, and in mild PHP with concurrent vitamin D deficiency.

Neonatal severe hyperparathyroidism (NSHP) presents in the first week of life with anorexia, constipation, hypotonia and respiratory distress.

There is severe hypercalcaemia (total calcium concentration 3.5–7.7 mmol/L), often with hyper-magnesaemia. PTH can be significantly elevated. Skeletal radiology shows demineralisation and typical features of severe hyperparathyroidism. As NSHP can result from homozygous or compound heterozygous inheritance of FHH alleles, there may be a history or biochemical evidence of FHH in one or both parents. However, NSHP can arise as a result of a de novo germ-line mutation in a child with normal parents.

Familial hyperparathyroidism-jaw tumour syndrome (FHP-JT)

FHP-JT describes the association of autosomal dominant familial hyperparathyroidism with ossifying tumours (fibromas) of the mandible and maxilla.[48] Polycystic kidney disease has also been described in kindreds with this condition. Hyperparathyroidism presents as in sporadic cases. Jaw and maxillary tumours can be occult, and may only be apparent on screening by orthopantomograph. The gene responsible for this condition (*HRPT2*) has been mapped to chromosome 1q21-31, and parathyroid tumours from patients with this condition show loss of heterozygosity at this locus. Increased awareness of this condition has led to its recognition as the underlying problem in kindreds previously thought to have isolated familial hyperparathyroidism.[49] Both somatic and germ-line mutations in *HRPT2* have been identified in patients with apparently sporadic parathyroid carcinoma, suggesting that some patients with this unusual tumour may represent a phenotypic variant of HPT-JT.[50]

Familial isolated hyperparathyroidism

Familial isolated hyperparathyroidism (FIHP) is an autosomal dominant disorder characterised by uniglandular or multiglandular hyperparathyroidism in the absence of other endocrine disease and without evidence of jaw tumours. Recent data suggest that at least 20% of kindreds thought to have FIHP have inactivating mutations in *MEN1*, suggesting that a significant proportion of FIHP may represent a distinct variant of MEN 1. Further analysis of the *MEN1* promoter (to exclude promoter region mutations) and exon dosage may increase this proportion. Whether more intensive surveillance will detect other features of MEN 1 in these kindreds over time remains unclear.[33] FIHP in some kindreds may thus be a prelude to MEN 1, a distinct variant of MEN 1, or the result of a mutation in a different gene.

MANAGEMENT

Parathyroid surgery should be avoided in FHH, as the hypercalcaemia persists after parathyroidectomy. Efforts should therefore be made to exclude this diagnosis in all patients presenting with hypercalcaemia. Once FHH is diagnosed, it should be treated conservatively without intervention. Appropriate counselling as to the risk of NSHP in offspring should be given. Genetic testing for specific calcium receptor mutations may be useful in certain situations.

NSHP is managed by rigorous rehydration, inhibition of bone resorption with bisphosphonates, and respiratory support in the initial phase. Failure to respond should lead to total parathyroidectomy in the first month of life. Milder forms of the disease may stabilise with medical therapy alone, with progression to a phase resembling FHH after several months.

Hyperparathyroidism in patients with FHP-JT syndrome and FIHP should be managed surgically in the same manner as sporadic disease. Family members should be offered biochemical screening for hyperparathyroidism and radiological screening for mandibular and maxillary tumours. Hypercalcaemic patients with a family history of multiglandular hyperparathyroidism should be offered total parathyroidectomy. Affected members of apparent FIHP kindreds should be offered genetic testing for *MEN1* gene mutations and orthopantomography. Additional studies of other members of affected kindreds can be considered if a positive diagnosis of an alternative syndrome (MEN 1 or FHP-JT) is found in an index case.

Familial non-medullary thyroid cancer syndromes

COWDEN'S SYNDROME

Presentation

Cowden's syndrome (CS) is an autosomal dominant inherited cancer syndrome characterised by the development of multiple hamartomas (benign tumours comprised of disorganised elements of a particular organ) in multiple systems derived from all three germ-cell layers, together with a predisposition to breast and non-medullary thyroid cancer. Most cases of CS are likely to be sporadic, with estimates of familial cases ranging from 10 to 50%.

The International Cowden Syndrome Consortium has defined operational criteria for the diagnosis of CS (**Box 4.1**). In the absence of a family history of CS, a diagnosis can be made on mucocutaneous findings alone if any of the following criteria are met:

- Six or more facial papules of which at least three are trichilemmoma.
- Facial papules and oral mucosal papillomatosis.
- Oral mucosal papillomatosis and acral keratoses.

Box 4.1 • International Cowden Syndrome Consortium operational criteria for the diagnosis of Cowden syndrome, 1996

Pathognomonic criteria (mucocutaneous lesions)
• Facial trichilemmomas
• Acral keratoses
• Papillomatous papules
• Mucosal lesions

Major criteria
• Breast carcinoma
• Thyroid carcinoma
• Macrocephaly greater than 97th centile
• Lhermitte–Duclos disease (LDD)

Minor criteria
• Thyroid adenoma or multinodular goitre
• Mental retardation
• GI hamartomas
• Fibrocystic disease of the breast
• Lipomas
• Hamartomas
• Reproductive tract tumours or malformation (e.g. uterine fibroadenomas)

- The presence of at least six palmoplantar keratoses.

In the absence of a family history and mucocutaneous signs, a diagnosis of CS can be made if two major criteria (at least one of which is macrocephaly or LDD) or one major together with three minor criteria are present. If there is a family history of CS, the diagnosis can be made if the pathognomonic mucocutaneous criteria are present; a single major criterion is present; or two minor criteria are present.

Expression of CS is varied. Penetration is age-dependent, increasing from less than 10% under the age of 20 years to nearly 100% for cutaneous stigmata by the third decade. Thyroid abnormalities occur in 50–67% of CS patients, with 3–10% of patients developing thyroid cancer (generally follicular). A diagnosis of CS may therefore be made in a patient presenting with thyroid disease (in the presence of other stigmata or relevant history), or may develop in a patient known to have CS who is under endocrine surveillance.

Management

Patients presenting with a thyroid abnormality (goitre or nodule) should be investigated and managed along standard lines. Once a diagnosis of CS has been made, individuals and affected relatives should have endocrine screening with thyroid palpation as part of an annual medical review. The value of routine ultrasound surveillance of the thyroid has not been established. If a family-specific mutation has been identified, screening of other family members for that mutation is of value. If such a mutation cannot be identified and the family fit the criteria established for the diagnosis of CS, predictive testing based on analysis of the *PTEN* gene is not possible. If the family in question is sufficiently large, linkage studies using markers flanking *PTEN* can be considered. The prevalence of germ-line mutations in *PTEN* in kindreds with a high incidence of thyroid cancer but without other criteria for the diagnosis of CS is less than 2%.

FAMILIAL PAPILLARY THYROID CANCER

Presentation

Between 3 and 13% of patients with papillary thyroid cancer (PTC) have a relative affected by the disease. The basis for this familial clustering is unclear. The disease can be multifocal.

Management

It has been suggested that when two or more family members are identified with PTC, first- and second-degree relatives should be screened clinically for the disease. The onset, frequency, optimum duration, role of ultrasound screening and ultimate cost-effectiveness of this approach remain to be established. Because the disease can be multifocal, total thyroidectomy rather than hemithyroidectomy is recommended when PTC is suspected in this context.

FAMILIAL ADENOMATOUS POLYPOSIS: GARDNER'S SYNDROME

Presentation

Gardner's syndrome (GS) is an autosomal dominant disorder characterised by the occurrence of multiple gastrointestinal adenomatous polyps in association with osteomas, epidermoid cysts, desmoid tumours and retinal pigmentation. Hepatoblastomas and adenomas of the upper gastrointestinal tract and pancreas are more unusual components of the syndrome. GS is more common in women, with a 1:16 male to female gender ratio. Expression is variable, though the disease is usually penetrant in the third decade. GS is associated with an increased risk of thyroid neoplasia. As with CS, a diagnosis of GS may therefore be made in a patient presenting with thyroid disease and an appropriate personal or family history, or be made in a patient known to have GS who is undergoing endocrine surveillance.

Management

The role of clinical and/or ultrasound surveillance remains to be established. As disease can be multi-centric, total thyroidectomy should be considered as an option for primary surgery in those GS patients who develop thyroid disease.

Familial non-MEN 2 phaeochromocytoma

VON HIPPEL–LINDAU DISEASE

von Hippel–Lindau (VHL) disease is an autosomal dominant familial syndrome characterised by the

Table 4.3 • Clinical characteristics of von Hippel–Lindau (VHL) disease: age at presentation and frequency of expression

Tumour	Age at presentation (years)	Frequency of expression (%)
Retinal haemangioblastoma	1–67	25–60
Cerebellar haemangioblastoma	9–78	44–72
Brainstem haemangioblastoma	12–46	10–25
Spinal cord haemangioblastoma	12–66	13–50
CNS haemangioblastoma (miscellaneous)		<1
Renal cell carcinoma or cysts	16–67	25–60
Phaeochromocytoma	5–58	10–20
Pancreatic tumour or cysts	5–70	35–70
Endolymphatic sac tumours	12–50	10
Epididymal cystadenoma	Unknown	25–60
Broad ligament cystadenoma	Unknown	Unknown

asynchronous and metachronous development of multiple benign and malignant tumours.[51] Key features are central nervous system haemangioblastoma, renal cell carcinoma, and phaeochromocytoma. A number of additional lesions are recognised (**Table 4.3**). VHL disease results from a germ-line mutation in the *VHL* tumour suppressor gene situated at the chromosomal locus 3p25-26. The products of the *VHL* gene (a 213 amino acid 18-kDa protein; and a truncated 160 amino acid 18-kDa protein arising from an alternative translational start site) are important components in the pathway targeting intracellular proteins for degradation via proteasomes. VHL disease has two major endocrine manifestations: phaeochromocytoma and pancreatic islet-cell tumours.[52]

Presentation

VHL disease has been divided into four subtypes on the basis of clinical presentation, as depicted in **Box 4.2**. To date, endolymphatic sac tumours and cystadenomas of the epididymis and broad ligament have not been assigned to a specific disease subtype. There is a phenotype-genotype correlation in VHL disease. As such, expression of subtype phenotype is consistent within a given kindred.

Phaeochromocytoma associated with VHL disease is pathologically distinct from that occurring as part of MEN 2. Tumours have a thick vascular

Box 4.2 • Subtypes of von Hippel–Lindau disease according to clinical presentation

Type 1

- Retinal haemangioblastoma
- CNS haemangioblastoma
- Renal cell carcinoma
- Pancreatic tumours and pancreatic cysts

Type 2a

- Phaeochromocytoma
- Retinal haemangioblastoma
- CNS haemangioblastoma

Type 2b

- Phaeochromocytoma
- Retinal haemangioblastoma
- CNS haemangioblastoma
- Renal cell carcinoma
- Pancreatic tumours and pancreatic cysts

Type 2c

- Phaeochromocytoma only

capsule, and contain small to medium-sized tumour cells interspersed with multiple small blood vessels. There is no evidence of adrenomedullary hyperplasia outwith the tumour, as can be found in MEN 2.[53] Clinical presentation of phaeochromocytoma is similar to that in sporadic and other familial forms. However, compared with tumours associated with MEN 2, patients presenting with phaeochromocytoma as part of VHL disease have fewer symptoms. This clinical observation correlates with lower tumour catecholamine content and reduced expression of tyrosine hydroxylase.[54] Increasingly, presentation is with asymptomatic disease detected through routine biochemical and radiological screening. Tumours can be multiple and extra-adrenal.

Diagnosis

Diagnosis of phaeochromocytoma in VHL disease follows the principles established in sporadic and other forms of familial disease: clinical suspicion, biochemical testing and radiological localisation. Phaeochromocytoma associated with VHL disease has a predominantly noradrenergic phenotype. Urine catecholamine excretion can be normal, as can plasma metanephrines. A combination of elevated plasma normetanephrines together with normal plasma metanephrines is highly suggestive of VHL-associated phaeochromocytoma.[54] Local-isation of biochemical disease can employ MRI, CT and radioisotope scanning. Adrenal and extra-adrenal masses detected on routine radiological surveillance for renal cell carcinoma should trigger appropriate testing to exclude phaeochromo-cytoma, with initial biochemical testing followed by further complementary radiological or radioisotope studies.

Treatment

Surgical and non-surgical treatments for phaeo-chromocytoma in VHL disease follow the same principles as outlined in sporadic and other forms of the tumour (see Chapter 3).

Surveillance and screening

Patients with VHL disease type 2 require annual biochemical screening for phaeochromocytoma with a combination of urine and plasma metanephrines and normetanephrines. Elevated screening tests should trigger verification of the result, and then appropriate localisation studies with MRI followed by radioisotope scanning if data are equivocal. Use of MRI in this context reduces lifetime radiation exposure in the context of regular screening for renal and pancreatic disease.

Index cases should be offered genetic testing. These data may help to guide subtype classification and will facilitate genetic screening in the kindred. Although it has been proposed that screening apparent sporadic cases of phaeochromocytoma for germ-line VHL mutations is not worthwhile, recent data have challenged this assumption.[47] Comparisons of the relative effectiveness of molecular and clinical approaches in this situation are required.

PANCREATIC NEUROENDOCRINE TUMOURS IN VHL DISEASE

Pancreatic neuroendocrine tumours associated with VHL disease are usually detected during radio-logical surveillance (CT and MRI). Though they may demonstrate immunopositivity for a variety of pancreatic hormones and neuroendocrine markers, they are clinically silent. Endoscopic ultrasound and ^{111}In-labelled somatostatin scintigraphy can be helpful in differentiating neuroendocrine tumours from pancreatic cysts and cystadenomas, which also occur in VHL disease. Surgical excision has been recommended on the following bases:

1. Absence of metastatic disease.
2. Tumour larger than 3 cm in the body or tail of pancreas.
3. Tumour larger than 2 cm in head of pancreas.
4. Independent of tumour size if the patient is undergoing laparotomy for other reasons.

Those tumours below the threshold for surgery should be monitored radiologically at regular (initially annual) intervals.

Familial paraganglioma syndromes

Familial paraganglioma syndromes are autosomal dominant disorders characterised by the develop-ment of multiple and metachronous para-gangliomas. Parent-of-origin influences may appear to distort the autosomal dominant picture. Familial paraganglioma should be considered in any patient presenting with phaeochromocytoma or paraganglioma in which there is a family history of a similar tumour. Although unusual, familial paraganglioma syndromes have recently gained increased interest because of developments in understanding their genetic basis.

PRESENTATION

Familial paraganglioma syndromes can present with tumour in the head and neck, chest or abdomen. Not all paragangliomas are secretory. Only 5% of those occurring in the head and neck (such as those arising from the carotid body) are thought to secrete catecholamines and thus present with local symptoms. Functional paragangliomas and phaeochromocytomas present in the same manner as in sporadic disease, though the development of effective screening programmes in affected kindreds is likely to lead to increasing detection in the asymptomatic phase.

Patients with familial paraganglioma due to mutations in the genes encoding succinate dehydrogenase subunits B and D (SDHB, SDHD), can develop both phaeochromocytoma and paraganglioma. Familial paraganglioma due to mutations in the gene encoding SDHC present with non-functioning head and neck tumours. Penetrance of SDHD mutations is dependent upon parent of origin. The disease is not expressed if the mutation is inherited from the mother.[24]

MANAGEMENT

Functional tumours should be removed if possible. Partially excised locally aggressive and metastatic disease may benefit from treatment with ^{131}I-metaiodobenzylguanidine (MIBG).[55] Excision of nonfunctional tumours should be considered if there are significant local symptoms, or radiological evidence of growth on serial monitoring. The metachronous nature of the condition means that recurrences and the development of additional tumours are common.

Patients with SDHB and SDHD mutations should undergo annual biochemical screening for functional tumours with timed overnight urine collections for catecholamines. Members of the kindred at risk of the condition should also undergo biochemical

surveillance until inheritance patterns have been confirmed. Non-functional tumours are only detectable through clinical and radiological assessment. Optimum strategies for imaging these patients are not yet established.

Index cases should be offered genetic testing for SDH complex mutations. This helps in defining the risk of functional tumour to the patient (SDHC mutations) and in developing genetic screening programmes for other members of the kindred. It is thought that SDH gene mutations are found in only 10% of patients presenting with apparent sporadic paraganglioma.[56]

Neurofibromatosis type 1 (NF1)

NF1 is an autosomal dominant multisystem disorder with predominant neurological, cutaneous, ophthalmic and skeletal manifestations. Prevalence is estimated at 1/3500. Fifty percent of cases are sporadic, and the disease is usually 100% penetrant by 5 years of age. Phaeochromocytoma occurs in approximately 1% of patients with NF1. An increased risk of carcinoid tumour is also reported. NF type 2 is not associated with phaeochromocytoma.

PRESENTATION

Two or more of the following criteria are required for a diagnosis of NF1:

- Six or more café-au-lait macules >5 mm prepubertal or >15 mm postpubertal.
- Axillary or inguinal freckling.
- Two or more neurofibromas or a single plexiform neurofibroma.
- Two or more Lisch nodules.
- Optic pathway glioma.
- Sphenoid wing dysplasia, thinning of long cortical bones or pseudoarthrosis.
- A first-degree relative with NF1.

Phaeochromocytoma in NF-1 can present in the same manner as sporadic disease, or be detected on routine endocrine surveillance. Patients with NF1 are also at risk of renal artery stenosis. Hypertension is therefore neither sensitive nor specific as a sign of phaeochromocytoma in NF1.

MANAGEMENT

Management should follow the same principles as that of sporadic disease (see Chapter 3). Patients with NF1 should have annual biochemical screening for phaeochromocytoma with analysis of timed overnight urine catecholamine production.

Familial adrenocortical disease

CARNEY SYNDROME

Carney syndrome is a multiple neoplasia syndrome with cardiac, cutaneous, endocrine and nervous system manifestations.[57] It is inherited in an autosomal dominant manner. Fifty percent of affected kindreds harbour an inactivating mutation in the tumour suppressor gene *PRKAR1A*, which codes for the type 1α regulatory subunit of protein kinase A.[58]

Presentation

Carney syndrome can present with single or multiple, synchronous or metachronous clinical and pathological features, each of which are unusual in isolation:

- Spotty pigmentation: hypermelanosis; lentigines; blue naevi; combined naevi.
- Myxomas: cardiac (any chamber and possibly multiple); cutaneous; breast; oral cavity.
- Endocrinopathy: Cushing's syndrome due to primary pigmented nodular adrenal disease; GH-secreting pituitary tumour; large-cell Sertoli cell tumour of testis; Leydig cell tumour; thyroid tumours; ovarian cysts.
- Psammomatous melanotic schwannoma: sympathetic chain; gastrointestinal tract.
- Ductal adenoma of breast.

ACTH-independent Cushing's syndrome is the most common endocrinopathy in Carney syndrome, and is present in up to 30% of cases. The underlying pathology, primary pigmented nodular adrenal hyperplasia (PPNAD), rarely occurs outside the disease. The adrenal glands are not enlarged and contain multiple pigmented nodules scattered throughout a characteristically atrophic cortex. These nodules may be visible on preoperative imaging. Acromegaly develops in 10% of cases and has been mainly due to pituitary macroadenoma. Prospective screening may alter this pattern. Testicular tumours occur in 30% of affected males, and may lead to precocious puberty. Thyroid and ovarian tumours also develop with increased frequency.

Management

Individual features of the syndrome should be managed as in sporadic disease. Presentation of cortisol excess may be atypical and indolent. Diagnosis of Carney syndrome should trigger periodic clinical, biochemical and radiological screening for additional features with the aim of reducing associated morbidity. Genetic testing is not widely available, placing the emphasis on careful clinical review of affected kindreds.

Familial hyperaldosteronism

Familial hyperaldosteronism type 1 (FHA1) and type 2 (FHA2) are rare autosomal dominant disorders of aldosterone excess.

PRESENTATION

FHA1 constitutes 1–3% of all cases of primary hyperaldosteronism.[59] Unlike other forms of hyperaldosteronism, it is present from birth and has no gender bias. It is characterised by moderate to severe hypertension and elevated aldosterone/renin ratios (though this is not specific). Many patients are normokalaemic. The diagnosis should be considered in any patient presenting with hypertension under the age of 25 years. A strong family history of hypertension is not always apparent. There may be a prominent family history of haemorrhagic stroke. Many patients do not respond to conventional antihypertensive agents, or develop hypokalaemia on potassium-wasting diuretics. Diagnosis is supported by suppression of aldosterone to undetectable levels during a low-dose dexamethasone suppression test (0.5 mg dexamethasone 6-hourly for 48 hours). Blood pressure may fall during the test.

FHA2 is not suppressible by dexamethasone and is mechanistically distinct from FHA1, though its precise molecular basis remains unclear. It is clinically, biochemically and pathologically indistinguishable from non-familial primary hyperaldosteronism.[60]

MANAGEMENT

Traditional therapy for FHA1 has been with gluco-corticoids to suppress adrenocorticotropin drive to the chimaeric 11-β-hydroxylase-aldosterone synthase gene. Longstanding hypertension may not respond fully to this approach. Moreover, excessive suppression with glucocorticoids may result in comorbidity, especially in young children. Mineralo-corticoid antagonists and dihydropyridine calcium-channel blockers are alternative approaches.

Management of FHA2 should follow the same principles as that of primary hyperaldosteronism, balancing surgical and medical approaches dependent upon localisation studies against the response to antihypertensive therapy with amiloride, mineralo-corticoid antagonists and/or dihydropyridine calcium-channel blockers (See Chapter 3).

Key points

- Inherited endocrine syndromes are rare.
- Multiple endocrine glands are often involved, either synchronously or consecutively.
- A multidisciplinary approach to these conditions involving endocrinologist, geneticist and endocrine surgeon is essential.
- Prophylactic surgery in at-risk individuals on the basis of genetic predisposition testing is an acceptable way to manage these patients.

REFERENCES

1. Mallick UK, Lucraft H, Proud G et al. Optimizing the management of differentiated thyroid cancer. Clin Oncol 2000; 12:363–4.

2. Clinical Genetics Society of the UK. The genetic testing of children. Report of a working party. J Med Genet 1994; 31:785–97.

3. Chandrasekharappa SC, Guru SC, Mannickam P et al. Positional cloning of the gene for multiple endocrine neoplasia type 1. Science 1997; 276:404–6.

4. Kaji H, Canaff L, Lebrun JJ et al. Inactivation of menin, a Smad3-interacting protein, blocks trans-forming growth factor type beta signalling. Proc Natl Acad Sci USA 2001; 98:3837–42.

5. Agarwal SK, Kester MB, Deblenko LV et al. Germline mutations of the men1 gene in familial multiple endocrine neoplasia type 1 and related states. Hum Mol Genet 1997; 6(7):1169–75.

6. Ullrich A, Schlessinger J. Signal transduction by receptors with tyrosine kinase activity. Cell 1990; 61:203–12.

7. Eng C, Clayton D, Schuffenecker I et al. The relationship between specific RET proto-oncogene mutations and disease phenotype in multiple endocrine neoplasia type 2. JAMA 1996; 276(19):1575–9.

8. Santoro M, Carlomango F, Romano A et al. Activation of RET as a dominant transforming gene by germ-line mutations of MEN2A and MEN2B. Science 1995; 267:381–3.

9. Hanssen AMN, Fryns JP. Syndrome of the month: Cowden syndrome. J Med Genet 1995; 32:117–19.

10. Schrager CA, Schneider D, Gruener AC et al. Clinical and pathological features of breast disease in Cowden's syndrome: an under recognised syndrome with an increased risk of breast cancer. Hum Pathol 1998; (1):47–53.

11. Gujrati M, Thomas C, Zelby A et al. Bannayan Zonana syndrome: A rare autosomal dominant syn-drome with multiple lipomas and haemangiomas: a case report and review of the literature. Surg Neurol 1998; 50:164–8.

12. Celebi JT, Tsou HC, Chen FF et al. Phenotypic findings of Cowden syndrome and Bannayan–Zonaz syndrome in a family associated with a single germline mutation in PTEN. J Med Genet 1999; (36):360–4.

13. Li D-M, Sun H. PTEN/MMAC1/TEP1 suppresses the tumorigenicity and induces G1 cell cycle arrest in human glioblastoma cells. Proc Natl Acad Sci USA 1998; 95:15406–11.

14. Bulow C, Bulow S, Group LCP. Is screening for thyroid carcinoma indicated in familial adenomatous polyposis. Int J Colorectal Dis 1997; 12:240–2.

15. Marx SJ, Spiegel AM, Brown EM et al. Family studies in patients with primary parathyroid hyperplasia. Am J Med 1997; 62:698–706.

16. Perrier ND, Villablanca A, Larsson C et al. Genetic screening for MEN-1 mutations in families presenting with familial primary hyperparathyroidism. World J Surg 2002; 26:907–13.

17. Friedrich CA. Genotype-phenotype correlation in von Hippel Lindau syndrome. Hum Mol Genet 2001; 10(7):763–7.

18. Weinstein LS, Shenker A, Gejman PV et al. Activating mutations of the stimulatory G protein in the McCune–Albright syndrome. N Engl J Med 1991; 325:1688–91.

19. Maher ER, Iselius L, Yates JRW et al. Von Hippel Lindau disease: a genetic study. J Med Genet 1991; 28:443–7.

20. Swinburn BA, Yeong ML, Lane MR et al. Neuro-fibromatosis associated with somatostatinoma: a report of two patients. Clin Endocrinol 1998; (28):353–9.

21. Clayton-Smith J. Genomic imprinting as a cause of disease. Br Med J 2003; 327:1121–2.

22. Maher ER, Eng C. The pressure rises: update on the genetics of phaeochromocytoma. Hum Mol Genet 2002; 11(20):2347–54.

23. Astuti D, Latif F, Dallol A et al. Gene mutations in the succinate dehydrogenase subunit SDHB cause susceptibility to familial phaeochromocytoma and to familial paraganglioma. Am J Hum Genet 2002; (69):49–54

24. Astuti D, Douglas F, Lennard TWJ et al. Germline SDHD mutation in familial phaeochromocytoma. Lancet 2001; 357:1181–2.

25. Anderson R. A familial instance of appendiceal carcinoid. Am J Surg 1966; 111:738–40.

26. Guo SS, Wu AY, Sawicki MP. Deletion of chromosome 1, but not mutation of MEN-1, predicts prognosis in sporadic pancreatic endocrine tumours. World J Surg 2002; 26:843–7.

27. Bordi C, Azzonzi C, D'Adda T et al. Pancreatic polypeptide-related tumors. Peptides 2002; 23:339–48.

28. Verges B, Boureille F, Goudet P et al. Pituitary disease in MEN type 1 (MEN1): data from the France-Belgium MEN1 multicenter study. J Clin Endocrinol Metab 2002; 87:457–65.

29. Stratakis CA, Schussheim DH, Freedman SM et al. Pituitary macroadenoma in a 5-year old: an early expression of multiple endocrine neoplasia type 1. J Clin Endocrinol Metab 2000; 85:4776–80.

30. Gibril F, Chen Y-J, Schrump D et al. Prospective study of thymic carcinoids in patients with multiple endocrine neoplasia type 1. J Clin Endocrinol Metab 2003; 88:1066–81.

31. Langer P, Cupisti K, Bartsch DK et al. Adrenal involvement in MEN type 1. World J Surg 2002; 26:891–6.

32. Burgess JR, Harle RA, Tucker P et al. Adrenal lesions in a large kindred with multiple endocrine neoplasia type 1. Arch Surg 1996; 131:699–702.

33. Brandi LB, Gagel RF, Angeli A et al. Guidelines for the diagnosis and therapy of MEN type 1 and type 2. J Clin Endocrinol Metab 2001; 86:5658–71.

34. Hai N, Aoki N, Shimatsu A et al. Clinical features of multiple endocrine neoplasia type 1 (MEN1) phenocopy without germline MEN1 gene mutations: analysis of 20 Japanese sporadic cases without MEN1. Clin Endocrinol 2000; 52:509–18.

35. Dean PG, van Heerden JA, Farley DR et al. Are patients with multiple endocrine neoplasia type 1 prone to premature death? World J Surg 2000; 24:1437–41.

36. Skogseid B. Multiple endocrine neoplasia type 1. Br J Surg 2003; 90:383–5.

37. Arnalsteen LC, Alesina PF, Quiereux JL et al. Long term results of less than total parathyroidectomy for hyperparathyroidism in multiple endocrine neoplasia type 1. Surgery 2002; 132:1119–24.

38. Norton JA, Fraker DL, Alexander HR et al. Surgery to cure the Zollinger–Ellison syndrome. N Engl J Med 1999; 341:644–53.

39. Norton JA, Alexander HR, Fraker DL et al. Comparison of surgical results in patients with advanced and limited disease with multiple endocrine neoplasia type 1 and Zollinger–Ellison syndrome. Ann Surg 2001; 234:495–505.

40. Gibril F, Venzon DJ, Ojeaburu JV et al. Prospective study of the natural history of gastrinoma in patients with MEN1: definition of an aggressive and a nonaggressive form. J Clin Endocrinol Metab 2001; 86:5282–93.

41. Gauger PG, Scheiman JM, Wamsteker E-J et al. Endoscopic ultrasound helps to identify and resect MEN-1 endocrine pancreatic tumours at an early stage. Br J Surg 2003; 90:748–54.

42. Machens A, Nicolli-Sire P, Hoegel J et al. Early malignant progression of hereditary medullary thyroid cancer. N Engl J Med 2003; 349:1517–25.

43. Kahraman T, de Groot JWB, Rou WEC et al. Acceptable age for prophylactic surgery in children with multiple endocrine neoplasia type 2a. Eur J Surg Oncol 2003; 29:331–5.

44. Sherman SI. Thyroid carcinoma. Lancet 2003, 361:501–11.

45. Gourgiotis L, Sarlis NJ, Reynolds JC et al. Localization of medullary thyroid carcinoma metastasis in a multiple endocrine neoplasia type 2A patient by 6-[18F]-fluorodopamine positron emission tomography. J Clin Endocrinol Metab 2003; 88:637–41.

46. Peaston RT, Lennard TWJ, Lai LC. Overnight excretion of urinary catecholamines and metabolites in the detection of phaeochromocytoma. J Clin Endocrinol Metab 1996; 81:1378–84.

47. Neumann HPH, Bausch B, McWhinney SR et al. Germ-line mutations in non-syndromic phaeo-chromocytoma. N Engl.J Med 2002; 346:1459–66.

48. Chen JD, Morrison C, Zhang C et al. Hyper-parathyroidism-jaw tumour syndrome. J Int Med 2003; 253:634–42.

49. Cetani F, Pardi E, Giovannetti A et al. Genetic analysis of the MEN1 and HPRT2 locus in two Italian kindreds with familial isolated hyper-parathyroidism. Clin Endocrinol 2002; 56:457–64.

50. Shattuck TM, Valimaki S, Obara T et al. Somatic and germ-line mutations of the *HRPT2* gene in sporadic parathyroid carcinoma. N Engl J Med 2003; 349:1722–9.

51. Lonser RR, Glen GM, Walther M et al. Von Hippel–Lindau disease. Lancet 2003; 361:2059–67.

52. Hes FJ, Hoppener JWM, Lips CJM. Phaeochromocytoma in von Hippel–Lindau disease. J Clin Endocrinol Metab 2003; 88:969–74.

53. Koch CA, Mauro D, Walhter MM et al. Phaeochromocytoma in von Hippel–Lindau disease: distinct histopathologic phenotype compared to phaeochromocytoma in multiple endocrine neoplasia type 2. Endocr Pathol 2002; 13:17–27.

54. Eisenhofer G, Walther MM, Huynh T-T et al. Phaeochromocytomas in von Hippel–Lindau syndrome and multiple endocrine neoplasia type 2 display distinct biochemical and clinical phenotypes. J Clin Endocrinol Metab 2001; 86:1999–2008.

55. Kaltsas GA, Mukherjee JJ, Foley R et al. Treatment of metastatic phaeochromocytoma with ^{131}I-meta-iodobenzylguanidine (MIBG). Endocrinologist 2003; 13:321–33.

56. Baysal BE, Willet-Brozick JE, Lawrence EC et al. Prevalence of SDHB, SDHC and SDHD germline mutations in clinic patients with head and neck paragangliomas. J Med Genet 2002; 39:178–83.

57. Carney JA. Discovery of the Carney complex, a familial lentiginosis-multiple endocrine neoplasia syndrome: a medical odyssey. Endocrinologist 2003; 13:23–30.

58. Stratakis CA, Kirschner LS, Carney JA. Clinical and molecular features of the Carney complex: diagnostic criteria and recommendations for patient evaluation. J Clin Endocrinol Metab 2001; 86:4041–6.

59. Jackson RV, Lafferty A, Torpy DJ et al. New genetic insights in familial hyperaldosteronism. Ann NY Acad Sci 2002; 970:77–88.

60. Stowasser M, Gunasekera TG, Gordon R. Familial varieties of primary aldosteronism. Clin Exp Pharmacol Phys 2001; 28:1087–90.

Five

Endocrine tumours of the pancreas

Jeffrey A. Norton

INTRODUCTION

Pancreatic endocrine neoplasms consist predominantly of gastrinomas and insulinomas, but a variety of other rarer tumours also occur (**Table 5.1**). All of these tumours arise from neuroendocrine cells, display characteristic ultrastructural features and biochemically consist of amine precursor uptake and decarboxylation cells (APUDomas). Pancreatic endocrine tumours, as a group, are different from most other neoplasms because they commonly produce physiologically uncontrolled levels of hormones, each of which may cause a clinical syndrome. Identification of the clinical syndrome and detection of the hormone proteins produced allows the classification of pancreatic endocrine tumours into specific types. Potentially life-threatening situations caused by hormone overproduction are a major reason to identify and resect these neoplasms. Some tumours may not secrete any immunohistochemically detectable or clinically relevant peptides and only cause symptoms by mass effect. Additionally, except for insulinomas, pancreatic endocrine neoplasms are malignant in most cases. Although pancreatic endocrine tumours are malignant, they are low-grade such that aggressive surgical extirpation is beneficial in most instances.

INSULINOMA

Endogenous hyperinsulinism was first described in 1927, and was the first syndrome of excessive pancreatic hormone production to be recognised.[1] Hyperinsulinaemia and consequent hypoglycaemia is the major cause of morbidity and potential mortality associated with insulinoma, a neoplasm arising from the pancreatic insulin-producing β cells. Insulinoma occurs in approximately one person per million population per year (**Table 5.1**).[1] The hyperinsulinaemic hypoglycaemia is not well controlled by medical therapy, and surgery has remained the cornerstone of treatment over the past 70 years. Insulinomas are unique among pancreatic endocrine tumours because 90% of insulinomas are benign, solitary growths that occur uniformly throughout and almost exclusively within the pancreas, without evidence of local invasion or loco-regional lymph node metastases.[2] However, the tumour may be as small as 6 mm in diameter and is usually less than 2 cm in size, which makes localisation difficult in many cases.[3]

Presentation

Excessive and physiologically uncontrolled secretion of insulin by the tumour causes periods of acute

Table 5.1 • Features of endocrine tumours of the pancreas

Tumour	Incidence (people/million/year)	Hormone secreted	Signs or symptoms	Diagnosis	Location (%) Duodenum	Location (%) Pancreas	Malignant (%)	MEN 1 (%)
Gastrinoma	0.1–3	Gastrin	Ulcer pain, diarrhoea, oesophagitis	Fasting serum gastrin >100 pg/mL Basal acid outpur >15 mEq/h	38	62	60–90	20
Insulinoma	0.8	Insulin	Hypoglycaemia	Standard fasting test	0	>99	5	5–10
VIPoma		Vasoactive polypeptide (VIP)	Watery diarrhoea, hypokalaemia, hypochlorhydria	Fasting plasma VIP >250 pg/h	15	85	60	<5
Glucagonoma		Glucagon	Rash, weight loss, malnutrition, diabetes	Fasting plasma glucagon >500 pg/h	0	>99	70	<5
Somatostatinoma		Somatostatin	Diabetes, cholelithlasis, steatorrhoea	Increased fasting plasma somatostatin concentration	50	50	70	<5
GRFoma	0.2	Growth hormone-releasing factor (GRF)	Acromegaly	Increased fasting plasma GRF concentration	0	100	30	30
ACTHoma		Adrenocorticotropic hormone (ACTH)	Cushing's syndrome	24-hour urinary free cortisol >100 µg, plasma ACTH >50 pg/h no dexamethasone suppression, **no CRH suppression**	0	100	100	<5
PTH-like-oma		Parathyroid hormone (PTH)-like factor	Hypercalcaemia, bone pain	Serum calcium >11mg/dL, serum PTH undetectable, increased serum PTH-like factor	0	100	100	<5
Neurotensinoma		Neurotensin	Tachycardia, hypotension, hypokalaemia	Increased fasting plasma neurotensin concentration	0	100	>80	<5
Non-functioning (PPoma)		Pancreatic polypeptide (PP) neurone-specific enolase	Pain, bleeding mass	Increased plasma PP concentration, increased neurone-specific enolase concentration	0	>99	>60	80–100

symptomatic hypoglycaemia, which results in patient presentation for medical evaluation. Acute neuroglycopenia induces anxiety, dizziness, obtundation, confusion, unconsciousness, personality changes and seizures.[3] Symptoms commonly occur during early morning hours, when glucose reserves are low after a period of overnight fasting and endogenous insulin overproduction continues. Patients may present when food intake is decreased to reduce weight, as most patients (80%) experience major weight gain. A majority (60–75%) of patients are women and many have undergone extensive psychiatric evaluation. Many patients will have been diagnosed with a neurological condition such as seizure disorders, cerebrovascular accidents or transient ischaemic attacks.[4] Potentially life-threatening symptoms may be present for several years before the correct diagnosis is considered.[3] Insulinomas during pregnancy have been reported and are usually managed medically until the fetus can be delivered and the pregnancy is concluded.[5] In a review of 59 patients with insulinoma, the interval from the onset of symptoms to the time of diagnosis ranged from 1 month to 30 years, with the median time to diagnosis being 2 years.[4] Because insulinoma is rare and neuroglycopenic symptoms are relatively non-specific, a high index of suspicion for insulinoma is necessary when other explanations for these symptoms are not evident. The recognition of symptomatic patients and the liberal use of simple and precise biochemical tests results in accurate diagnosis of insulinoma prior to life-threatening sequelae.

SCREENING FOR MEN 1

Approximately 5–10% of patients with insulinoma also have multiple endocrine neoplasia type 1 (MEN 1; **Table 5.1**) (see Chapter 4). These patients must be recognised because they frequently have multiple pancreatic tumours and this greatly influences operative management.[6] MEN 1 is inherited as an autosomal dominant disease, and tumours develop in several endocrine organs. Sporadic primary hyperparathyroidism (PHP) due to multiglandular disease in patients youger than age 40 years may be the first organ manifestation of MEN 1 despite a negative family history, and these patients should be screened for pancreatic endocrine tumours.[7] Virtually all (96%) MEN 1 patients have four-gland parathyroid hyperplasia, up to 75% develop pancreatic islet cell tumours, and pituitary tumours (usually prolactinomas) occur in less than 50% of patients. Functional pancreatic tumours are most commonly gastrinomas, with insulinomas occurring second in frequency.[1] A recent study of 109 affected individuals from 24 kindreds with MEN 1 showed that primary hyperparathyroidism occurred in 74%, pancreatic endocrine tumours in 51% and pituitary tumours in 35%.[8] Islet cell tumours of different types may occur simultaneously in a patient with MEN 1. Patients may also have thyroid adenomas, adrenocortical tumours, carcinoid tumours and lipomas.

Questions should be directed at other possible manifestations of the syndrome and a family history of endocrine tumours. If the clinical history is equivocal or suspicious for MEN 1, then the measurement of serum concentrations of calcium, prolactin, chromogranin A and pancreatic poly-peptide may help to confirm or exclude MEN 1. Screening of other family members for features of MEN 1 is indicated when a patient is suspected to have MEN 1. The *MEN1* gene has been cloned and mapped to the long arm of chromosome 11 (locus 11q13); it encodes a 610-amino-acid protein termed menin.[9,10] Early studies have shown menin to be a nuclear protein.[11] The exact functional role of menin has not been confirmed, but recent research supports a tumour suppressor function of *MEN1*, and germline *MEN1* mutations have been identified in most MEN 1 families.[11,12] Although the exact function of menin is still unknown, overexpression of menin inhibits proliferation of *ras*-transformed NIH3T3 cells. Since menin interacts with proteins from both the transforming growth factor β (TGF-β) and AP-1 signalling pathways, it is thought that its tumour suppressor function works through either of these two pathways.[13] Genetic counselling and screening should be provided to family members to identify those individuals who are carriers of the mutant gene and have a high risk of developing the disease. These patients should enter a clinical screening programme, which can enable earlier detection and treatment of MEN 1-associated tumours and prompt treatment of hyperparathyroidism.[12,14] Standardised meal tests have been used to screen patients at risk for MEN 1 for pancreatico-duodenal neuroendocrine tumours.[15] However, the standardised meal test has not been as sensitive as measuring serum levels of pancreatic polypeptide and gastrin. Serum levels of chromogranin A may also be used.

Diagnosis

The classic diagnostic triad, proposed by Whipple in 1935 based on his observations in 32 patients, consists of symptoms of hypoglycaemia during a fast, a concomitant blood glucose concentration less than 3 mmol/L and relief of the hypoglycaemic symptoms after glucose administration.[1] Symptomatic patients with suspected insulinoma may first be instructed to undergo an overnight fast in an outpatient setting, during which time the development of any symptoms can be recorded and the serum glucose and insulin concentrations measured. The development of symptoms during fasting hypoglycaemia strongly suggests an insulinoma.

'Factitious hypoglycaemia', in which exogenous insulin or oral hypoglycaemic drugs are administered clandestinely, may present with exactly the same symptoms as an insulinoma and may lead to an inappropriate diagnosis.[16] Factitious hypoglycaemia may be suspected more often in a patient with relatives who are diabetic or in a young woman associated with the medical profession, such as a nurse. The diagnosis of insulinoma must be reached (excluding factitious hypoglycaemia) in each patient by using the 72-hour supervised standard fasting test in a hospital setting with appropriate biochemical measurements prior to tumour localisation or surgery. Urinary sulphonylurea concentrations (to exclude oral hypoglycaemic drugs) should be measured by gas chromatography-mass spectroscopy; they are undetectable in patients with insulinoma. Anti-insulin antibodies should not be detectable in those with insulinoma, and C-peptide concentrations are increased in equimolar concentrations with insulin in true insulinoma cases. Insulinoma may be difficult to diagnose in patients with renal failure because they may develop hypoglycaemia for other reasons, but it still has been reported to occur.[17]

SUPERVISED STANDARD FASTING TEST

The standard fasting test is carried out in a hospital setting and begins with a baseline examination in which recent memory, calculations and coordination

are documented. An intravenous catheter with a heparin lock is then placed, and the patient is allowed to drink only non-caloric beverages. Close observation is necessary. Blood is collected every 6 hours for measurement of serum glucose and immunoreactive insulin concentrations. As the blood glucose level falls below 3 mmol/L, blood samples are collected more frequently (every hour or less), and the patient is observed more closely. When neuroglycopenic symptoms appear, blood is collected immediately for determination of serum insulin, glucose, C-peptide and proinsulin concentrations. Glucose is then administered, and the fast is terminated. If a patient remains symptom-free for the entire 72 hours, the test is terminated and the above blood concentrations are measured.

Neuroglycopenic symptoms manifest in approximately 60% of patients with insulinomas within 24 hours after fasting begins,[1] and nearly all patients with insulinomas have symptoms by 72 hours.[18] Approximately 16% of patients with insulinoma develop symptoms when the blood glucose concentration is greater than 2.5 mmol/L.[3] The blood glucose concentration eventually decreases below 2.5 mmol/L in approximately 85% of patients with insulinomas during the 72-hour fast (**Table 5.2, Fig. 5.1**). The most definitive diagnostic biochemical test for insulinoma is an inappropriately increased plasma immunoreactive insulin concentration above 5 μU/mL at the time of documented hypoglycaemia and symptoms.[18] The plasma insulin concentration is usually greater than 10 μU/mL in most patients (**Fig. 5.1**).[3] Although prolonged maximal stimulation of insulin secretion in normal subjects does not cause the release of the insulin precursor molecule, proinsulin, some insulinomas secrete large amounts of uncleaved proinsulin. Patients with high proinsulin-producing tumours may remain euglycaemic and asymptomatic for longer periods during the fast because proinsulin is not biologically active. The proinsulin-like component (PLC) is measured at the time of symptomatic hypoglycaemia and termination of the fast. A value greater than 25% or an increased PLC:total immunoreactive insulin ratio is abnormal and consistent with the diagnosis of insulinoma.[3,18] Some data suggest that an increased PLC value may also be an indication of malignancy,[18] but this has not been substantiated by other groups. Hypersecretion of endogenous insulin also results

Table 5.2 • Standard fasting test results and the differentiation of insulinoma from factitious hypoglycaemia

Blood measurement	Fasting normal range	Result with Insulinoma	Result with factitious hypoglycaemia	Test sensitivity (%)
Glucose	90–150 mg/dL	<40 mg/dL	<40 mg/dL	99
Immunoreactive insulin (IRI)	<5 µU/mL	Increased	Increased (usually >10 µU/mL)	100
C-peptide	<1.7 ng/mL	Increased	Normal range	78
Direct proinsulin-like component (PLC)	<0.2 ng/mL	Increased	Normal range	85
PLC/total IRI	<25%	Increased	Normal range	87

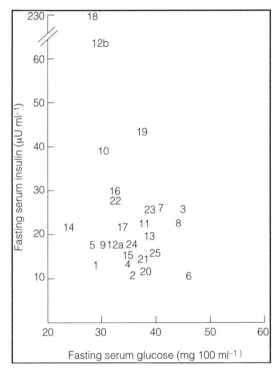

Figure 5.1 • Serum glucose and insulin concentrations at time of development of neuroglycopenic symptoms and termination of fast in 25 patients with insulinoma. Each number represents a patient. All patients had a serum insulin concentration >5 µU/mL, whereas 21 patients had a serum glucose concentration <49 mg/dL. Each patient had an insulinoma resected. From Doherty GM, Doppman JL, Shawker TH et al. Results of a prospective strategy to diagnose, localize and resect insulinomas. Surgery 1991; 110:989–97, with permission.

in increases of the circulating concentration of C-peptide, a biologically inactive by-product of enzymatic insulin cleavage from the precursor proinsulin molecule. Most patients with insulinomas have C-peptide concentrations greater than 1.7 ng/mL (**Fig. 5.2**).[3]

To exclude definitively factitious hypoglycaemia, sulphonylurea concentrations in the blood from oral hypoglycaemic drugs should be measured. Human antibodies to animal insulin are detectable if the patient is not receiving recombinant human insulin. Increased serum concentrations of proinsulin or C-peptide during hypoglycaemia effectively excludes the diagnosis of factitious hypoglycaemia because exogenously administered insulin does not contain these proteins and actually suppresses their endogenous production. However, approximately 13–22% of patients with insulinoma do not have increased serum proinsulin or C-peptide concentrations, and a supervised fast prohibiting exogenous insulin administration remains the best test to diagnose insulinoma and conclusively exclude factitious hypoglycaemia. The biochemical parameters measured during the standard fasting test cannot discriminate between patients with MEN 1 and ones with sporadic insulinoma.[18]

NESIDIOBLASTOSIS

Because of differences in their surgical management, insulinoma must be distinguished from nesidioblastosis, a congenital islet cell dysmaturation or malregulation that occurs in infants and causes hyperinsulinaemic hypoglycaemia. Age at the time of presentation is the most important distinguishing

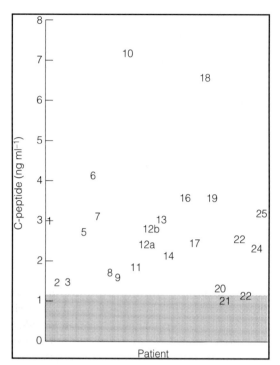

Figure 5.2 • Serum C-peptide concentrations at time of development of neuroglycopenic symptoms and termination of fast in 25 patients with insulinoma. Shaded area is normal range. Twenty-three of 25 patients had increased concentrations. From Doherty GM, Doppman JL, Shawker TH et al. Results of a prospective strategy to diagnose, localize and resect insulinomas. Surgery 1991; 110:989–97, with permission.

factor. Nesidioblastosis occurs most commonly in children under the age of 18 months. Although the existence of adult nesidioblastosis remains plausible,[19] the diagnosis of nesidioblastosis in an adult should be critically suspect because islet cell hyperplasia may be present in the pancreas of patients with insulinoma and an occult insulinoma may be missed in this situation.[1,20] In a review of over 300 cases of hyperinsulinaemic hypoglycaemia at the Mayo Clinic since 1927, only five adult patients had a reasonably confirmed diagnosis of nesidioblastosis.[21] Case reports continue to identify nesidioblastosis as a cause of hypoglycaemia.[22] However, many experts warn against the presumed diagnosis of nesidioblastosis in adults with hypoglycaemia as nesidioblastosis in adults does not exist and this may decrease the ability to find the insulinoma.[23] Biochemical tests (blood glucose, immunoreactive insulin and C-peptide) do not reliably distinguish

hyperinsulinaemic hypoglycaemia caused by an insulinoma from that attributed to nesidioblastosis. Thus, children symptomatic after age 18 months must be evaluated to exclude an insulinoma, which must be localised and resected as for an adult. Approximately half of infants with nesidioblastosis require a spleen-preserving near-total pancreatectomy, in which 95% of the pancreas is removed, because this disorder affects the entire pancreas diffusely.[24,25]

Management

MEDICAL MANAGEMENT OF HYPOGLYCAEMIA

Medical management should prevent hypoglycaemia caused by the hyperinsulinism so that symptoms and life-threatening sequelae are avoided. In patients with acute hypoglycaemia, blood glucose concentrations are normalised initially with an intravenous glucose infusion. To prevent hypoglycaemic episodes during diagnosis, tumour localisation and the preoperative period, euglycaemia is maintained by giving frequent feeds of a high-carbohydrate diet, including a night meal. Cornstarch may be added to food for prolonged slow absorption. For patients who continue to become hypoglycaemic between feedings, diazoxide may be added to the treatment regimen at a dose of 400–600 mg orally each day. Diazoxide inhibits insulin release in approximately 50% of patients with insulinoma; however, side effects of oedema, weight gain and hirsutism occur in 50% of patients, and nausea occurs in over 10%.[21] Diazoxide should be discontinued 1 week prior to surgery to avoid intraoperative hypotension. Calcium-channel blockers or phenytoin may also suppress insulin production in some patients. The short-term use of octreotide preoperatively may be beneficial if the patient is not responding well to traditional medical management and surgery is delayed for tumour localisation. Long-term control of hypoglycaemic symptoms with medical management has generally been ineffective for patients with insulinoma. Knowledge of the patient's response to medical management is important for the surgeon so that the urgency and potential benefits of surgery can be determined.[26]

Octreotide is a synthetic, long-acting (half life >100 min) analogue of the naturally occurring hormone somatostatin.[26] Octreotide binds to and activates somatostatin receptors on cells expressing them, inhibiting the secretion of many gastro-intestinal peptides. Octreotide may be useful for treating symptoms caused by VIPomas and carcinoid tumours but is not recommended for insulinomas because its efficacy in inhibiting insulin release is unpredictable.[27,28] The usefulness of radiolabelled octreotide in imaging insulinomas and in treating metastatic islet cell tumours has been equally dis-appointing.[29] Therefore, long-term medical manage-ment of hypoglycaemia in patients with insulinomas generally is reserved for the few patients (<5%) with unlocalised, unresected tumours after thorough preoperative testing and exploratory laparotomy and for patients with metastatic, unresectable malignant insulinoma.[28] Patients with malignant insulinomas and refractory hypoglycaemia may even require the placement of implantable glucose pumps for continuous glucose infusions.[21]

PREOPERATIVE TUMOUR LOCALISATION

After definitive diagnosis the tumour must be localised and the presence of unresectable metastatic disease excluded. Accurate tumour localisation is the most difficult aspect of management because the tumours are usually very small and solitary.

Non-invasive imaging studies

An initial attempt should be made to localise the tumour and identify metastatic disease by using non-invasive tests. The least expensive and invasive imaging modality for the pancreas is transabdominal ultrasonography, in which an insulinoma appears as a sonolucent mass on a background of 'echodense' normal pancreas. However, the ability to image the pancreas is severely limited by obesity and over-lying bowel gas and overall test sensitivity is only 0–25% in most studies (Table 5.3).[3,30–32] Further, a new ultrasound study called echo-enhanced power Doppler sonography has been used to image pan-creatic neuroendocrine tumours based on increased blood flow. In a preliminary study of 190 patients, it has a sensitivity of 94% and a specificity of 96%, suggesting that it will have value.[33]

Computed tomography (CT) and magnetic resonance imaging (MRI) (Table 5.3) are able to identify pancreatic tumours as small as 1 cm in diameter. For CT, oral contrast should be administered to differentiate bowel and to define more clearly the pancreas, and thin slices of the peripancreatic area – at most 5 mm apart – should be obtained.[34] The administration of intravenous contrast may cause a tumour blush owing to increased vascularity. The sensitivity of CT for insulinoma ranges between 11 and 40% in most series.[3,30–32,35,36] MRI may image an islet cell tumour based on increased signal intensity (brightness) on T2-weighted images. The sensitivity of MRI is equivalent to that of CT[3,30,31] and, as expected, the accuracy of both CT and MRI increases with larger tumour size, achieving a sensitivity of 100% as tumour size increases to 6 cm.[37]

Malignant insulinomas are almost always very large (>4 cm) and are easily imaged by CT or MRI. The extent of bulky metastatic tumour deposits and hepatic metastases are also usually readily identifi-able by CT or MRI. Metastases should be identified preoperatively so that the operative approach can be planned, or, in the case of unresectability, unnecessary surgery avoided.

Somatostatin receptor scintigraphy (SRS), or octreoscan, is a relatively new modality, which utilises octreotide labelled with a radioactive tracer and given intravenously (Table 5.3). The radio-labelled octreotide binds to tumours with somato-statin receptors, causing the tumour to appear as a 'hotspot' on whole-body gamma camera scintigraphy.[38] Thus, SRS depends on the ability of a particular islet cell tumour to express somato-statin receptors.[39] Some islet cell tumours, such as gastrinomas, express somatostatin receptors and are nearly always (80%) imaged by labelled octreotide. However, less than 50% of insulinomas are imaged by SRS[38,39] because they do not consistently express high levels of somatostatin receptors. However, when SRS was combined with endoscopic ultrasound (EUS), the sensitivity for insulinoma was 94% (15 of 16 tumors).[40] SRS has also been shown to be much better than meta-iodo benzylguanidine (MIBG) scan for localising pancreatic neuroendocrine tumors.[41] Thus SRS is not recommended for localising insulinomas; however, it may be useful when combined with EUS and it is useful for all other pancreatic neuroendocrine tumours. An initial report of radioiodinated vasoactive intestinal poly-peptide (VIP) scanning[42] suggested that it may be

Table 5.3 • Sensitivities of localisation studies for insulinomas and gastrinomas

Study	Insulinoma	% of tumours localised			
		Gastrinoma			
		Overall	Pancreas	Duodenum	Liver metastases
PREOPERATIVE					
Non-invasive					
Transabdominal ultrasonography	0–25	20–30			14
Abdominal computed tomography	11–40	50	80	35	50
Abdominal magnetic resonance imaging	11–43	25			83
Octreoscan	0–50	88			
Invasive					
Endoscopic ultrasonography	70–90	85	88–100	<5	<5
Selective arteriography	40–70	68		34	86
+ calcium stimulation	88–94	–	–	–	–
+ secretin injection	–	90–100			
Portal venous sampling	67–80	70–90			
Unlocalised primary tumour	10–20	15			
INTRAOPERATIVE					
Palpation	65	65	91	60	
Intraoperative ultrasonography	75–100	83	95	58	
Endoscopic transillumination	–	–	–	70	
Duodenotomy	–	–	–	100	
Unlocalised primary tumour	1	5			

useful but experience is presently too limited to consistently recommend its use.

Invasive localising procedures

Approximately 50% of patients have small (<2 cm) insulinomas that are not detected by non-invasive imaging tests, and a variety of more sensitive invasive tests are used to localise the tumour preoperatively. Endoscopic ultrasonography (EUS) is safe and highly effective in experienced hands and may replace the routine use of other preoperative localisation studies.[43–45] An endoscope is passed into the duodenum and a balloon is inflated against the intestinal wall with saline. A 5–10-MHz transducer is used to generate an image of the pancreas through the intestinal and stomach walls. Tumours as small as 2–3 mm in diameter can be identified in the pancreatic head by moving the transducer through the duodenum at the junction of the pancreas. The endoscope must be passed well into the third portion of the duodenum to adequately visualise the uncinate process. Insulinomas in the pancreatic body and tail are imaged by positioning the transducer in the stomach and scanning through its posterior wall. Sensitivity for EUS ranges from 70 to 90% and specificity is near 100% (**Table 5.3**).[44,46–48] It more accurately detects tumours in the head of the pancreas (as compared with tumours in the body and tail) because the head can be viewed through three angles (from the third portion of the duodenum, through the bulb of the duodenum and through the stomach) whereas the body and tail can only be viewed through the stomach. A case-control study evaluating the cost-effectiveness of EUS on preoperative localisation of pancreatic endocrine tumours showed a greater than US$2000 cost saving per patient for pre-operative localisation studies, mainly because of the reduced need for angiograms and venous sampling procedures.[49] Total surgical and anaesthesia times were also reduced in the EUS group. EUS is cost-effective when used early in the preoperative localisation strategy and may avoid unnecessary morbidity associated with more invasive tests.[49]

Despite the tremendous potential and proven benefit of EUS for insulinoma, there are some limitations. First, there may be false positives, which include accessory spleens and intrapancreatic lymph nodes. Further, EUS is limited in assessment of malignancy, identification of pedunculated tumours, evaluation of the pancreatic tail, and differentiation of large tumours from the pancreatic parenchyma.[50]

In patients with negative results after non-invasive imaging studies or EUS, a regional localisation study – either calcium arteriography or portal venous sampling (PVS) – may be obtained. These two studies rely on the functional activity of the insulinoma (i.e. excessive insulin production) and not on the ability to image the tumour (i.e. tumour size). The calcium arteriogram is the most informa-tive preoperative test for localising insulinomas. It is replacing PVS as the invasive localising study of

choice.[30] Calcium provocation may identify the region of the pancreas containing the tumour (head, body or tail). Arteries that perfuse the pancreatic head (gastroduodenal artery and superior mesenteric artery) and the body/tail (splenic artery) are selectively catheterised sequentially, and a small amount of calcium gluconate (0.025 mEq Ca^{2+}/kg bodyweight) is injected into each artery during different runs. A catheter positioned in the right hepatic vein is used to collect blood for measure-ment of insulin concentrations 30–60 seconds after the calcium injection. Calcium stimulates a marked increase in insulin secretion from the insulinoma. A greater than twofold increase in the hepatic vein insulin concentration indicates localisation of the tumour to the area of the pancreas being perfused by the injected artery (**Fig. 5.3**). Additionally, injec-tion of contrast may reveal a tumour blush, con-firming the location of the insulinoma by imaging the tumour. It may be necessary to obtain multiple views (including oblique images) to evaluate lesions obscured by vessels and bones. This test therefore combines the functionality advantage of PVS with the more exact localisation capability of an arteriogram. These combined features are especially useful in patients with MEN 1 who may have multiple functional islet cell tumours. The reported sensitivity of calcium stimulation is between 88 and 94% and few false-positive results occur (**Table 5.3**).[30,51,52] This has been confirmed by another recent prospective study that demonstrated

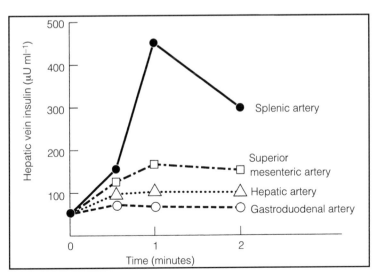

Figure 5.3 • Calcium angiogram in a patient with an insulinoma localised to the pancreatic tail. Intra-arterial calcium was selectively injected into splenic, superior mesenteric, hepatic and gastroduodenal arteries in four different runs. Blood samples were taken serially from hepatic vein and insulin concentrations measured at 0, 1 and 2 minutes before and after calcium injection. After injection into the splenic artery there was a rapid marked increase in hepatic vein insulin concentrations at 1 and 2 minutes. This finding localised the insulinoma to the pancreatic tail.

that calcium angiogram correctly localised the insulinoma in 11 of 11 patients and it was much more sensitive than the other studies used.[53]

PVS is performed by measuring insulin concentrations in the portal vein and its tributaries.[30] A catheter is passed through the liver into the portal vein. It may be associated with complications, including haemobilia and haemorrhage.[54] It is more costly because approximately 20 blood samples are assayed for insulin concentration. Sensitivity ranges from 67 to 80% (**Table 5.3**) and there are few false positives.[3,30–32] Because the calcium angiogram provides similar information, can image the tumour and is less costly and invasive, it should replace PVS for invasive localisation.

A small proportion of insulinomas remain unlocalised even after the results of all localisation studies are obtained, and such tumours are therefore considered occult. When the diagnosis is certain on the basis of the results of the fast, surgical exploration with careful inspection, palpation and intraoperative ultrasonography (IOUS) of the pancreas is still indicated. Most of these patients (>90%) will still have an insulinoma identified and removed by experienced surgeons.[1,55] Retrospective reviews have shown that the combination of surgical exploration with IOUS will identify almost all insulinomas.[56–60]

OPERATIVE MANAGEMENT

Surgery is the only curative therapy for insulinoma. Blind pancreatic resection is no longer indicated, and IOUS should be used to identify clearly the tumour to preserve as much normal pancreatic tissue as possible. Accurate preoperative localisation correlates with a high probability of cure. However, even with successful preoperative localisation, a careful pancreatic exploration should be performed at the time of surgery, including palpation and IOUS. The possibility of multiple insulinomas or a false-positive result with a preoperative localisation test may result in surgical failure. IOUS also helps to define the relationship of the tumour to the common bile duct, pancreatic duct, portal vein and adjacent blood vessels. When preoperative localisation studies are inconclusive, adequate mobilisation of the pancreas with the use of IOUS results in successful identification and resection of the insulinoma in nearly all cases.

Operative approach

Pneumococcal, meningococcal and *Haemophilus* influenza vaccination is used preoperatively if it is thought that a distal pancreatectomy with splenectomy is necessary. The prophylactic use of octreotide preoperatively to reduce fistulas and pseudocysts has not been proven to be beneficial.[61] A standard midline laparotomy or bilateral subcostal incision is recommended to give adequate exposure to the abdomen, which is facilitated by a fixed upper abdominal retractor. The entire abdomen, including regional lymph nodes, is initially inspected for potential metastases, which occur in 10% of sporadic cases. Metastatic insulinoma deposits on the surface of the liver typically appear as firm nodules. IOUS with a 5-MHz transducer may be helpful in identifying deep hepatic metastases.

Suspicious hepatic lesions that are small and peripheral should be excised by wedge resection, and larger or deeper lesions should be biopsied. Samples are sent for immediate frozen-section analysis to exclude tumour. In general, resection of localised tumour metastases is indicated to decrease symptoms associated with hyperinsulinaemia, which may be poorly controlled long term by medical means. To expose adequately the pancreas, the hepatic and splenic flexures of the colon are mobilised out of the upper abdomen, and the gastrocolic ligament is divided to open the lesser sac.

Pancreatic mobilisation

In contradistinction to gastrinomas, virtually all insulinomas are located within the pancreas and are uniformly distributed throughout the entire gland.[3] Therefore, the head, body and tail of the pancreas must be sufficiently mobilised to permit evaluation of the entire organ. This requires an extended Kocher manoeuvre to lift adequately the head of the pancreas out of the retroperitoneum and division of attachments at the inferior and posterior border of the pancreas, to permit evaluation of the posterior body and tail (**Fig. 5.4**). Because the head of the pancreas is thick, small tumours that are centrally located may not be easily palpated. The entire pancreatic head must be sufficiently mobilised so that the posterior surface can be adequately examined visually and palpated between the thumb and forefinger. The splenic ligaments may be divided to

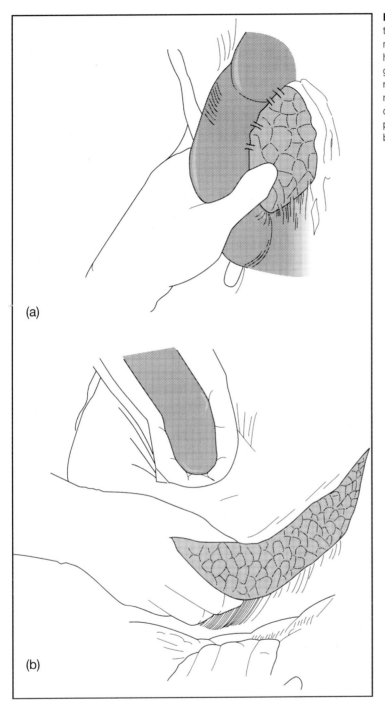

Figure 5.4 • Operative manoeuvres to identify insulinoma. **(a)** Kocher manoeuvre with careful palpation of head of pancreas. **(b)** Opening gastrocolic ligament, superior retraction of stomach, inferior retraction of transverse colon and careful palpation of body and tail of pancreas after incision along inferior border.

completely mobilise the spleen out of the retro-peritoneum for full examination and palpation of the pancreatic tail.

Intraoperative manoeuvres to find insulinoma

Direct inspection of the entire pancreatic surface is carried out first because an insulinoma may appear as a brownish-red purple mass, like a cherry. Most insulinomas are encompassed by pancreatic parenchyma and may not be directly visible, but careful palpation of the pancreas between the thumb and forefinger may identify some of these. The tumour feels like a firm, nodular and discrete mass. Approximately 65% of insulinomas may be identified by the traditional operative manoeuvres of inspection and palpation.[3] Tumours are more difficult to identify when the pancreas is scarred from previous surgery or alcoholism and when tumours arise centrally within the thick pancreatic head.

IOUS is the best intraoperative method to find and remove insulinoma. It is performed by placing the transducer on the surface of the pancreas, which is covered in a pool of saline to maximise image quality. A 10-MHz or 7.5-MHz real-time probe is used, which has a short focal length and high resolution. An insulinoma appears as a sonolucent mass with margins distinct from the uniform, more echodense pancreatic parenchyma (**Fig. 5.5**).

IOUS can localise an occult insulinoma that has not been identified preoperatively[62] and can identify tumours that are not visible or palpable (**Fig. 5.5**).[3,55] It is particularly helpful in evaluation of the pancreatic head. In conjunction with simultaneous palpation, ultrasonography further clarifies lesions.[55] The sensitivity for detecting insulinomas using IOUS is greater than 75%[32,35] and approaches 100% (**Table 5.3**).[3,30] A study of 37 consecutive patients showed that intraoperative ultrasound correctly idetified 35 (95%) and the two tumours that were missed were in the pancreatic tail.[63]

Insulinoma resection

Enucleation means excision only of the adenoma with minimal normal pancreatic tissue. It is currently the operation of choice for benign insulinomas. With the use of preoperative localisation and IOUS, blind distal pancreatectomy is no longer advocated. Tumour size, location and surrounding anatomy determine whether enucleation or pancreatic resection is performed. It is important to consider the relationship of the tumour to the pancreatic duct by imaging both structures with IOUS prior to tumour excision. Small tumours that are separated from the pancreatic duct and major vessels by normal pancreas can be safely enucleated (**Fig. 5.5**). IOUS allows a precise, safe tumour enucleation and helps plan the shortest, most direct route to the tumour while avoiding the pancreatic duct. If a clear margin of normal pancreatic tissue does not exist between the insulinoma and other structures, then a spleen-preserving distal or subtotal pancreatectomy is advised.[3,62,63] Ductal injury in an attempt to resect a tumour in close proximity to the pancreatic duct results in significant postoperative morbidity. Evidence of malignancy, such as involvement of peripancreatic lymph nodes or tumour invasion, mandates pancreatic resection and not enucleation.[55] Large tumour size may also be an indication for pancreatic resection. Rarely, pancreatico-duodenectomy is indicated if enucleation cannot be performed safely. A study reviewing 50 patients treated by pancreatico-duodenectomy for periampullary neuroendocrine tumours showed a postoperative mortality rate of 2%, with no postoperative deaths occurring after 1967.[64] Rapid intraoperative insulin assay has been used by one group to determine the outcome of surgery during the surgery. It correctly predicted outcome in six consecutive patients (five true positives and one true negative).[65] However, this is a preliminary study and frozen-section diagnosis of

Figure 5.5 • Intraoperative ultrasonography of insulinoma (arrow). The insulinoma appears sonolucent compared with more echodense pancreas. This tumour measures 1 cm in diameter and was not palpable within the pancreatic head.

neuroendocrine tumour is traditionally used as the endpoint of surgery.

Studies suggest that insulinomas can now be removed by minimally invasive methods. This is greatly facilitated by laparoscopic ultrasonography. In a recent study, six of seven patients could have the insulinoma removed laparoscopically and had less operative pain and shorter length of stay than those done through an open operation.[66] Another report confirms this but with fewer patients.[67]

INSULINOMA AND MEN 1

Approximately 10% of insulinomas occur in the setting of MEN 1 syndrome, and 20% of patients with MEN 1 develop insulinomas. Insulinomas in MEN 1 syndrome may be multiple and may occur simultaneously and diffusely throughout the pancreas.[68] The goal of treatment is to ameliorate the hypoglycaemia by eliminating the source of insulin hypersecretion. Difficulty arises in identifying which tumour or tumours produce the excessive insulin, but there is usually a dominant large tumour (>3 cm) that is readily identified on abdominal CT.[69] An invasive regional localisation test such as the calcium angiogram is indicated to determine if the imaged tumour is responsible for the excessive secretion of insulin. Other small islet cell tumours may also be identified, but these tumours are most likely clinically insignificant. If the dominant insulinoma(s) arises within the body or tail of the pancreas, then a subtotal or distal pancreatectomy is indicated because multiple other islet cell tumours are virtually always present.[70] A tumour that arises in the head of the pancreas is enucleated, if possible, or alternatively resected by pancreatico-duodenectomy. The use of calcium angiogram can determine the region of the pancreas that contains the insulinoma. Intraoperative measurements of insulin concentration can accurately predict the completeness of surgery.[65,71] Medical management for this condition is reserved for those occasional patients who have failed surgical therapy, those who are poor surgical risks or those in whom a single source of hyperinsulinism cannot be found.[72]

LAPAROSCOPIC SURGERY

Laparoscopic surgery offers many advantages to patients, including decreased hospital stay, reduced pain, smaller incisions and a shorter recovery period. There is an ever-widening array of procedures that can now be safely performed laparoscopically with very successful results. Because insulinomas are usually small, benign and almost always located within the pancreas, laparoscopic surgery with laparoscopic IOUS is a logical approach to treat these patients. There are several successful case reports of laparoscopic enucleation of pancreatic insulinomas and laparoscopic distal pancreatectomies.[66,67,73–78] Operative times ranged from 180 to 360 minutes for those operations that were successfully completed laparoscopically. Complications included pancreatic fistula, and some procedures required conversion to open surgery. Minimally invasive surgery for pancreatic insulinomas is feasible in the hands of the experienced surgeon but requires a well-localised tumour on preoperative imaging studies.

Outcome

Most patients with insulinoma are cured of hypo-glycaemia and return to a normal, fully functional lifestyle. Appropriate localisation of sporadic insulinoma and surgical resection of all adeno-matous tissue results in a cure rate of greater than 95%.[3,35,63] Virtually all patients with benign, sporadic insulinomas are cured of their disease and have a normal long-term survival (**Table 5.4**).[63,77] Symptoms resolve postoperatively and the fasting serum concentration of glucose normalises.[3] Although successful resection of the tumour(s) responsible for hyperinsulinism renders most MEN 1 patients asymptomatic postoperatively,[69] persistent or recurrent hypoglycaemia owing to a missed insulinoma or metastatic disease from the original tumour may develop.[1]

In general, pancreatic surgery for insulinoma should have an associated morbidity rate less than 20% and a mortality rate approaching 0%.[1] Potential complications specifically associated with pancreatic surgery include fistula, pseudocyst, pancreatitis and abscess. Octreotide reduces the amount of pancreatic drainage[26] but has not been shown to reduce complications.[61,78] The use of IOUS decreases complications from ductal injury.

GASTRINOMA

Each year, approximately 0.1–3 people per million population develop gastrinoma, the second most common pancreatic endocrine tumour (**Table 5.1**).[79]

Table 5.4 • Results of recent series for insulinoma and localized gastrinoma

Series	n	Tumour found (%)	Initial remission (%)
Insulinoma			
Brown et al.[51]	36	100	100
Huai et al.[57]	28	100	100
Hashimoto and Walsh[58]	21	95	94
Lo et al.[60]	27	100	96
Doherty et al.[3]	25	96	96
Grant et al.[35]	36	100	97
Hiramoto et al.[63]	37	37	100
Gastrinoma			
Norton et al.[112]	123	86/100[a]	51[b]
Mignon et al.[158]	125	81	26
Howard et al.[110]	11	91	82
Thompson et al.[108]	5	100	100

[a]Gastrinomas were found in 86% of initial explorations and 100% of subsequent explorations.
[b]5-year-disease-free survival was maintained at 49%

The clinical features of this tumour were first described by Zollinger and Ellison in 1955.[80] Because of an increased awareness of Zollinger–Ellison syndrome (ZES) and the widespread availability of accurate immunoassays to measure serum concentrations of gastrin, gastrinoma is increasingly diagnosed and treated at an early stage of disease. However, the mean time from symptoms to diagnosis is 8 years in many studies so that improvements in detection are needed.

Patient presentation

Gastrinomas secrete excessive amounts of the hormone gastrin, which may cause epigastric abdominal pain, diarrhoea and oesophagitis. The most common symptoms are those of peptic ulcer disease. Diarrhoea, caused by gastrin-induced hypersecretion and increased bowel motility, is the second most common symptom and may be the only manifestation of ZES in 20% of patients.

Oesophagitis with or without stricture occurs with more severe forms of the syndrome. Approximately 20% of patients with ZES will have it as part of MEN 1,[1] and this syndrome must always be excluded. A significant family history of ulcers, peptic ulceration occurring at a young age, and peptic ulcers in association with hyperparathyroidism and/or nephrolithiasis all may be indicative of MEN 1. These patients may also have multiple subcutaneous lipomas.

As a result of increased serum gastrin concentrations, the gastric chief cells are under constant stimulation to produce acid, which causes peptic ulceration and epigastric abdominal pain in 80% of patients with ZES. Approximately 0.1–1% of patients who present with peptic ulcer disease have ZES.[79]

Patients with ZES usually have a solitary ulcer in the proximal duodenum, similar to patients with peptic ulcer disease unrelated to gastrinoma, and 'typical' ulceration does not exclude ZES. All patients with peptic ulcer disease severe enough to require surgery should be screened preoperatively for gastrinoma by obtaining a fasting serum gastrin concentration. Recurrent ulceration after appropriate medical treatment or after acid-reducing surgical procedures, or peptic ulceration in multiple locations or unusual locations such as distal duodenum or jejunum, should all raise suspicion of ZES. Patients with ZES may present with a perforated ulcer, which may occur in the jejunum. Not all patients with ZES have peptic ulcer disease, and 20% of patients with ZES have no evidence of peptic ulceration at the time of presentation.[81]

Diagnosis

The evaluation of a patient in whom ZES is suspected begins by obtaining a fasting serum concentration of gastrin (**Fig. 5.6**). Hypergastrinaemia occurs in almost all patients with ZES and is defined as a serum gastrin concentration >100 pg/mL.[82] Therefore, a normal fasting serum gastrin concentration effectively excludes ZES. Antacid medications like histamine receptor antagonists or proton-pump inhibitors may cause a false-positive increase in serum gastrin concentration, and those medicines should be withheld for 3 days before measurement of the serum gastrin concentration.

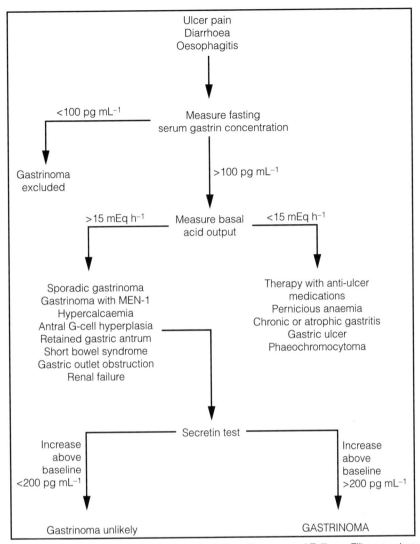

Figure 5.6 • Flow diagram for diagnosis and evaluation of patients with suspected Zollinger–Ellison syndrome (gastrinoma).

Achlorhydria is a common cause of hyper-gastrinaemia, and gastric acid secretion is measured to exclude this condition (**Fig. 5.6**). A basal acid output (BAO) greater than 15 mEq/h (>5 mEq/h in patients who have undergone previous acid-reducing operations) is abnormal and occurs in 98% of patients with ZES. Measurement of gastric pH is a simpler but less accurate indicator of gastric acid hypersecretion. A gastric pH >3 essentially excludes ZES, whereas a pH ≤2 is consistent with ZES.

An increased fasting serum gastrin concentration (>100 pg/mL) and abnormally elevated BAO (>15 mEq/L) establish the diagnosis of ZES. Many

patients with ZES have gastric acid hypersecretion and minimally increased fasting serum gastrin con-centrations (100–1000 pg/mL). For these patients, the secretin stimulation test is the provocative test of choice.[1] The secretin test is carried out after an overnight fast; secretin, 2 U/kg i.v. injection, is administered, and blood samples are collected immediately before and at 2, 5, 10 and 15 minutes after giving the secretin. A 200 pg/mL increase of gastrin concentration above baseline is diagnostic of ZES. The test sensitivity is not 100%, and approximately 15% of patients with gastrinoma may have a negative secretin test.

Management

MEDICAL CONTROL OF GASTRIC ACID HYPERSECRETION

The management of patients with gastrinoma consists of two phases: control of the symptoms associated with acid hypersecretion and removal of the tumour, which is potentially malignant and life-threatening. The development of H_2-receptor antagonists and Na^+/K^+-ATPase inhibitors (proton-pump inhibitors, PPI) has made medical control of gastric acid hypersecretion possible in all patients. Patients with ZES typically require 2–5 times the usual dose of anti-ulcer medications to keep the BAO <15 mEq/h. Omeprazole at 20–40 mg p.o. twice a day will usually control acid hypersecretion. Patients who have reflux oesophagitis or who have had prior operations to reduce acid secretion, such as subtotal gastrectomy, should have the acid output maintained at <5 mEq/h. An intravenous form of PPI called pantoprazole is now available in the US, and it should be administered at the same dose throughout the perioperative period. If acid hypersecretion is controlled, epigastric discomfort resolves and ulcers heal in virtually all patients.[83,84] Because of the recent advances in the medical treatment of peptic ulcer disease, total gastrectomy is not indicated in patients with gastrinoma.

Adequate medical control of gastric acid hypersecretion with resolution of symptoms and decreased ulcerogenic complications has resulted in increased concern about the potential malignancy of the primary tumour. The most important determinant of long-term survival in patients with ZES is the growth of the primary tumour and its metastatic spread.[84] Tumour progression accounted for most deaths when patients were followed long term.[84] Development of liver metastases is associated with subsequent death from tumour, and surgical resection of the primary can reduce the incidence of liver metastases. Hepatic metastases developed in only 3% of patients with gastrinoma treated by surgical excision of the primary compared with 23% managed without surgery.[85] Therefore, the current goal of surgery for ZES has shifted away from controlling gastric-acid hypersecretion to aggressive resection of the primary tumour as well as localised metastatic disease. Surgical intervention can obviate the need for long-term medical therapy,

which is important since experimental rodent studies suggest that the long-term use of omeprazole is associated with the development of gastric carcinoid tumours.[86] The author has recently diagnosed diffuse malignant gastric carcinoids in five patients with ZES and MEN 1 who have been taking omeprazole for 10 years. It is imperative that such patients are monitored with periodic endoscopy to screen for the development of carcinoid tumours.

The natural history of longstanding ZES in patients in whom the excessive acid secretion is controlled is largely unclear, primarily because effective medical therapy is relatively new. A longitudinal study of 212 patients with ZES and well-controlled acid secretion showed that none of these patients died of acid-related complications.[87] This study evaluated the long-term clinical course of patients with gastrinoma. Pancreatic location of tumour and a tumour diameter >3 cm were found to be associated with an increased risk of death from gastrinoma, and higher serum gastrin concentrations correlated with more malignant disease and a shortened survival time.[87] Extensive liver metastases had increased negative effects on survival, as did the development of bone metastases or ectopic Cushing's syndrome. These results lend further support to early surgical intervention (as surgery decreases the rate of development of liver metastases), as well as aggressive surgical therapy of limited hepatic metastases.[87,88]

PREOPERATIVE TUMOUR LOCALISATION

In contradistinction to insulinoma, gastrinoma is malignant in 60–90% of patients.[2] Duodenal gastrinomas as small as 2 mm in diameter may have associated regional lymph node metastases.[89] At the time of diagnosis, approximately 25–40% of patients have liver metastases.[90,91] Imaging studies must carefully assess the liver, and all patients with ZES should undergo preoperative testing to localise the tumour and to define the extent of disease so that appropriate surgical treatment can be undertaken.

Non-invasive tumour-localising studies

Initial tumour localisation studies should be non-invasive, should attempt to image the primary tumour and should adequately assess the liver for metastases. As with localising insulinoma, abdominal ultrasonography has a low sensitivity of only 20–30% for gastrinoma (**Table 5.3**). Abdominal CT detects approximately 50% of gastrinomas overall, but sensitivity depends greatly on tumour size, tumour location and the presence of metastases.[92] Gastrinomas >3 cm in diameter are reliably detected by CT, whereas tumours <1 cm in diameter are rarely detected (**Fig. 5.7**).

Primary gastrinomas that arise within the pancreas are identified much more reliably than those in extrapancreatic, extrahepatic locations (80% vs. 35%). CT scanning identifies 50% of liver metastases. Abdominal MRI has a low sensitivity (25%) in localising primary gastrinomas but is the study of choice to show hepatic metastases (**Table 5.3**). Gastrinoma metastases in the liver appear bright on dynamic T2-weighted images and show a distinct ring with gadolinium enhancement.[93] MRI is especially useful to differentiate gastrinoma metastases within the liver from haemangiomas.

Studies indicate that somatostatin receptor scintigraphy (SRS) significantly improves the preoperative localisation of gastrinomas.[94] SRS images gastrinomas on the basis of the density of somatostatin type 2 receptors. Because a high proportion of gastrinomas have these type 2 receptors, approximately 80% of primary tumours can be identified, and the true extent of metastatic disease is delineated more accurately than by CT or MRI.[95] SRS is now the non-invasive imaging modality of choice for gastrinomas (**Fig. 5.7**). SRS is better than MRI and CT combined. Further, the sensitivity of SRS for gastrinomas may be improved by EUS – the combination identified 17 of 18 tumours in one study.[40]

Several prospective studies have evaluated the utility of SRS compared with conventional studies. In a prospective study of 35 patients, SRS had a greater sensitivity than all other conventional

Figure 5.7 • **(a)** Computed tomography scan and **(b)** somatostatin receptor scintigraphy preoperatively identified large gastrinomas in this patient.

studies combined (angiography, MRI, CT, ultra-sonography).[96] The rate of detection correlated closely with tumour size: 30% of gastrinomas <1.1 cm in diameter and 96% of those >2 cm were detected. A positive SRS study strongly predicts the presence of tumour, but the high negative predictive value (33–100%) cautions against excluding a tumour on the basis of a negative study.[97] Another prospective study in 146 patients found a sensitivity of 71%, specificity of 86%, positive predictive value of 85% and a negative predictive value of 52%. These 146 patients underwent 480 SRS studies, with a false-positive localisation rate of 12%. Extra-abdominal false-positive localisation studies were more common than intra-abdominal false-positive scans and were attributed to thyroid, breast or granulomatous lung disease.[98] The most common causes of false-positive intra-abdominal SRS scans were accessory spleens, localisation to prior operative sites and renal parapelvic cysts. Only 2.7% of these false-positive studies actually altered management, suggesting the importance of a high awareness of other potential causes for a positive SRS scan in the clinical setting.

Invasive tumour-localising modalities

Although non-invasive imaging studies are important as initial tests to exclude gross hepatic metastases and unresectable disease, these studies may fail to image the primary gastrinoma. Invasive modalities may be useful to localise accurately the primary tumour prior to surgery. EUS has a reported sensitivity of 85% for detecting gastrinomas and a specificity of 95% (**Table 5.3**).[44,47,48] Tumours in the pancreas as small as 2–3 mm may be imaged. Duodenal gastrinomas can be visualised as a submucosal mass with EUS (**Fig. 5.8**). The ability to detect duodenal wall gastrinomas directly has been disappointing, and liver metastases are not reliably imaged. The combination of EUS and SRS for gastrinomas has been found to be 93% in a small series of patients.[99]

Previously the best imaging modality to localise a primary gastrinoma was selective angiography. Angiograms are obtained by selectively catheterising gastroduodenal, hepatic, superior mesenteric and splenic arteries. A hypervascular tumour 'blush' is characteristically observed in the location of the gastrinoma (**Fig. 5.9**). Sensitivity is 68% overall for

Figure 5.8 • View of duodenal wall gastrinoma through endoscope. The tumour appears as a small submucosal mass, which was biopsied and confirmed as a gastrinoma.

extrahepatic gastrinomas and 86% for hepatic metastases, but only 34% for duodenal gastrinomas (**Table 5.3**).[100,101] Tumours <1–2 cm are less reliably detected. Selective arterial secretin injection (SASI) during angiography, and collection of blood samples from a hepatic vein as well as a peripheral vein for measurement of the gastrin concentration, increases the sensitivity for localising the primary tumour to 90–100%, with a specificity of virtually 100% (**Fig. 5.9**).[102] Injection of secretin into the artery supplying the gastrinoma causes an increase in the hepatic vein gastrin concentration by >80 pg/mL in 40 s. In this way the gastrinoma can be localised to either the head, body/tail of the pancreas or the liver. Gastrinomas are usually only found in the gastroduodenal artery territory and occult tumours are usually in the gastrinoma triangle. PVS for gastrin is similar and provides regional localisation, with similar sensitivity to the SASI test. Neither study is particularly useful in patients with ZES because gradients are nearly always found in the gastrinoma triangle.

SURGERY FOR TUMOUR ERADICATION

If preoperative imaging studies reveal no evidence of unresectable metastatic disease, then patients with sporadic gastrinoma and acceptable risks

(a)

(a)

(b)

Figure 5.9 • Secretin angiogram in patient with Zollinger–Ellison syndrome and gastrinoma localised to duodenum. **(a)** Results of secretin injection of selective arteries that perfuse the pancreas and duodenum (gastroduodenal artery, hepatic artery, superior mesenteric artery, splenic artery). Gastrin concentrations were measured in the hepatic vein before secretin injection and at intervals after secretin injection. **(b)** When secretin was injected into the gastroduodenal artery gastrinoma was visualised in the wall of the duodenum as a 'blush' (arrow), and the hepatic vein gastrin concentrations were most increased **(a)**.

should undergo abdominal exploration for tumour resection and possible cure.

Operative approach

Vaccination against encapsulated bacteria is required preoperatively. The surgeon should be prepared for hepatic resection if unsuspected liver metastases are identified intraoperatively. An upper abdominal incision that provides adequate exposure for exploration of the entire pancreas, regional lymph nodes and liver is necessary. The abdomen is initially inspected for metastases, with particular attention to possible ectopic sites of tumour such as the ovaries, jejunum and omentum. The entire surface of the liver is then palpated for metastatic lesions. Metastases typically appear tan in colour and feel firm. Deep hepatic metastases may be identified by using IOUS with a 5-MHz transducer. All suspicious hepatic lesions must be either excised or biopsied to exclude malignant gastrinoma. In general, liver metastases that are not identified preoperatively by abdominal MRI or SRS are small and potentially resectable at the time of operation. Similarly, hilar, coeliac and peripancreatic regional lymph nodes are carefully sampled for metastatic disease.

Intraoperative manoeuvres to find the primary gastrinoma

Successful intraoperative localisation and resection of tumours may be extremely challenging because gastrinomas only 2 mm in diameter may reside in the wall of the duodenum. There is also a high rate of associated lymph node metastases and a possible occurrence of primary gastrinomas within lymph nodes with no other identifiable primary tumour.[103,104] The initial finding of a single involved lymph node may, therefore, represent a primary tumour or metastatic disease from a very small, unlocalised primary tumour. Preoperative studies, such as SRS, accurately localise the primary gastrinoma and metastases and greatly facilitate the operative management, allowing a surgical approach directed to the area containing the tumour. Intraoperative localisation is still necessary because 20–40% of patients in whom the tumour is not apparent with preoperative studies will still have tumour identified at surgery. A potentially useful new tool is the measurement of intraoperative gastrin concentrations. In a series of 20 patients, this test had an accuracy of 94% in predicting the successful removal of all gastrin-secreting tumours.[105] Both the positive predictive value and specificity were 100%, and the negative predictive value 88%, with a sensitivity of 91%. Although involving only a small series of patients, the study showed that intraoperative measurements of gastrin concentration may provide an additional tool to help guide complete resection.

Successful tumour identification requires knowledge of where primary gastrinomas arise. The so-called 'gastrinoma triangle', bounded by the neck and body of the pancreas medially, the junction of the cystic and common bile ducts superiorly, and the second and third portions of the duodenum inferiorly, contains more than 80% of primary gastrinomas.[106] In this region, most gastrinomas arise within the duodenum. The head of the pancreas and duodenum are first exposed by mobilising the hepatic flexure of the colon out of the upper abdomen and dividing the gastrocolic ligament to open the lesser sac. A Kocher manoeuvre is performed to lift the head of the pancreas out of the retroperitoneum. The entire pancreatic surface is carefully examined visually and palpated between the thumb and forefinger (**Fig. 5.4**). IOUS is very useful for localising intrapancreatic gastrinomas (**Table 5.3**). The body and tail of the pancreas may be mobilised and similarly examined after dividing the inferior and posterior pancreatic attachments to find the few gastrinomas that may arise in the distal pancreas.

Primary gastrinomas have increasingly been recognised as occurring in extrapancreatic locations.[106–108] IOUS is poor at detecting gastrinomas within the duodenum (**Table 5.3**), and the surgeon must rely more on inspection, palpation and duodenotomy to find these tumours.[55] In 50% of patients, the gastrinoma is located in the submucosa of the duodenum. Duodenal gastrinomas are usually very small – <6 mm – and are difficult to palpate. Endoscopic transillumination of the duo-

denum may allow small duodenal tumours to be seen and guide precise tumour resection.[109] The gastrinoma appears as a dark, opaque shadow surrounded by the semitransparent red glow of the duodenal wall. If the tumour is not localised by endoscopic transillumination, then duodenotomy is recommended to allow direct inspection and exploration of the duodenal mucosa. Duodenal wall gastrinomas occur in greatest density more proximally in the duodenum (**Fig. 5.10**). Tumours are detected most usually by duodenotomy, followed by intraoperative endoscopy with transillumination and least often by palpation (**Fig. 5.10**). Regional lymph nodes should be systematically sampled, as lymph node metastases may be inapparent at exploration and will be found in 55% of patients with duodenal tumours. Gastrinomas can be found by an experienced surgeon in >95% of patients (**Table 5.4**).[108,110–112] Further, duodenotomy is associated with a higher rate of finding gastrinoma and a higher rate of cure.[111]

Approximately 5–24% of gastrinomas are found in extrapancreatic, extraintestinal lymph nodes only,

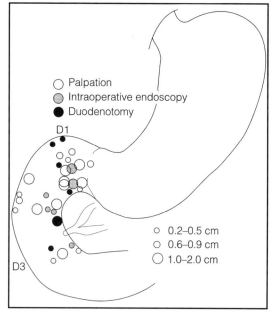

Figure 5.10 • Density of duodenal gastrinomas found at surgery and method of operative identification. Gastrinomas within the wall of the duodenum are most common in the first portion (D1) and decrease in density distally (D3). Duodenotomy identified the most tumours, followed by intraoperative endoscopy and then palpation.

with no apparent primary pancreatic or duodenal tumour.[104,113–116] Whether these represent primary tumours or metastases from occult pancreatic or intestinal primary tumours is controversial. Primary tumours as small as 2 mm may have associated lymph node metastases[89] and are easily missed intraoperatively without meticulous exploration. There are many reported patients without previous gastric or pancreatic resections who seem to be biochemically cured after the excision of only lymph nodes containing gastrinoma.[104,115–117] Peripancreatic lymph nodes from patients undergoing Whipple resection for non-endocrine tumour may contain cells that stain positive for neuroendocrine markers, giving a plausible explanation for lymph node primary gastrinoma.[103] A prospective study found eight patients to have extrapancreatic, extraduodenal, extralymphatic primary gastrinomas. These tumours were located in the liver (three patients), common bile duct (one), jejunum (one), omentum (one), pylorus (one) and ovary (one).[118] A gastrinoma has been reported in the interventricular septum of the heart.[119] It is reasonable to conclude the operation if careful exploration, including examination of the duodenum with duodenotomy, does not reveal a primary tumour, all involved lymph nodes have been resected and other ectopic sites have been examined carefully.

Tumour resection

As described for insulinoma, tumour enucleation remains the procedure of choice for resecting sporadic gastrinomas. Tumours that arise within the pancreas and that are not near the pancreatic duct or major vessels are safely enucleated. Large pancreatic tumours with vital structures in close proximity must be removed by pancreatic resection. Duodenal gastrinomas may be precisely resected using endoscopic transillumination of the duodenum.[109] Some normal duodenal wall around the tumour is removed, but as much of the duodenal wall as possible is preserved to allow a nonconstricting closure. Special attention is paid to avoid the ampulla of Vater. Involved regional lymph nodes should be excised. Although most gastrinomas are malignant, performing a more radical pancreatic resection that includes regional lymph nodes (e.g. pancreatico-duodenectomy) is currently not indicated. Small tumours can be easily

enucleated and because of the slow progression of disease, symptomatic relief with medical treatment is easily achieved. Pancreatico-duodenectomy (Whipple procedure) can be performed with acceptable morbidity and mortality and may be indicated for patients with larger, locally aggressive tumours.[64] Further, the morbidity and mortality of a Whipple operation for smaller and less malignant tumours are decreasing making this a potentially acceptable operative procedure for locally advanced gastrinomas and other islet cell tumours.[120]

The presence of lymph node metastases at the time of operation should not discourage an aggressive surgical approach to remove all gross tumour. Gastrinoma is associated with lymph node involvement in 50–80% of patients and, unlike many other types of cancer, lymph node involvement alone without hepatic or distant metastases does not seem to decrease survival.[2,121,122] Resection of all apparent tumour to eradicate disease increases disease-free survival and may extend overall survival. The development of hepatic and distant metastatic disease occurs in 25–90% of patients and is the most common cause of morbidity and mortality associated with tumour.[81,101,122,123] Patients should be carefully followed by screening for recurrent disease because if a patient develops an increased serum gastrin concentration in conjunction with a tumour that has been imaged, re-operation should be considered. Approximately one-third of these patients can be rendered free of disease.[124]

GASTRINOMA AND MEN 1

In a recent study of 107 patients with ZES and MEN 1, 60% had pituitary tumours, 45% adrenal disease, 30% had carcinoid tumours, 94% had primary hyperparathyroidism, 6% thyroid disease, and 5% had lipomas. Importantly, 25% lacked a family history of MEN 1.[125] Parathyroidectomy should be performed first in patients with MEN 1 who have hyperparathyroidism and ZES because normalisation of the serum calcium concentration usually results in a marked decrease in serum gastrin, allowing better medical control of the symptoms of ZES.[126] Whether patients should undergo abdominal exploration is controversial. Earlier surgical series suggest that resecting gastrinoma does not cure these patients of ZES. Some studies suggest that aggressive surgical approaches may result in normalisation of serum gastrin concentrations in MEN 1 patients.[127] However, prospective studies with strict criteria for cure indicate that no patients with ZES and MEN 1 are cured. All patients with MEN 1 and ZES should undergo SASI to determine the pancreatic region of the tumour secreting gastrin and then undergo surgery to resect the primary tumour and metastases. Tumours that are ≥3 cm usually have lymph node metastases.[128] Preoperative abdominal CT is necessary to identify hepatic metastases and plan surgical resection. SRS is also useful in determining the true extent of disease. In patients with MEN 1, 70% of gastrinomas are found within the duodenum, and approximately 50% of patients may have multiple duodenal tumours.[128] We advocate performing routine duodenotomy and peripancreatic lymph node sampling whenever a duodenal gastrinoma is found in a patient with MEN 1, as well as enucleation of palpable tumours in the pancreas.[127]

The appropriate extent of surgical resection in patients with ZES and MEN 1 is controversial because these tumours are uncommon and only a few studies have enough patients to allow for an analysis of surgical outcome. Thompson argues for an aggressive surgical approach.[129,130] In a series of 34 patients with ZES and MEN 1 who had undergone surgery, 68% remained eugastrinaemic, with a 15-year survival rate of 94%. He recommends performing a distal pancreatectomy (because of the concomitant neuroendocrine tumours in the neck, body and tail of the pancreas in these patients), enucleation of any tumours in the pancreatic head or uncinate process, duodenotomy and exision of any tumours from the first to fourth portions of the duodenum, and a peripancreatic lymph node dissection in those patients with a duodenal tumour or a pancreatic tumour >3 cm in diameter.[129,130] We, however, found that patients with MEN 1 and ZES rarely became free of disease despite extensive duodenal exploration, with only 16% of patients free of disease immediately after surgery and only 6% at 5 years.[112] This is in contrast to a surgical cure of approximately 40% of patients with sporadic gastrinomas.[112]

There is also controversy over the role of enteropancreatic surgery for asymptomatic patients with MEN 1. Opinions differ about the size of tumour that warrants surgery, with some setting the threshold at 1 cm and others at 3 cm. Some believe that the goal of surgery is cancer prevention and that surgery should be performed when the diagnosis is certain regardless of the size of imageable tumour. The standard surgical procedure involves distal pancreatic resection and intraoperative ultrasound for enucleation of tumours within the pancreatic head and duodenal submucosa. If the main tumour burden is localised to the pancreatic head and is bulky in nature, a Whipple pancreaticoduodenectomy may be considered.[131]

Outcome

The overall survival for patients with sporadic gastrinoma not metastatic to the liver is >90% at 5 years and >85% at 10 years (Table 5.4). An immediate postoperative cure rate of 60% can be obtained if all tumour is identified and resected, and over 30% of these patients remain free of disease at 5-year follow-up.[112] Patients with liver metastases at presentation have an overall survival of only 20–38%.[122]

OTHER RARE ENDOCRINE TUMOURS OF THE PANCREAS

Other pancreatic endocrine tumours include vasoactive intestinal peptide (VIP)-oma, glucagonoma, somatostatinoma, growth hormone-releasing factor (GRF)-oma, adrenocorticotropic hormone (ACTH)-oma, parathyroid hormone (PTH)-likeoma, neurotensinoma and non-functional islet cell tumour or pancreatic peptide (PP)-oma (Table 5.1).[108] These neoplasms occur in less than 0.2 persons per million per year. In general, these tumours resemble gastrinoma in that all are associated with a high incidence of malignancy. Each can also arise in association with MEN 1, including GRFoma (30%) and PPoma (80–100%). The hormones, symptoms and signs, diagnostic tests, sites of occurrence, proportions malignant and frequency of associated MEN 1 for each tumour are given in Table 5.1.

Glucagonomas produce a characteristic rash called necrolytic migratory erythema (NME).[132,133] These patients commonly have type 2 diabetes mellitus, weight loss, anaemia, stomatitis, glossitis, thromboembolism, and other gastrointestinal and neuropsychiatric symptoms. The rash is secondary to severe hypoaminoacidaemia and zinc deficiency.[132,133] These tumours are commonly malignant and not resectable for cure. However, in some instances all tumour can be removed surgically, which leads to complete amelioration of all signs and symptoms (**Fig. 5.11**).

PPomas produce pancreatic polypeptide and neurone-specific enolase, which have no clinically appreciable biological activity, and therefore patients do not present with a typical hormonal syndrome. Symptoms arise because of mass effect and include abdominal pain, gastrointestinal bleeding and obstruction. Diagnosis may only be made after palpation of an abdominal mass or incidental identification of a pancreatic mass on imaging studies. Malignant spread to lymph nodes or liver is common and related to tumour size (>50% for tumours >3 cm).

For all of these tumours, preoperative abdominal CT is necessary in attempting to localise the primary tumour and to exclude liver metastases.[128] The goals of surgical treatment are to control symptoms caused by excessive hormone production and to potentially cure or decrease disease bulk.

Figure 5.11 • 3-D pancreatic protocol CT scan of a glucagonoma within the body of the pancreas (arrows). The tumour was abutting the superior mesenteric vein and causing obstruction of the pancreatic duct with atrophy of the tail of the pancreas.

The only potentially curative treatment for malignant endocrine tumours is surgical resection.[134–138] Patients with extensive bilobar hepatic metastases are typically not candidates for surgery, and symptoms may respond to chemotherapy, interferon α or octreotide.[134]

OCCULT PANCREATIC ENDOCRINE TUMOURS

An 'occult' islet cell tumour is an unlocalised tumour that occurs in a patient with a definitively diagnosed clinical hormonal syndrome, such as fasting hyperinsulinaemic hypoglycaemia or ZES. The tumour is biochemically proven, but its anatomical site remains unclear. Approximately 10–20% of insulinomas and 15% of gastrinomas are occult. Patients with insulinoma should undergo a regional localisation study, such as the calcium angiogram, preoperatively in an attempt to localise the tumour to a specific anatomical area (**Fig. 5.3**). Patients with occult gastrinomas need not undergo a regional localisation study as these tumours are nearly always in the duodenum within the gastrinoma triangle. Exploratory laparotomy is then the last resort to identify the location of the tumour and to resect it. Surgery should not be performed in patients with insulinoma unless IOUS is available, given its advantages in finding small tumours within the pancreas (**Fig. 5.5**).[1] Surgery in patients with occult gastrinoma should focus on the duodenum, including transillumination and duodenotomy (**Fig. 5.10**).

Abdominal exploration by an experienced pancreatic endocrine surgeon, knowledge of the sites of occurrence of specific tumours and the use of IOUS results in identification and removal of the tumour in all but a few patients. In the rare instance that a tumour remains unlocalised and unresected after thorough exploration, the decision whether to perform a pancreatectomy depends on the particular patient's response to medical management and the results of the preoperative regional localisation study. Pancreatic resection is not indicated if the patient's hormonal syndrome can be well controlled by medical management. When medical management is unsatisfactory, the only alternative is to perform a pancreatectomy on the basis of the regional localisation data. Blind pancreatectomy is never indicated.

MALIGNANT PANCREATIC ENDOCRINE TUMOURS

With improvements in the medical management of syndromes of hormonal excess, growth and metastatic spread of primary islet cell tumours has increasingly become more problematic. Except for insulinomas, which are malignant in only 5–10% of cases, more than 60% of pancreatic endocrine tumours overall are malignant.[134,137,138] Data concerning the management of these patients are mainly derived from experience with malignant gastrinomas, which occur more commonly than other more obscure pancreatic neuroendocrine tumours.

No diagnostic histological criteria from examination of tumour biopsy samples or resected primary tumours exist to define malignancy for pancreatic endocrine tumours. Malignancy is definitively established with surgical exploration and histological evidence of tumour remote from the primary lesion, usually in peripancreatic lymph nodes or the liver. Recurrence of tumour at a location distant from a resected primary tumour site also definitively indicates malignancy. Gross invasion of blood vessels, surrounding tissues or adjacent organs usually suggests a malignant tumour.[135] IOUS showing a pancreatic tumour with indistinct margins may imply local invasion and malignancy.[62] Very large tumours (>5 cm) have an increased risk of being malignant.[2] Tumour DNA ploidy and tumoral growth fraction determined by flow cytometry may provide an indication of biological behaviour of some of these tumours. Because islet cell tumours generally grow slowly, metastases may not become evident until years after the initial primary tumour resection.

Evaluation of metastatic disease

Evaluation of a patient with a malignant neuroendocrine tumour begins by assessing the extent of disease using radiological imaging studies. SRS seems to be the single best imaging study to select patients for aggressive surgery to remove metastatic disease.[1] If the tumour binds this isotope, then disease anywhere in the body can be identified. Miliary or extensive bilobar hepatic disease and distant metastases are considered inoperable and, if identified preoperatively, can prevent unnecessary surgery. CT or MRI may identify disease in the chest and abdomen. Specific complaints of bone pain are elicited and, if present, evaluated with bone scan and radiography.

Malignant primary insulinomas are relatively large (≈6 cm) and can usually be readily detected by non-invasive imaging studies.[55] Gastrinomas may metastasise to regional lymph nodes when only millimetres in size. In one study, duodenal primary gastrinomas have been found to have a higher incidence of lymph node metastases (55%) than pancreatic gastrinomas (22%).[1] Some suggest that rare gastrinomas to the left of the superior mesenteric artery in the pancreatic tail are always malignant and more commonly produce liver metastases. Metastatic tumour must be distinguished from multiple tumours, which occur simultaneously. If multiple insulinomas or gastrinomas are found in a patient, then MEN 1 should be suspected.

Surgical management

Pancreatic neuroendocrine carcinomas have a better prognosis than adenocarcinoma of the exocrine pancreas and are often managed with aggressive surgical resection.[94] Surgery is undertaken to decrease tumour bulk so that hormonal syndromes are more effectively controlled by medical management, to relieve symptoms of mass effect, and/or to eliminate cancerous tissue and improve disease-free or overall survival. Preoperative staging studies are important to exclude patients from surgery who would not benefit from resection. Recent studies demonstrate that CT combined with preoperative laparoscopy predicts the ability to completely remove all tumour better than CT alone. The predictive value for tumour resectability was 74% for CT alone and 95% for CT followed by diagnostic laparoscopy.[139]

Limited metastases as well as the primary tumour should be resected to adequately debulk tumour and to eliminate the hormonal syndrome.[140] Some patients with MEN 1 and ZES have had more aggressive tumours, as evidenced by larger size, liver metastases and higher serum levels of gastrin.[141] Resection of advanced disease, even in MEN 1 patients, has been done safely and is suggested to improve survival.[142] Incomplete tumour resection may not improve the ability to control the hormonal syndrome medically. For medically fit patients with metastatic insulinoma in whom hypoglycaemia is poorly controlled by medical management, tumour debulking may control symptoms for prolonged time periods, even in the setting of distant metastases.[81] Approximately 50% of patients with metastatic insulinoma undergoing resection have complete biochemical remission.[143] Surgical resection of the primary tumour, and aggressive resection of liver metastases are both asscociated with prolonged survival in many studies.[144]

Although treatment is generally palliative and not curative for patients with locally advanced tumours and limited metastatic disease, surgery may be the only therapy that effectively ameliorates life-threatening symptoms. It may increase survival because these tumours are generally indolent, slow-growing neoplasms.[143–145] Limited regional metastatic disease can often be successfully resected and may be curative if no liver metastases are present.[140] This type of aggressive re-operative surgery can be done with acceptable morbidity (30%) and minimal mortality (0% in one series).[146] Complete resection of localised or regional nodal metastases with negative margins at the initial surgery provides the highest probability of cure.[1] Although disease-free survival is prolonged in most patients, most eventually develop recurrent tumour.

Approximately 30% of patients with metastatic insulinoma can undergo complete resection of tumour.[143,145] Median survival is increased from 11 months in patients with metastatic insulinoma who cannot undergo resection to 4 years in those in whom tumour debulking is possible.[122] Palliative re-resection of recurrent tumour extends median survival from 11–19 months to 4 years.[147] Surgery may also be the most effective treatment for patients with metastatic gastrinoma if most or all of the tumour can be resected.[1] Aggressive resection of liver metastases of gastrinoma, considered resectable by preoperative radiological imaging studies, improves 5-year survival from 28% in patients with inoperable metastases to 79–85%.[140,148] Surgical resection of other liver metastatic neuroendocrine tumours besides gastrinoma is also associated with a 5-year survival of 73%.[149,150]

Patients with solitary, localised metastatic disease benefit most. Recurrence of disease in more than one lobe of the liver may be treated by hepatic arterial embolisation or orthotopic liver transplant. Laparoscopic radiofrequency ablation (RFA) is a novel, minimally invasive method of providing effective cytoreduction of neuroendocrine tumours metastatic to the liver.[151] The lesion control rate with RFA is approximately 90% and the complications and mortality rates are low.[152] Cryoablation is similar and it can reduce symptoms and help with the medical management of the excessive hormonal secretion, but in general the lesion control rate is not as good and in most series is approximately 33% compared with 90% for RFA.[153] Patients may also have symptoms, such as obstruction secondary to mass effect from the size or location of the tumour, or gastrointestinal bleeding from direct tumour invasion into adjacent bowel, which are effectively eliminated by resection of the tumour.[140] Pain secondary to neural invasion may be effectively palliated by percutaneous coeliac axis nerve block.

Non-surgical management

Symptoms from extensive metastases may respond to chemotherapy or octreotide, but these treatments are not curative.[1] Combination chemotherapy with streptozocin and 5-fluorouracil is the most effective regimen for metastatic insulinoma, producing at least a partial response in 60% of patients. Doxorubicin may also be used. Patients with metastatic gastrinoma are treated with streptozocin, doxorubicin and/or 5-fluorouracil. Treatment with octreotide results in unpredictable responses, causing decreased tumour growth in some patients and having no effect in others.[123,154] The addition of interferon α to octreotide therapy may benefit a subgroup of patients with advanced metastatic disease that is unresponsive to octreotide monotherapy.[155] Dacarbazine may be effective in controlling the clinical and biochemical manifestations of gastrinoma.[156] Cryosurgery may be a useful adjuvant in patients with refractory hepatic neuroendocrine metastases. Cryosurgery can relieve symptoms and causes a reduction in tumour markers, which may allow a better response to subsequent systemic therapy.[157] Octreotide may ameliorate symptoms, especially in patients with malignant VIPoma (**Fig. 5.12**), and when symptoms are adequately controlled, patients can live comfortably and productively for many years with metastatic disease.

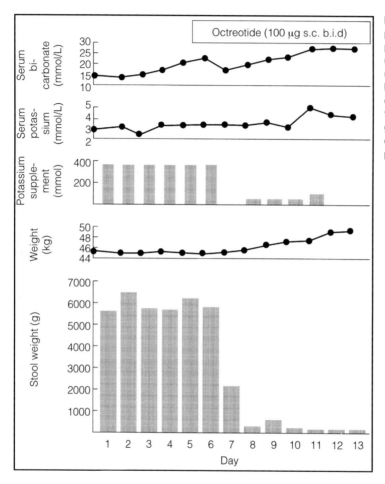

Figure 5.12 • Use of octreotide in patient with metastatic VIPoma. The patient had voluminous diarrhoea (5–6 kg/day) and hypokalaemia (serum K^+= 3 mmol/L) and required large potassium supplements. After octreotide 100 μg b.i.d. was started, the diarrhoea stopped, the patient gained weight and the serum concentrations of bicarbonate and potassium normalised.

155

REFERENCES

1. Norton JA. Neuroendocrine tumors of the pancreas and duodenum. Curr Probl Surg 1994; 31:77–164.

2. Peplinski GR, Norton JA. Gastrointestinal endocrine cancers and nodal metastases: biological significance and therapeutic implications. Surg Oncol Clin North Am 1996; 5:159–71.

3. Doherty GM, Doppman JL, Shawker TH et al. Results of a prospective strategy to diagnose, localize and resect insulinomas. Surgery 1991; 110:989–97.

Excellent paper about the results of diagnostic testing for insulinoma in 25 consecutive patients with the tumour.

4. Dizon AM, Kowalyk S, Hoogwerf BJ. Neuroglycopenic and other symptoms in patients with insulinomas. Am J Med 1999; 106:307–10.

5. Takacs CA, Krivak TC, Napolitano PG. Insulinoma in pregnancy: a case report and review of the literature. Obstet Gynecol Surv 2002; 57:229–35.

6. Thompson NW, Lloyd RV, Nishiyama RH et al. MEN I pancreas: a histological and immunohistochemical study. World J Surg 1984; 8:561–74.

7. Langer P, Wild A, Hall A et al. Prevalence of multiple endocrine neoplasia type 1 in young patients with apparently sporadic primary hyperparathyroidism or pancreaticoduodenal endocrine tumours. Br J Surg 2003; 90:1599–603.

8. Kouvaraki MA, Lee J E, Shapiro SE et al. Genotype-phenotype analysis in multiple endocrine neoplasia type 1. Arch Surg 2002; 137:641–7.

9. Chandrasekharappa SC, Guru SC, Manickam P et al. Positional cloning of the gene for multiple endocrine neoplasia-type 1. Science 1997; 276:404–7.

Outstanding scientific work in which the gene for menin, MEN 1 was cloned.

10. Lemmens I, Van de Ven WJM, Kas K et al. Identification of the multiple endocrine neoplasia type 1 (MEN1) gene. Hum Mol Genet 1997; 6:1169–75.

11. Marx SJ, Agarwal SK, Heppner C et al. The gene for multiple endocrine neoplasia type 1 – recent findings. Bone 1999; 25:119–22.

12. Bartsch D, Kopp I, Bergenfelz A et al. MEN1 gene mutations in 12 MEN1 families and their associated tumors. Eur J Endocrinol 1998; 139:416–20.

13. Guo SS, Sawicki MP. Molecular and genetic mechanisms of tumorigenesis in multiple endocrine neoplasia type-1. Mol Endocrinol 2001; 15:1653–64.

14. Burgess JR, Greenaway TM, Parameswaran V et al. Enteropancreatic malignancy associated with multiple endocrine neoplasia type 1. Cancer 1998; 83:428–34.

15. Langer P, Wild A, Celik L et al. Prospective controlled trial of a standardized meal stimulation test in the detection of pancreaticoduodenal endocrine tumors in patients with multiple endocrine neoplasia type 1. Br J Surg 2001; 88:1403–7.

16. Grunberger G, Weiner JL, Silverman R et al. Factitious hypoglycemia due to surreptitious administration of insulin: diagnosis, treatment and long-term follow-up. Ann Intern Med 1988; 108:252–7.

Critical paper that describes the results in patients with factitious hypoglycaemia.

17. Basu A, Sheehan MT, Thompson GB et al. Insulinoma in chronic renal failure. J Clin Endocrinol Metab 2002; 87:4889–91.

18. Gorden P, Skarulis MC, Roach P et al. Plasma proinsulin-like component in insulinoma: a 25-year experience. J Clin Endocrinol Metab 1995; 80:2884–7.

19. Farley DR, van Heerden JA, Myers JL. Adult pancreatic nesidioblastosis: unusual presentations of a rare entity. Arch Surg 1994; 129:329–32.

20. Goudswaard WB, Houthoff HJ, Koudstaal J et al. Nesidioblastosis and endocrine hyperplasia of the pancreas: a secondary phenomenon. Hum Pathol 1986; 17:46–54.

21. Grant CS. Insulinoma. Surg Oncol Clin North Am 1998; 7:819–44.

22. Nakano K, Mizuta A, Oohashi S et al. Nesidioblastosis with glucagon-reactive islet cell hyperplasia: a case report. Pancreas 2003; 26:402–7.

23. Hirshberg B, Alexander HR, Bartlett DL et al. Nesidioblastosis in adults: a clinical enigma. J Clin Endocrinol Metab 2001; 86:2329.

24. Thornton PS, Alter CA, Katz LE et al. Short- and long-term use of octreotide in the treatment of congenital hyperinsulinism. J Pediatr 1993; 123:637–43.

25. Glaser B, Hirsch HJ, Landau H. Persistent hyperinsulinemic hypoglycemia of infancy: long-term octreotide treatment without pancreatectomy. J Pediatr 1993; 123:644–50.

26. Gorden P, Comi RJ, Maton PN et al. Somatostatin and somatostatin analogue (SMS 201-995) in treatment of hormone-secreting tumors of the pituitary and gastrointestinal tract and non-neoplastic diseases of the gut. Ann Intern Med 1989; 110:35–50.

27. Arnold R, Frank M, Kajdan U. Management of gastroenteropancreatic endocrine tumors: the place of somatostatin analogues. Digestion 1994; 55(suppl. 3):107–13.

28. von Eyben FE, Grodum E, Gjessing HJ et al. Metabolic remission with octreotide in patients with insulinoma. J Intern Med 1994; 235:245–8.

29. Arnold R, Neuhaus C, Benning R et al. Somato-statin analog sandostatin and inhibition of tumor growth in patients with metastatic endocrine gastroenteropancreatic tumors. World J Surg 1993; 17:511–19.

30. Doppman JL, Chang R, Fraker DL et al. Local-ization of insulinomas to regions of the pancreas by intra-arterial stimulation with calcium. Ann Intern Med 1995; 123:269–73.

31. Vinik AI, Delbridge L, Moattari R et al. Trans-hepatic portal vein catheterization for local-ization of insulinomas: a ten-year experience. Surgery 1991; 109:1–11.

32. Gianello P, Gigot JF, Berthet F et al. Pre- and intraoperative localization of insulinomas: report of 22 observations. World J Surg 1988; 12:389–97.

33. Rickes S, Unkrodt K, Ocran K et al. Differ-entiation of neuroendocrine tumors from other pancreatic lesions by echo-enhanced power doppler sonography and somatostatin receptor scintigraphy. Pancreas 2003; 26:76–81.

34. Fraker DL, Norton JA. Localization and resection of insulinomas and gastrinomas. JAMA 1988; 259:3601–5.

35. Grant CS, van Heerden J, Charboneau JW et al. Insulinoma: the value of intraoperative ultra-sonography. Arch Surg 1988; 123:843–8.

36. Rodallec M, Vilgrain V, Zins M et al. Helical CT of pancreatic endocrine tumours. J Comp Assist Tomography 2002: 26:728–33.

37. Boukhman MP, Karam JM, Shaver J et al. Localization of insulinomas. Arch Surg 1999; 134:818–23.

38. Lamberts SW, Bakker WH, Reubi JC et al. Somatostatin receptor imaging in the local-ization of endocrine tumors. N Engl J Med 1990; 323:1246–9.

Original description of somatostatin receptor scintigraphy (SRS).

39. Lamberts SW, Hofland LJ, van Koetsveld PM et al. Parallel in vivo and in vitro detection of functional somatostatin receptors in human endocrine pancreatic tumors: consequences with regard to diagnosis, localization and therapy. J Clin Endocrinol Metab 1990; 71:566–74.

40. Mirallie E, Pattou F, Maunoury V et al. Non-invasive imaging of insulinomas and gastrinomas with endoscopic ultrasonography and somato-statin receptor scintigraphy. Br J Surg 2001; 88:1272–6.

41. Kaltsas G, Korbonits M, Heintz E et al. Comparison of somatostatin analog and meta-iodobenzylguanidine radionuclides in the diagnosis and localisation of advanced neuro-endocrine tumors. J Clin Endo Metabol 2001; 86:895–902.

42. Virgolini I, Raderer M, Kurtaran A et al. Vasoactive intestinal peptide-receptor imaging for the localization of intestinal adenocarcinomas and endocrine tumors. N Engl J Med 1994; 331:1116–21.

43. Owens LV, Huth JF, Cance WG. Insulinoma: pitfalls in preoperative localization. Eur J Surg Oncol 1995; 21:326–8.

44. Thompson NW, Czako PF, Fritts LL et al. Role of endoscopic ultrasonography in the localization of insulinomas and gastrinomas. Surgery 1994; 116:1131–8.

45. Bottger TC, Junginger T. Is preoperative radiographic localization of islet cell tumors in patients with insulinoma necessary? World J Surg 1993; 17:427–32.

46. Heyder N. Localization of an insulinoma by ultrasonic endoscopy. N Engl J Med 1985; 312:860–1.

47. Glover JR, Shorvon PJ, Lees WR. Endoscopic ultrasound for localization of islet cell tumors. Gut 1992; 33:108–10.

48. Rosch T, Lightdale CJ, Botet JF et al. Localization of pancreatic endocrine tumors by endoscopic ultrasonography. N Engl J Med 1992; 326:1721–6.

Initial description of endoscopic ultrasound for the localisation of pancreatic endocrine tumours.

49. Bansal R, Tierney W, Carpenter S et al. Cost effectiveness of EUS for preoperative localization of pancreatic endocrine tumors. Gastrointest Endosc 1999; 49:19–25.

50. Richards M, Gauger PG, Thompson NW et al. Pitfalls in the surgical treatment of insulinoma. Surgery 2002; 132:1040–9.

51. Brown CK, Barlett DL, Doppman JL et al. Intra-arterial calcium stimulation and intraoperative

ultrasonography in the localization and resection of insulinomas. Surgery 1997; 122:1189–94.

52. Cohen MS, Picus D, Lairmore TC et al. Prospective study of provocative angiograms to localize functional islet cell tumors of the pancreas. Surgery 1997; 122:1091–100.

53. Brandle M, Pfammatter T, Spinas GA et al. Assessment of selective arterial calcium stimulation and hepatic venous sampling to localize insulin secreting tumours. Clin Endo 2001; 55:357–62.

54. Miller DL, Doppman JL, Metz DC et al. Zollinger–Ellison syndrome: technique, results, and complications of portal venous sampling. Radiology 1992; 182:235–41.

55. Norton JA, Cromack DT, Shawker TH et al. Intraoperative ultrasonographic localization of islet cell tumors. Ann Surg 1988; 207:160–8.

56. Boukhman MP, Karam JH, Shaver J et al. Insulinoma – experience from 1950 to 1995. West J Med 1998; 169:98–104.

57. Huai J, Zhang W, Niu H et al. Localization and surgical treatment of pancreatic insulinomas guided by intraoperative ultrasound. Am J Surg 1998; 175:18–21.

58. Hashimoto LA, Walsh RM. Preoperative localization of insulinomas is not necessary. J Am Coll Surg 1999; 189:368–73.

59. Norton JA. Intraoperative methods to stage and localize pancreatic and duodenal tumors. Ann Oncol 1999; 10(suppl. 4):182–4S.

60. Lo C, Lam K, Kung AWC et al. Pancreatic insulinomas – a 15-year experience. Arch Surg 1997; 132:926–30.

61. Buchler M, Friess H, Klempa I et al. Role of octreotide in the prevention of postoperative complications following pancreatic resection. Am J Surg 1992; 163:125–31.

62. Norton JA, Sigel B, Baker AR et al. Localization of an occult insulinoma by intraoperative ultra-sonography. Surgery 1985; 97:381–4.

63. Hiramoto JA, Feldstein VA, LaBerge JM et al. Intraoperative ultrasound and preoperative localisation detects all occult insulinomas. Arch Surg 2001; 136:1020–6.

    Results with intra-arterial calcium stimulation test and intraoperative ultrasound for localisation of insulinoma and successful surgical outcome.

64. Phan GQ, Yeo CJ, Cameron JL et al. Pancreatico-duodenectomy for selected periampullary neuro-endocrine tumors: fifty patients. Surgery 1997; 122:989–97.

65. Carneiro DM, Levi JU, Irvin GL. Rapid insulin assay for intraoperative confirmation of com-plete resection of insulinoma. Surgery 2002; 132:937–43.

66. Iihara M, Kanbe M, Okamoto T et al. Laparoscopic ultrasonography for resection of insulinomas. Surgery 2001; 130:1086–92.

67. Park AE, Heniford T. Therapeutic laparoscopy of the pancreas. Ann Surg 2002; 236:149–58.

68. Demeure MJ, Klonoff DC, Karam JH et al. Insulinomas associated with multiple endocrine neoplasia type 1: the need for a different surgical approach. Surgery 1991; 110:998–1004.

69. Sheppard BC, Norton JA, Doppman JL et al. Management of islet cell tumors in patients with multiple endocrine neoplasia: a prospective study. Surgery 1989; 106:1108–18.

70. O'Riordain DS, O'Brien T, van Heerden JA et al. Surgical management of insulinoma associated with multiple endocrine neoplasia type I. World J Surg 1994; 18:488–93.

71. Prove C, Pattou F, Carnaille B et al. Intra-operative insulin measurement during surgical management of insulinomas. World J Surg 1998; 22:1218–24.

72. Veldhuis JD, Norton JA, Wells SA et al. Thera-peutic controversy: surgical versus medical management of multiple endocrine neoplasia (MEN) type 1. J Clin Endocrinol Metab 1997; 82:357–64.

73. Dexter SPL, Martin IG, Leindler L et al. Laparoscopic enucleation of a solitary pancreatic insulinoma. Surg Endosc 1999; 13: 406–8.

74. Yoshida T, Bandoh T, Ninomiya K et al. Lapar-oscopic enucleation of a pancreatic insulinoma: report of a case. Surg Today 1998; 28:1188–91.

75. Vezakis A, Davides D, Larvin M et al. Laparoscopic surgery combined with preser-vation of the spleen for distal pancreatic tumors. Surg Endosc 1999; 13:26–9.

76. Gagner M, Pomp A, Herrera MF. Early experience with laparoscopic resections of islet cell tumors. Surgery 1996; 120:1051–4.

77. Service FJ, McMahon MM, O'Brien PC et al. Functioning insulinoma – incidence, recurrence, and long-term survival of patients: a 60-year study. Mayo Clin Proc 1991; 66:711–19.

78. Lange JR, Steinberg S, Doherty GM et al. A randomized prospective trial of postoperative somatostatin analogue in patients with neuro-endocrine tumors of the pancreas. Surgery 1992; 112:1033–8.

79. Eriksson B, Oberg K, Skogseid B. Neuro-endocrine pancreatic tumors: clinical findings in a prospective study of 84 patients. Acta Oncol 1989; 28:373–7.

80. Zollinger RM, Ellison EH. Primary peptic ulceration of the jejunum associated with islet cell tumors of the pancreas. Ann Surg 1955; 142:709–28.

81. Norton JA, Doppman JL, Jensen RT. Curative resection in Zollinger–Ellison syndrome: results of a 10 year prospective study. Ann Surg 1992; 215:8–18.

82. Wolfe MM, Jensen RT. Zollinger–Ellison syndrome, current concepts in diagnosis and management. N Engl J Med 1987; 317:1200–9.

83. Fox PS, Hofmann JW, DeCosse JJ et al. The influence of total gastrectomy on survival in malignant Zollinger–Ellison tumors. Ann Surg 1974; 180:558–66.

84. Zollinger RM, Ellison EC, O'Dorsio TM et al. Thirty years' experience with gastrinoma. World J Surg 1984; 8:427–35.

85. Fraker DL, Norton JA, Alexander HR et al. Surgery in Zollinger–Ellison syndrome alters the natural history of gastrinoma. Ann Surg 1994; 220:320–30.

86. Larsson H, Carlsson E, Matsson H. Plasma gastrin and gastric enterochromaffin cell activation and proliferation – studies with omeprazole and ranitidine in intact and adrenalectomized rats. Gastroenterology 1986; 90:391–9.

87. Yu F, Venzon DJ, Serrano J et al. Prospective study of the clinical course, prognostic factors, causes of death, and survival in patients with long-standing Zollinger–Ellison syndrome. J Clin Oncol 1999; 17:615–30.

88. Norton JA. Gastrinoma – advances in localization and treatment. Surg Oncol Clin North Am 1998; 7:845–61.

89. Thompson NW, Pasieka J, Fukuuchi A. Duodenal gastrinomas, duodenotomy, and duodenal exploration in the surgical management of Zollinger–Ellison syndrome. World J Surg 1993; 17: 455–62.

90. Sutliff VE, Doppman JL, Gibril F et al. Growth of newly diagnosed, untreated metastatic gastrinomas and predictors of growth patterns. J Clin Oncol 1997; 15:2420–31.

91. von Schrenck T, Howard JM, Doppman JL et al. Prospective study of chemotherapy in patients with metastatic gastrinoma. Gastroenterology 1988; 94:1326–34.

92. Wank SA, Doppman HL, Miller DL et al. Prospective study of the ability of computerized axial tomography to localize gastrinomas in patients with Zollinger–Ellison syndrome. Gastroenterology 1987; 92:905–12.

93. Semelka RC, Cumming MJ, Shoenut JP et al. Islet cell tumors: comparison of dynamic contrast-enhanced CT and MR imaging with dynamic gadolinium enhancement and fat suppression. Radiology 1993; 186:799–802.

94. Schirmer WJ, Melvin WS, Rush RM et al. ^{111}In-pentetreotide scanning versus conventional imaging techniques for the localization of gastrinoma. Surgery 1995; 118:1105–13.

95. Gibril F, Reynolds JC, Doppman JL et al. Somatostatin receptor scintigraphy: its sensitivity compared with that of other imaging methods in detecting primary and metastatic gastrinomas. Ann Intern Med 1996; 125:26–34.

96. Alexander HR, Fraker DL, Norton JA et al. Prospective study of somatostatin receptor scintigraphy and its effect on operative outcome in patients with Zollinger–Ellison syndrome. Ann Surg 1998; 228:228–38.

97. Meko JB, Doherty GM, Siegel BA et al. Evaluation of somatostatin-receptor scintigraphy for detecting neuroendocrine tumors. Surgery 1996; 120:975–84.

98. Gibril F, Reynolds JC, Chen CC et al. Specificity of somatostatin receptor scintigraphy: a prospective study and effects of false-positive localizations on management in patients with gastrinomas. J Nucl Med 1999; 40:539–53.

99. Proye C, Malvaux P, Pattou F et al. Noninvasive imaging of insulinomas and gastrinomas with endoscopic ultrasonography and somatostatin receptor scintigraphy. Surgery 1998; 124:1134–44.

100. Maton PN, Miller DL, Doppman HL et al. Role of selective angiography in the management of Zollinger–Ellison syndrome. Gastroenterology 1987; 92:913–19.

101. Thom AK, Norton JA, Axiotis CA et al. Location, incidence and malignant potential of duodenal gastrinomas. Surgery 1991; 110:1086–93.

102. Imamura M, Takahashi K. Use of selective arterial secretin injection test to guide surgery in patients with Zollinger–Ellison syndrome. World J Surg 1993; 17:433–8.

103. Perrier ND, Batts KP, Thompson GB et al. An immunohistochemical survey for neuro-endocrine cells in regional pancreatic lymph nodes – a plausible explanation for primary nodal gastrinomas. Surgery 1995; 118:957–65.

104. Norton JA, Alexander HR, Fraker DL et al. Possible primary lymph node gastrinomas: occurrence, natural history and predictive factors. Ann Surg 2003; 237:650–9.

105. Proye C, Pattou F, Carnaille B et al. Intra-operative gastrin measurements during surgical management of patients with gastrinomas: experience with 20 cases. World J Surg 1998; 22:643–50.

106. Stabile BE, Morrow DJ, Passaro E. The gastrinoma triangle: operative implications. Am J Surg 1984; 147:25–31.

107. Pipeleers-Marichal M, Donow C, Heitz PU et al. Pathologic aspects of gastrinomas in patients with Zollinger–Ellison syndrome with and without multiple endocrine neoplasia type I. World J Surg 1993; 17:481–8.

108. Thompson NW, Vinik AI, Eckhauser FE. Micro-gastrinomas of the duodenum. Ann Surg 1989; 209:396–404.

109. Frucht H, Norton JA, London JF et al. Detection of duodenal gastrinomas by operative endo-scopic transillumination, a prospective study. Gastroenterology 1990; 99:1622–7.

110. Howard TJ, Zinner MJ, Stabile BE et al. Gastrinoma excision for cure. Ann Surg 1990; 211:9–14.

111. Norton JA, Alexander HR, Fraker DL et al. Does the use of routine duodenotomy affect rate of cure, development of liver metastases, or survival in patients with Zollinger–Ellison syndrome? Ann Surg 2004 (in press).

Demonstrates that duodenotomy not only finds more gastrinomas, but increases the rate of cure.

112. Norton JA, Fraker DL, Alexander HR et al. Surgery to cure the Zollinger–Ellison syndrome. N Engl J Med 1999; 341:635–44.

Results of a prospective surgical trial to cure ZES.

113. Norton JA. Advances in the management of Zollinger–Ellison syndrome. Adv Surg 1994; 27:129–59.

114. Wolfe MM, Alexander RW, McGuigan JE. Extrapancreatic, extraintestinal gastrinoma: effective treatment by surgery. N Engl J Med 1982; 306:1533–6.

115. Norton JA, Doppman JL, Collen MJ et al. Prospective study of gastrinoma localization and resection in patients with Zollinger–Ellison syndrome. Ann Surg 1986; 204:468–79.

116. Bornman PC, Marks IN, Mee AS et al. Favourable response to conservative surgery for extra-pancreatic gastrinoma with lymph node metastases. Br J Surg 1987; 74:198–201.

117. Richardson CT, Peters MN, Feldman M. Treatment of Zollinger–Ellison syndrome with exploratory laparotomy, proximal gastric vagotomy, and H_2-receptor antagonists. Gastroenterology 1985; 89:357–67.

118. Wu PC, Alexander HR, Bartlett DL et al. A prospective analysis of the frequency, location, and curability of ectopic (nonpancreatico-duodenal, nonnodal) gastrinoma. Surgery 1997; 122:1176–82.

119. Noda S, Norton JA, Jensen RT et al. Surgical resection of intracardiac gastrinoma. Ann Thoracic Surg 1999; 67:532–3.

120. Ahn YJ, Kim SW, Park YC et al. Duodenal-preserving resection of the head of the pancreas and the pancreatic head resection with second-portion duodenectomy for benign lesions, low-grade malignancies, and early carcinoma involving the periampullary region. Arch Surg 2003; 138:162–8.

121. Kisker O, Bastian D, Bartsch D et al. Localization, malignant potential, and surgical management of gastrinomas. World J Surg 1998; 22:651–8.

122. Ellison EC. Forty year appraisal of gastrinoma: back to the future. Ann Surg 1995; 222: 11–21.

123. Norton JA, Sugarbaker PH, Doppman JL et al. Aggressive resection of metastatic disease in selected patients with malignant gastrinoma. Ann Surg 1986; 203:352–9.

124. Jaskowiak NT, Fraker DL, Alexander R et al. Is reoperation for gastrinoma excision indicated in Zollinger–Ellison syndrome? Surgery 1996; 120:1055–63.

125. Gibril F, Schumann M, Pace A et al. Multiple endocrine neoplasia type 1 and Zollinger–Ellison syndrome: a prospective study of 107 cases and comparison with 1009 cases from the literature. Medicine 2004; 83:43–83.

126. Norton JA, Cornelius MJ, Doppman JL et al. Effect of parathyroidectomy in patients with hyperparathyroidism, Zollinger–Ellison syn-drome, and multiple endocrine neoplasia type 1: a prospective study. Surgery 1987; 102:958–66.

127. Thompson NW. Surgical treatment of the endocrine pancreas and Zollinger–Ellison syndrome in the MEN I syndrome. Henry Ford Hosp Med J 1992; 40:195–8.

128. Macfarlane MP, Fraker DL, Alexander HR et al. A prospective study of surgical resection of duo-denal and pancreatic gastrinomas in MEN-1. Surgery 1995; 118:973–9.

129. Thompson NW. Current concepts in the surgical management of multiple endocrine neoplasia

type 1 pancreatic-duodenal disease. Results in the treatment of 40 patients with Zollinger–Ellison syndrome, hypoglycaemia or both. J Intern Med 1998; 243:495–500.

130. Thompson NW. Management of pancreatic endocrine tumors in patients with multiple endocrine neoplasia type I. Surg Oncol Clin North Am 1998; 7:881–91.

131. Brandi ML, Gagel RF, Angeli A et al. Consensus guidelines for diagnosis and therapy of MEN type 1 and type 2. J Clin Endocrinol Metab 2001; 86:5658–71.

132. Bornman PC, Beckingham IJ. ABC of diseases of liver, pancreas, and biliary system. Pancreatic tumors. Br Med J 2001; 322:721–3.

133. Chastain MA. The glucagonoma syndrome: a review of its features and discussion of new perspectives. Am J Med Sci 2001; 321:306–20.

134. Vinik AI, Strodel WE, Eckhauser FE et al. Somatostatinomas, PPomas, neurotensinomas. Semin Oncol 1987; 14:263.

135. Verner JV, Morrison AB. Endocrine pancreatic islet disease with diarrhea: report of a case due to diffuse hyperplasia of no beta islet tissue with a review of 54 additional cases. Arch Intern Med 1974; 133:492–9.

136. Capella C, Polak JM, Butta R et al. Morphologic patterns and diagnostic criteria of VIP-producing endocrine tumors. A histologic, histochemical, ultrastructural and biochemical study of 32 cases. Cancer 1983; 52:1860.

137. Caplan PH, Koob L, Abellera RM et al. Cure of acromegaly by operative removal of an islet cell tumor of the pancreas. Am J Med 1978; 64:874.

138. Bresler L, Boissel P, Conroy T et al. Pancreatic islet cell carcinoma with hypercalcemia: complete remission 5 years after surgical excision and chemotherapy. Am J Gastroenterol 1991; 86:635.

139. Hochwald SN, Weiser MR, Colleoni R et al. Laparoscopy predicts metastatic disease and spares laparotomy in selected patients with pancreatic nonfunctioning islet cell tumors. Ann Surg Oncol 2001; 8:249–53.

140. Danforth DN, Gorden P, Brennan MF. Metastatic insulin secreting carcinoma of the pancreas. Clinical course and the role of surgery. Surgery 1984; 96:1027–36.

141. Gibril F, Venzon DJ, Ojeaburu JV et al. Prospective study of the natural history of gastrinoma in patients with MEN1: definition of an aggressive and a nonaggressive form. J Clin Endocrinol Metab 2001; 86:5282–93.

142. Norton JA, Alexander HR, Fraker DL et al. Comparison of surgical results in patients with advanced and limited disease with multiple endocrine neoplasia type 1 and Zollinger–Ellison syndrome. Ann Surg 2001; 4:495–506.

143. Rothmund M, Stinner B, Arnold R. Endocrine pancreatic carcinoma. Eur J Surg Oncol 1991; 17:191–9.

144. Chu Q, Hill HC, Douglass HO et al. Predictive factors associated with long-term survival in patients with neuroendocrine tumors of the pancreas. Ann Surg Oncol 2002; 9:855–62.

145. Modlin IM, Lewis JJ, Ahlman H et al. Management of unresectable malignant endocrine tumors of the pancreas. Surg Gynecol Obstet 1993; 176:507–18.

146. Norton JA, Kivlen M, Li M et al. Morbidity and mortality of aggressive resection in patients with advanced neuroendocrine tumors. Arch Surg 2003; 138:859–66.

147. Zogakis TG, Norton JA. Palliative operations for patients with unresectable endocrine neoplasia. Surg Clin North Am 1995; 75:525–38.

148. Norton JA, Doherty GM, Fraker DL et al. Surgical treatment of localized gastrinoma within the liver: a prospective study. Surgery 1998; 124:1145–52.

149. Norton JA, Warren RS, Kelly MG et al. Aggressive surgery for metastatic liver neuroendocrine tumors. Surgery 2003; 134:1057–63.

150. Sarmiento JM, Que FG, Florencia G et al. Concurrent resections of pancreatic islet cell cancers with synchronous hepatic metastases: outcomes of an aggressive approach. Surgery 2002; 132:976–83.

151. Siperstein AE, Rogers SJ, Hansen PD et al. Laparoscopic thermal ablation of hepatic neuroendocrine tumor metastases. Surgery 1997; 122:1147–55.

152. Mulier S, Mulier P, Ni Y et al. Complications of radiofrequency coagulation of liver tumors. Brit J Surg 2002; 89:1206–22.

153. Sheen AJ, Poston J, Sherlock DJ. Cryotherapeutic ablation of liver tumours. Brit J Surg 2002; 89:1396–401.

154. Mozell E, Woltering EA, O'Dorisio TM et al. Effect of somatostatin analog on peptide release and tumor growth in the Zollinger–Ellison syndrome. Surg Gynecol Obstet 1990; 170:476–84.

155. Frank M, Klose KJ, Wied M et al. Combination therapy with octreotide and alpha-interferon: effect on tumor growth in metastatic endocrine

gastroenteropancreatic tumors. Am J Gastroenterol 1999; 94:1381–7.

156. Ohshio G, Hosotani R, Imamura M et al. Gastrinoma with multiple liver metastases: effectiveness of dacarbazine (DTIC) therapy. J Hepatobiliary Pancreat Surg 1998; 5:339–43.

157. Bilchik AJ, Sarantou T, Foshag LJ et al. Cryosurgical palliation of metastatic neuroendocrine tumors resistant to conventional therapy. Surgery 1997; 122:1040–8.

158. Mignon M, Ruszniewski R, Haffan S et al. Current approach to the management of the tumoral process in patients with gastrinoma. World J Surg 1986; 10:702–9.

Six

Gastrointestinal carcinoids

Göran Åkerström,
Per Hellman and
Ola Hessman

INTRODUCTION

In 1907 Oberndorfer first used the name carcinoid to describe rare ileal tumours with less malignant behaviour than common large bowel carcinomas. Subsequently it has become a common name for tumours derived from a widely distributed neuro-endocrine cell system, with a typical positive silver staining reaction termed argyrophilia. The carcinoids have been classified according to embryological origin into **foregut carcinoids** (lungs, thymus, stomach, duodenum, pancreas), **midgut carcinoids** (small bowel to proximal colon) and **hindgut carcinoids** (distal colon and rectum), and each of these tumour groups have displayed variable staining character-istics and clinical features. The midgut carcinoids, originating from intestinal enterochromaffin (EC) cells have been named classical carcinoids because of their positive argentaffin silver staining reaction (positive Masson stain), due to serotonin production in the tumour cells.

Carcinoids are relatively rare neuroendocrine tumours with an incidence of 1.2–2.1 per 100 000 population per year.[1-3] Nearly 70% of carcinoids occur in the gastrointestinal tract (**Table 6.1**).[4] Many carcinoids may be clinically silent since subclinical carcinoids have been detected at autopsy with an incidence of 8.4%.[4] Appendiceal carcinoids have been common in autopsy studies and previous clinical series,[1] although recent reports indicate an

Table 6.1 • Distribution of carcinoid tumours by site[3]

Site	Occurrence (%)
Extra-gastrointestinal (lung, thymic, ovary, uterus)	33
Oesophagus	<1
Stomach	4
Duodenum/pancreas	2
Small intestine	32
Appendix	8
Colon	10
Rectum	11

increased proportion of pulmonary, small intestinal and gastric carcinoids, mainly due to increased awareness and improved detection.[2,3]

Under a new classification the term 'carcinoid tumours' is reserved for classical midgut carcinoid tumours secreting serotonin, often demonstrated by specific immunoreactivity. Other types of carcinoids are named neuroendocrine tumours of the respec-tive organ of origin. They are further classified into the categories well-differentiated neuroendocrine tumours, well-differentiated endocrine carcinoma, poorly differentiated endocrine carcinomas, and mixed exocrine-endocrine tumours (**Box 6.1**).[5-7]

The classification is based on histological appearance, mitotic index (number of mitoses per 2 mm^2 or ten high-power fields), and proliferation index established by Ki67/Mib-1 antibody staining (against proliferation antigen).[8] The well-differentiated tumours have a low rate of mitosis and low proliferation index (generally <2%). Most poorly differentiated tumours have an increased rate of mitosis and higher proliferation index of around 20–40%, but a subgroup has intermediate proliferation with an index of 5–15%, indicating variable rate of tumour progression. The Ki67 proliferation index has become of increased importance in clinical planning. Extensive surgery is more likely to be beneficial for differentiated tumours with low proliferation, in contrast to chemotherapy, which generally has little effect in low proliferating typical carcinoids. Chromogranin A and synaptophysin immunostains, which identify proteins of neurosecretory granules, are now commonly used instead of silver stains to identify the neuroendocrine tumours. Antibodies against cytosolic markers – neurone-specific enolase (NSE) and PGP9.5 – have also been used for identification of certain tumours, but have generally not been as specific.[9] For poorly differentiated lesions chromogranin staining may be variable and involve only subsets of cells. Synaptophysin reactivity alone in the absence of chromogranin staining may indicate an exocrine tumour with endocrine differentiation, or a so-called mixed exocrine-endocrine carcinoma. Dominant secretion (e.g. serotonin, histamine, gastrin, somatostatin) may also be detected in neuroendocrine tumours, and occasionally ectopic hormone production, such as adrenocorticotropic hormone (ACTH) and corticotropin-releasing factor (CRF), is seen. The latter two sometimes cause an ectopic Cushing's syndrome in association with foregut carcinoids (**Table 6.2**).[9]

This chapter will for clarity utilise the common older classification, and the term midgut carcinoids will mainly refer to the majority of jejunoileal tumours.

Box 6.1 • Alternative classification of endocrine tumours, including the carcinoids[5]

Well-differentiated neuroendocrine tumour (carcinoid)

Benign behaviour: confined to mucosa-submucosa, non-angioinvasive, ≤1 cm in size and non-functioning.

Uncertain behaviour: confined to mucosa-submucosa, >1 cm in size or angioinvasive.

Well-differentiated endocrine carcinoma (malignant carcinoid)

Low-grade malignant, deeply invasive (muscularis propria or beyond) or with metastases.

Non-functioning or **functioning**

Poorly differentiated endocrine carcinoma – small-cell carcinoma

High-grade malignant, usually non-functioning (occasionally with ectopic Cushing's syndrome).

Mixed exocrine-endocrine tumours

Table 6.2 • Classification of carcinoid tumours, hormone production and syndromes[9]

Category	Localisation	Hormone production*	Syndrome
Foregut carcinoids	Thymus	ACTH, CRF	Ectopic Cushing's syndrome, acromegaly, atypical carcinoid syndrome
	Lung	ACTH, CRF, ADH, GRH, gastrin, PP, hCG-α/β, serotonin	
	Stomach	Gastrin, histamine (serotonin)	Atypical carcinoid syndrome
	Duodenum	Gastrin, somatostatin	Zollinger–Ellison syndrome
	Pancreas	(Serotonin)	(Carcinoid syndrome)
Midgut carcinoids	Jejunum-ileum	Serotonin, NKA	Classical carcinoid syndrome
	Prox. colon	Substance P, bradykinin, prostaglandins	
	Appendix	No hormone production (serotonin)	(Carcinoid syndrome)
Hindgut carcinoids	Colon	PYY	
	Rectum	hCG-α/β	

*ACTH, adrenocorticotropic hormone; ADH, antidiuretic hormone (vasopressin); CRF, corticotropin-releasing factor; GRH, growth hormone; hCG, human choriogonadotropin (α/β subunits); NKA, neurokinin A; PP, pancreatic polypeptide; PYY, peptide YY.

Patients with any of the carcinoid tumours may be at increased risk for a second malignancy, mainly colorectal cancers, but also breast and prostate carcinoma, and although this has been disputed it should be considered during long-term patient follow-up.

OESOPHAGEAL CARCINOIDS

Oesophageal carcinoids are exceedingly rare, and occur with male predominance at an age of around 60 years.[10] Most tumours are found in the lower third of the oesophagus or in the gastro-oesophageal junction. Symptoms are non-specific and similar to adenocarcinoma or squamous carcinoma, and patients rarely exhibit a carcinoid syndrome. Lymph node metastases have been present at diagnosis in 50% of patients; survival correlates with stage of the disease, and overall is poor.

GASTRIC CARCINOIDS

Gastric carcinoids are rare tumours, constituting less than 1% of gastric neoplasms and approximately 4–5% of all carcinoids (**Table 6.1**).[3,10] Most of these tumours are derived from argyrophilic enterochromaffin-like (ECL) cells of the gastric fundus and corpus. The majority of gastric carcinoids occur secondary to hypergastrinaemia in patients with chronic atrophic gastritis (CAG). These carcinoids are typically multicentric and develop concomitant with ECL cell hyperplasia in the fundus and corpus, or occasionally in the transitional zone to the antrum[11] (**type 1 gastric carcinoids**). Similar non-antral and multicentric argyrophilic carcinoids and ECL cell hyperplasia have less frequently been diagnosed in patients with hypergastrinaemia and multiple endocrine neoplasia type 1 (MEN 1)-related Zollinger–Ellison syndrome (ZES) (**type 2 gastric carcinoids**). More uncommon are gastric carcinoids that develop as sporadic, generally solitary tumours, without concomitant argyrophilic cell hyperplasia (**type 3 gastric carcinoids**). The sporadic carcinoids are often larger when detected, and more frequently associated with metastases. Like the other gastric carcinoids, the sporadic tumours most often develop from ECL cells, but may also originate in argentaffin (serotonin-producing) cells, or contain a mixture with other endocrine cell types. The ECL cells have the ability to secrete histamine, and disseminated lesions of the solitary type may occasionally be associated with an atypical carcinoid syndrome. Exceptionally prepyloric or antral sporadic tumours may produce gastrin and should be named gastrinoma. Another group of gastric neuroendocrine tumours consists of undifferentiated tumours, composed of intermediate-size or small cells – **type 4 gastric carcinoids** (**poorly differentiated neuroendocrine carcinoma**).

The incidence of gastric carcinoids has increased, due to more frequent gastroscopic examinations, as during population screening for gastric cancer, or when screening studies have been performed in patients with atrophic gastritis or pernicious anemia.[11]

Histology

Different histological patterns have been defined in ECL hyperplasia, and used to depict the stepwise progression through dysplasia to formation of carcinoid tumours.[7,11–13] **Simple or diffuse hyperplasia** is defined as increased density of often hypertrophic, argyrophilic ECL cells; **linear hyperplasia** consists of ECL cell trabeculae along the basement membrane or gastric glands; **micronodular hyperplasia** depicts clusters or nodules of such cells, and is together with linear hyperplasia common in CAG patients with advanced hypergastrinaemia; **adenomatoid hyperplasia** consists of collections of several micronodules often found in cases with CAG or MEN 1-ZES.

Dysplastic or precarcinoid ECL cell lesions also appear with different histological patterns, but generally consist of larger collections of slightly atypical endocrine cells with enlarged nuclei and reduced reactivity for secretory granule markers. These lesions are non-invasive, and do not infiltrate beyond the muscularis mucosae, but constitute markers for neoplastic alterations, since they coexist with carcinoids in CAG and MEN 1-ZES.[14,15]

When nodules are larger than 0.5 mm the lesions are classified as **carcinoid tumours**. Gastric carcinoids are generally composed of regular-shaped tumour cells with round nuclei and mainly characterised by microlobules and trabeculae. In histological grading grades 1 and 2 correspond to 'typical' and 'atypical' carcinoids, and grade 3 to the poorly differentiated neuroendocrine carcinomas.[6] Mitoses are absent or rare in **grade 1** lesions, occur with cellular atypia in **grade 2**, and are abundant with poor differentiation, severe atypia, and cell necroses in **grade 3**.[6]

ECL cell tumours are strongly agyrophilic and immunoreactive to chromogranin A and histamine, and can be identified with the specific marker vesicular monoamine transporter isoform 2 (VMAT2).[16,17] Immunoreactivity to hormonal products such as serotonin, gastrin, somatostatin, pancreatic polypeptide (PP) or α-subunit of human choriogonadotropin (hCG-α) is absent or focal.[7] Grade 1 lesions with a proliferation index <1–2%, size less than 1 cm, and no invasion beyond the mucosa, are mostly benign, whereas tumours with histological grade 2 and 3, size ≥3 cm, and with higher mitotic and proliferation index (Ki67 >5%), are more commonly malignant.[6]

Type 1: gastric carcinoids associated with chronic atrophic gastritis

These tumours account for 70–80% of gastric carcinoids (**Table 6.3**). They occur occasionally in young individuals, but most commonly in older patients, with a mean age around 65 years, and there is a 3:1 female to male predominance.[18]

The carcinoids develop in patients with autoimmune CAG type A,[11,19,20] where atrophy of the fundic mucosa is accompanied by pentagastrin-resistant achlorhydria and vitamin B_{12} malabsorption. More than half of the patients also have pernicious anaemia (**Table 6.3**). Reduction of gastric acid and increase in pH stimulates gastrin secretion from gastrin (G) cells in the antrum, and the resulting hypergastrinaemia induces hyperplasia of the fundic ECL cells. Diffuse argyrophilic hyperplasia of the non-antral mucosa occurs in 65% of patients with CAG, and micronodular/adenomatoid hyperplasia in 30%, whereas the precarcinoid and dysplastic, enlarged micronodules develop mainly in patients with gross carcinoids. The tumour development progresses from the specified stages of hyperplasia, through dysplastic stages, to neoplastic intramucosal or invasive carcinoids.[13]

It is important to emphasise that, although CAG is common in elderly individuals, only a few affected patients (4–7%) ultimately develop gastric carcinoids. The tumours occur mainly in patients with a long duration of a markedly raised serum gastrin, and who have more prevalent hyperplastic changes. The CAG-associated carcinoids contain predominantly ECL cells, intermingled with other specific or poorly defined endocrine cells.

Table 6.3 • Gastric carcinoid tumours[10]

	Type 1 (70–80%)	Type 2 (6–8%)	Type 3 (20%)
Description	Chronic atrophic gastritis (type A), pernicious anaemia, autoimmune disorders	MEN 1-associated Zollinger–Ellison syndrome	Sporadic
Tumour site in stomach	Fundus and body	Fundus and body	Fundus, body and antrum
Characteristics	Usually multiple polyps (often <1 cm, occasionally 1–2 cm)	Usually multiple (<1–2 cm), occasionally larger	Single, solitary (2–5 cm)
Histopathology*/ gastric fundal biopsy	ECL-cell lesion; progression: hyperplasia-dysplasia-neoplasia	ECL-cell lesion; progression: hyperplasia-dysplasia-neoplasia	ECL-, EC- or other cells; normal adjacent mucosa
Biological behaviour	Slow growth, rarely metastasise	Usually slow growth, metastases relatively infrequent	Relatively aggressive, frequent metastases to regional nodes (55%) and liver (24%)
Plasma gastrin	Elevated	Elevated	Normal
Acid output	Low or absent	High	Normal or low

*EC, enterochromaffin; ECL, enterochromaffin-like.

The argyrophilic gastric carcinoids are predominantly located within the body or the fundus of the stomach or in the transitional zone to the antrum.[20–22] They are frequently multicentric, consisting of multiple, small gastric polyps and invariably associated with ECL cell hyperplasia and microscopic tumours. The number of gross lesions can, however, be limited and some tumours may thus appear as solitary. Individual tumours can present as broad-based, round polypoid lesions, reddish to yellowish, depending on the thickness of the covering mucosa. Some carcinoids can be flat and broad, or appear as discoloured spots or simply as slight mucosal protrusions. Only a few are ulcerated or bleeding. The number and size vary from innumerable pinpoint-size tumours to a few or solitary prominent lesions ranging from a few millimetres up to 1–1.5 cm, and only occasionally larger tumours (>2 cm). The tumours are generally benign, without signs of invasion beyond the submucosa. Infiltration of the muscularis propria is found in a minority (<10%).[18] The polypoid carcinoids may be difficult to distinguish from hyperplastic polyps, which are also more frequent in patients with CAG.

CAG-associated carcinoids have a lower incidence of metastases and more favourable outcome than other types of gastric carcinoids. Metastases to regional lymph nodes are found in less than 5%, and distant metastases in fewer than 2%.[18,23] However, earlier reports with a greater proportion of large lesions described more frequent metastases.[24] Disease-related deaths are rare.

Occasional CAG patients have harboured larger, considerably more invasive tumours, representing poorly differentiated neuroendocrine carcinomas or composite endocrine tumours/adenocarcinoma (see below). All these have an unfavourable prognosis.

Type 2: carcinoids associated with ZES in MEN 1 patients

These gastric carcinoids constitute 6–8%[10] of all gastric carcinoids, and are thus much less common than those associated with atrophic gastritis (Table 6.3). They occur in patients with MEN 1 and gastrin-producing tumours as a cause of ZES, with equal female:male distribution, at a mean age of 45–50 years.[21]

ECL cell hyperplasia is found in almost 80% of MEN 1 patients with ZES, and fundic gastric carcinoids develop in up to 15–30% of these patients.[18,25,26] In addition to the hyperplasia and dysplasia of ECL cells in the fundic mucosa, the oxyntic mucosal thickness is invariably increased, in contrast to the atrophy of type 1 lesions. These carcinoids also develop in a hyperplasia-dysplasia-neoplasia sequence, but have mainly been associated with diffuse hyperplasia and precarcinoid lesions, and less evident micronodular changes. However, gastric carcinoids in sporadic ZES have been rare, and only ZES in association with MEN 1 seems to promote growth of gastric carcinoids.[27] The MEN 1 syndrome is caused by an inherited mutation of the *MEN1* tumour suppressor gene located on chromosome 11q13.[28] As in other MEN 1 lesions, the gastric carcinoids in MEN 1 lose their single remaining functional copy of the *MEN1* gene by chromosomal deletions.[29] In MEN 1 patients without ZES, gastric carcinoids are extremely rare.[30] Thus, hypergastrinaemia seems to be required for development of gastric carcinoids from ECL hyperplasia. However, additional factors are obviously needed for tumour formation, since only around 5% of patients with hypergastrinaemia due to atrophic gastritis and few patients with sporadic ZES develop gastric carcinoids.[20,31–33]

The type 2 gastric carcinoids are located in the gastric body and fundus and have been composed mainly of ECL cells with occasional other cell types. They are most often multicentric and small (73% have been smaller than 1.5 cm), although often larger than type 1 tumours, with a size varying from 0.5 mm to 3–4 cm. Occasionally there are markedly larger tumours.[18] The malignant potential is intermediate between that of CAG-associated gastric carcinoids and sporadic carcinoids, and 90% will not have infiltrated beyond the submucosa. However, lymph node metastases have been present in up to 30% of the patients,[18] and distant metastases, assumed to originate from gastric carcinoids, have occurred in around 10%.[18,34] It needs to be emphasised that MEN 1 patients develop distant metastases from other MEN 1-associated tumours as well, and thus these may not always originate from the gastric carcinoids.[35] The overall prognosis will depend more on the other MEN 1 lesions, and the prognosis is usually rather favourable for the type 2 carcinoids.[27] However, rare cases of highly malignant neuroendocrine gastric carcinomas with poor prognosis have also occurred in some MEN 1 ZES patients.[30]

Type 3: sporadic carcinoid tumours

Tumours with no association to hypergastrinaemia account for 20% of the gastric carcinoids and have features that markedly differ from type 1 and type 2 lesions (**Table 6.3**).[21] They occur sporadically, are most often solitary, and grow much more aggressively. Many are already disseminated at diagnosis.[21] These carcinoids have a male predominance, with a male:female ratio of 3:1; mean age of presentation is reportedly around 50 years. The sporadic gastric carcinoids occur in non-atrophic gastric mucosa, without endocrine cell proliferation. Determination of serum calcium and examination of the family history may help exclude the MEN 1 syndrome, which should be suspected in all patients with foregut carcinoids unrelated to atrophic gastritis.

The sporadic tumours are often large; one-third exceed 2 cm (**Fig. 6.1**). Two-thirds of the lesions will have infiltrated the muscularis propria, and 50% invaded all layers of the gastric wall.[18] Some tumours occur in the antral, prepyloric regions, although the majority are located in the body and fundus of the stomach. Most tumours originate in argyrophilic ECL cells, but a mixture of other cell types and EC cells may be present, and are associated with a less favourable prognosis. Regional lymph node metastases have been described in 20–50% of the patients, and liver metastases have ultimately developed in two-thirds of the patients. Half of patients are alive after follow-up of 5 years,[18,23] but patients with distant metastases have a 10% 5-year survival.[3]

The sporadic carcinoids may have typical or atypical histology. Atypical implies marked nuclear pleomorphism with irregular hyperchromatic nuclei, increased number of mitoses, and frequent areas of necrosis. The atypical tumours are larger, more frequently invasive, and commonly associated with metastases at diagnosis.[6] A series of sporadic gastric carcinoids with atypical morphology reported a mean size of 5 cm and unfavourable survival.[36]

An **atypical carcinoid syndrome** has developed in 5–10% of the patients with sporadic gastric carcinoids, and has been associated with tumour release of histamine. The syndrome is characterised by bright-red cutaneous flushing, often with a patchy 'geographic' distribution, cutaneous oedema, intense itching, bronchospasm, salivary gland swelling, and lacrimation.[10,21] The atypical carcinoid syndrome is related to histamine secretion, and urinary estimates of the histamine metabolite methylimidazoleacetic acid (MelmAA) may serve as tumour marker. Most gastric carcinoid tumours are deficient in the enzyme L-amino acid-decarboxylase, and only a few patients have elevated levels of serotonin. Urinary excretion of the serotonin metabolite 5-hydroxyindoleacetic acid (5-HIAA) is therefore less appropriate as a tumour marker.[22] However, the precursor 5-hydroxytryptophan (5-HTP) may be excreted and partly decarboxylated in the kidney, and the patients with disseminated sporadic gastric carcinoids may exhibit some elevated urinary 5-HIAA values.

GASTRINOMA

Tumours with sparse staining for gastrin may occur in association with chronic atrophic gastritis. Tumours with intense positive staining for gastrin are rare in the stomach, and have been located in the antropyloric mucosa close to the duodenum. Few gastric carcinoids have caused hypergastrinaemia and peptic ulcer disease, but they still represent an exceptional but possible origin of gastrin excess and ZES.[22]

Figure 6.1 • Sporadic, solitary gastric carcinoid with lymph gland metastasis removed by gastric resection.

Type 4: poorly differentiated neuroendocrine carcinomas

The poorly differentiated neuroendocrine carcinomas are highly malignant neoplasms, with generally extensive local invasion and metastases already at diagnosis. They are not associated with the carcinoid syndrome, and occur at a mean age of 60–70 years, with male predominance.[18,37] Atrophic gastritis has been revealed in half of the patients, but is not believed to cause the tumour, since only a minority of patients have hypergastrinaemia.[18] The majority of tumours are located in the gastric corpus or fundus, but 10–20% may occur in the antrum.[18,37] The tumours are generally large, with median size of around 4–5 cm,[18] invariably deeply invading the gastric wall and associated with metastases. The majority of lesions appear as ulcerated tumours, and a quarter are fungating.[37] They all tend to be of histological grade 3, and often have solid structures with necroses, a high degree of atypia, frequent mitoses, and high proliferation index in Ki67 staining (generally around 20–40%). Almost all tumours show vascular and perineural invasion. In contrast to the well-differentiated gastric carcinoids, the poorly differentiated neuroendocrine carcinomas may have sparse immunoreactivity to chromogranin A, at least in the majority of tumour cells.[6] Immunoreactivity to synaptophysin (and possibly NSE or PGP9.5) may verify the neuroendocrine differentiation and separate these tumours from exocrine carcinomas. The prognosis is poor with a median survival of 8 months, albeit some individuals are reported to be still alive after follow-up of 10–15 years.[6,18,37]

The possibility of progression from well-differentiated gastric carcinoids, especially type 3 lesions, to neuroendocrine carcinomas has been suggested by a few cases with coexisting well- and poorly differentiated gastric neuroendocrine tumours.[6,7,30]

Aberration of the p53 tumour suppressor gene, and chromosomal deletion of the long arm of chromosome 18, have been common in poorly differentiated neuroendocrine carcinomas, and occasionally found also in type 3 sporadic gastric carcinoids.[6] These genetic defects occur in gastro-intestinal exocrine carcinomas and may promote aggressive tumour growth. Genetic studies of rare mixed neuroendocrine/exocrine gastric carcinomas have indicated that the endocrine tumour component may originate in adenocarcinoma cells.[38]

Clinical evaluation

SYMPTOMS AND PATIENT HISTORY

The majority of gastric carcinoids found in elderly patients with atrophic gastritis are detected incidentally by gastroscopy evaluation for anaemia or uncharacteristic abdominal symptoms, or by routine endoscopic screening. Minimal bleeding and anaemia may occur from these carcinoids, generally the larger, mainly sporadic carcinoids. The largest of these tumours may cause more obvious bleeding, and the poorly differentiated tumours especially may mimic gastric carcinoma, with gastric outlet obstruction. Some become apparent because of metastases, and a few disseminated sporadic carcinoids present with the atypical carcinoid syndrome.

Patient history should explore the presence of CAG or pernicious anaemia or MEN 1-related endocrinopathies (hyperparathyroidism, endocrine pancreatic or pituitary tumours) both in the patient and family members.

DIAGNOSIS

Diagnosis of CAG carcinoids is based on demonstration of high levels of serum gastrin, lack of gastric acid secretion, and demonstration of atrophy of the oxyntic mucosa, with concomitant ECL cell hyperplasia in mucosal biopsies from the fundus (Table 6.3). The serum levels of gastrin are also high in patients with MEN 1 gastrinomas, although these patients have contrasting high gastric acidity.

Thorough gastroscopic examination should be performed to evaluate multiplicity and size of the carcinoid tumours. Tumour biopsies should be stained with specific endocrine tumour markers and proliferation markers (chromogranin A, Ki67 staining), and should carefully investigate infiltrative depth, and possible vascular invasion. In addition, multiple biopsies from the fundus region, away from the tumour(s), are crucial to reveal concomitant ECL cell hyperplasia or dysplasia, the presence of atrophic gastritis, or the contrasting increased oxyntic mucosa thickness of rare MEN 1 ZES (**Table 6.3**). Multiple carcinoid polyps in the gastric fundus in an elderly individual is most likely to represent CAG-associated carcinoids, since MEN 1-associated carcinoids are rare. A larger, solitary tumour is more likely to be sporadic (**Fig. 6.1**), and the largest ulcerating and most prominent lesions may be poorly differentiated. Endoscopic ultrasound added to the gastroscopic examination may give information about infiltrative depth and reveal associated lesions in the pancreas or duodenum in MEN 1 patients, and possibly also show metastases to regional lymph nodes or the liver.[39]

Biochemical screening for other MEN 1 endocrinopathies should include analysis of serum calcium and parathyroid hormone, pituitary related hormones such as growth hormone, prolactin and insulin-like growth factor 1 (IGF-1), and pancreatic hormones (**Box 6.2**). For cases with the atypical carcinoid syndrome, screening should include urinary analysis of the histamine metabolite MelmAA.[11] Serum values of chromogranin A are generally raised in patients with CAG and ECL hyperplasia. These values are also the most important tumour markers, and since they tend to reflect the tumour load, they are often used to monitor patients undergoing treatment for advanced gastric carcinoids.[34,40]

Computed tomography (CT) with contrast enhancement is routinely performed for tumour delineation and to detect regional lymph node or liver metastases. Scintigraphy using ^{111}In-octreotide scintigraphy (OctreoScan) can often efficiently reveal metastatic spread from differentiated carcinoids.[41]

Box 6.2 • Biochemical screening for the MEN-1 syndrome (serum estimates)

- Serum calcium
- Parathyroid hormone
- Chromogranin A
- Pancreatic polypeptide (PP)
- Gastrin
- Insulin, proinsulin/glucose
- Glucagon
- Prolactin
- Somatomedin C (IGF-1)

Treatment

CAG-ASSOCIATED TYPE 1 GASTRIC CARCINOIDS

These may disappear spontaneously, and few show more marked progression.[22,31,42–44] Small, multicentric lesions may be followed with repeated endoscopy.

Carcinoids up to 1 cm are generally indolent, with minimal risk for invasion, and can be treated by endoscopic polypectomy, if histopathology excludes deep gastric wall invasion. Follow-up with gastroscopy is needed to exclude persistence or recurrence. Treatment of tumours measuring 1–2 cm has been equivocal because of low-grade malignancy, but surgical excision is often recommended, since this implies reduced risk of recurrence, and offers the possibility of removing regional lymph node metastases.[21–23,42] Tumours >2 cm should be removed surgically, generally by subtotal gastric resection. Gastrectomy is considered for rare invasive large tumours, or multifocal larger lesions if they appear difficult to excise with clear margins.

Antrectomy has been recommended for treatment of CAG-associated gastric carcinoids, with the aim of inhibiting antral overproduction of gastrin.[45,46] The antrectomy may cause regression of ECL dysplasia and small carcinoids, whereas large, invasive or metastatic lesions invariably remain unaffected.[45,47,48] Resection of the antrum may therefore be considered for multicentric or recurrent tumour, and is often combined with surgical excision of larger type 1 carcinoids, but results and morbidity of this versus repeated endoscopic excision remain unclear.[23,49]

MEN 1-RELATED TYPE 2 GASTRIC CARCINOIDS

These are more malignant than CAG-associated carcinoids. Surgical treatment should focus both on removal of the source of hypergastrinaemia and on excision of the gastric carcinoids. Concomitant exposure of both pancreas and duodenum, via duodenotomy, is done to locate both gastrinomas and possible MEN 1 pancreatic lesions, and 80% distal pancreatic resection is most often performed.[50] Gastric carcinoids per se may be treated as type 1 lesions, implying endoscopic removal of tumours smaller than 1 cm, but liberal surgical excision or gastric resection with regional lymph node clearance is advocated for larger tumours.[21]

Total gastrectomy may occasionally be required for larger tumours[51] although gastrin excess in MEN 1 gastrinoma is generally efficiently treated by proton-pump inhibitors.

SPORADIC TYPE 3 GASTRIC CARCINOIDS

These are even more malignant, with a high risk of metastases. Most tumours are large and require operative excision, often performed as gastric resection, combined with regional lymph node clearance. Tumours >2 cm or those with atypical histology or gastric wall invasion are most appropriately dealt with by gastrectomy.[22,23]

In cases with metastases, tumour debulking of lymph gland and liver metastases may alleviate symptoms of an associated carcinoid syndrome and apparently improve survival.[21] Hepatic metastases may be treated with liver resection, hepatic artery embolisation or chemoembolisation, and radio frequency (RF) ablation (see below). The somatostatin analogue octreotide may palliate symptoms in patients with the carcinoid syndrome. Chemotherapy is likely to be valuable when the proliferation index exceeds 5%, and has response rates of 20–40%. Chemotherapy can be combined with other treatment modalities.[52]

TYPE 4 POORLY DIFFERENTIATED NEUROENDOCRINE TUMOURS

These generally have a dismal prognosis, with a median survival of only 8 months.[6,18] The tumours are rarely suitable for radical surgery and recurrence should be checked for after gastric resection. However, aggressive surgery together with chemotherapy may be an option to consider, especially in patients with mixtures of well- and poorly differentiated tumours.[6]

DUODENAL CARCINOIDS

Carcinoids of the duodenum are rare, and comprise less than 2% of all gastrointestinal neuroendocrine

tumours.[22,53] Duodenal adenomas or adenocarcinomas are much more frequent. However, the endocrine tumours are important to recognise because of a possible association with hormonal or hereditary syndromes and the consequential requirements of treatment. Duodenal carcinoids are so rare that it is difficult to identify prognostic factors and decide optimal treatment on an evidence base.

Gastrinomas

Gastrinomas are the most prevalent and constitute 60% of the duodenal neuroendocrine tumours; the most common of these are argyrophil duodenal tumours with typical carcinoid features.[53,54] Most gastrinomas are located in the first and second parts of the duodenum. They are frequently small (often around 0.5 cm or smaller), with early metastases to regional lymph nodes reported in 30–70% of patients.[18,54–58] The regional lymph node metastases may be considerably larger than the primary tumours, which sometimes may be difficult to detect even at operation. There is generally considerable delay before liver metastases develop, and this is claimed to provide a favourable interval for surgical treatment.[57] One-third of duodenal gastrinomas are associated with clinical ZES; the remainder may be clinically silent and found fortuitously in surgical specimens by their intense gastrin immunoreactivity. It has been recognised that 40–60% of gastrinomas responsible for ZES are located within the duodenal submucosa.[55–58] MEN 1/ZES patients have, in nearly 90% of cases, multifocal duodenal gastrinomas.[59–61] The duodenal gastrinomas in ZES are slow-growing, indolent malignancies despite their tendency to spread with local lymph node metastases. Duodenal gastrinomas in ZES are rarely identified by endoscopy because of their small size, and they are also often difficult to visualise during surgery. Endoscopic transillumination has been advocated, but it is more efficient to perform a long duodenotomy, allowing discovery of gastrinomas after inversion and palpation of the duodenal mucosa.[55,60]

Duodenal tumours smaller than 5 mm can be enucleated with the overlying mucosa, larger tumours are excised with full thickness of the duodenal wall. Careful exploration is undertaken for the removal of lymph gland metastases around the pancreatic head. The duodenal gastrinoma has been considered as a potentially curable entity of ZES, especially for non-MEN 1 ZES. The prognosis is favourable after resection of duodenal gastrinomas in both sporadic and MEN 1/ZES patients, with survival reaching 60–85% after 10 years.[56,59]

Somatostatin-rich carcinoids

Carcinoids with somatostatin reactivity comprise 15–20% of duodenal neuroendocrine tumours. These tumours are most often clinically hormonally non-functioning.[53,54,62–64] They occur almost exclusively in the ampulla of Vater, causing obstructive jaundice, pancreatitis or bleeding. The tumours appear as 1–2-cm homogeneous ampulla nodules, which only occasionally are polypoid, larger or ulcerated. Regional lymph node or liver metastases are present in nearly 50% of patients. Unlike conventional carcinoids, these tumours have a glandular growth pattern and characteristically contain special laminated psammoma bodies. They are neither argyrophilic nor argentaffin but can be identified with special silver staining or chromogranin stain. One-third of these lesions are associated with von Recklinghausen's neurofibromatosis (neurofibromatosis type 1, NF1) and occasionally with phaeochromocytoma.[63] Depending on the size of the tumours and the age of the patient, the somatostatin-rich carcinoids may be locally excised or removed by pancreatico-duodenectomy.

Gangliocytic paragangliomas

Gangliocytic paragangliomas are rare tumours, occurring almost exclusively in the second portion of the duodenum, and are sometimes associated with neurofibromatosis (NF1).[54,65] The tumours consist of a mixture of paraganglioma, ganglioneuroma and carcinoid tissue with reactivity for somatostatin and PP. The tumours are generally benign, recognised only incidentally or because of bleeding, and have an excellent prognosis following surgical excision.

Other carcinoids

More unusual well-differentiated duodenal carcinoids may display reactivity for other hormones, such as calcitonin, pancreatic polypeptide (PP) and serotonin.[66,67] Most of these tumours are found in the proximal part of the duodenum as small polyps (<2 cm). Multiple tumours should raise suspicion of an associated MEN 1 syndrome. The majority of these tumours are low-grade malignant and often suitable for local surgical excision. Only rarely do large tumours require pancreatico-duodenectomy.

A distinct group of duodenal carcinoids without release or staining for hormones is also recognised. These tumours have a somewhat different biology and have less often metastasised than the gastrinomas and somatostatinomas.[68] Some of them are asymptomatic and incidentally found at endoscopic examination. Others present with non-specific abdominal symptoms, gastrointestinal bleeding, and sometimes with vomiting or weight loss.[68] Most tumours are located in the first portion of the duodenum, occasionally in the second part and rarely in the third portion (horizontal duodenum). The majority stain for chromogranin A, and some for synaptophysin and/or NSE.[68] Up to one-third of the patients have had other primary malignancies as well, including adenocarcinomas of the gastrointestinal tract, prostate or other organs.[68]

More than half of the tumours are smaller than 2 cm, and generally have a good prognosis after resection. Size >2 cm, invasion beyond the submucosa, or presence of mitotic figures are independent risk factors for metastases.[53] Tumours with these risk factors are likely to recur also after apparently curative surgery, even if no lymph node metastases have been detected, whereas lesions smaller than 2 cm rarely metastasise.[68]

Lesions smaller than 1 cm can possibly be endoscopically excised, but re-examination with follow-up endoscopy is required to ensure complete removal.[68] Tumours smaller than 2 cm, without signs of invasion of the muscularis, can be safely treated by open local excision. The treatment suggested for larger tumours is segmental resection or pancreatico-duodenectomy in order to decrease the risk of recurrence.[68] Periampullary tumours behave in a malignant fashion and need more radical surgery. Patients with metastasising duodenal carcinoids may survive for decades, substantiating that these neuroendocrine tumours are less aggressive than adenocarcinomas.

Neuroendocrine carcinomas

Poorly differentiated neuroendocrine carcinomas in the duodenum are exceptionally rare. Most occur in the ampulla of Vater, and the patients present with obstructive jaundice, and invariably with a rapidly fatal course.[22]

Pancreatic carcinoids

Pancreatic islet cell tumours, are generally classified according to their dominant hormone secretion, or depicted as clinically non-functioning if not associated with any clinical syndrome of hormone excess. These tumours should not be included among carcinoids in the presence of minimal serotonin immunoreactivity. Exceptionally endocrine tumours of the pancreas stain intensely for serotonin (and may also contain other biogenic amines).[22,69] They appear histologically as classical carcinoids, but few have been associated with the carcinoid syndrome. The tumours are managed surgically according to guidelines similar to those for other malignant endocrine pancreatic tumours. Hepatic metastases and a carcinoid syndrome may be treated with somatostatin analogues and interferon, or chemotherapy in the presence of higher proliferation rate.

JEJUNO-ILEAL/MIDGUT CARCINOIDS

The midgut carcinoids originate from intestinal enterochromaffin (EC) cells in intestinal crypts. They have been named classical carcinoids, and typically display both an argyrophilic and argentaffin silver staining reaction (positive Masson stain) due to serotonin production in the tumour cells.[70] The small-intestinal carcinoids have increased in frequency, and constitute around 32% of carcinoids.[2,3,10,27,70] Being the most common cause of the carcinoid syndrome, these tumours have often prevailed at referral centres, since this syndrome has required somewhat complicated and often combined medical and surgical treatment.[10,70] The small-intestinal carcinoids account for 25% of small-bowel neoplasms, and have been diagnosed at an average age of 65 years, with slight male predominance.

Morphological features

The primary small-intestinal carcinoid is most commonly located in the terminal parts of the ileum, often appearing as a small, flat and fibrotic submucosal tumour, measuring around 1 cm or less (**Fig. 6.2**),[70,71] occasionally with some central navelling. Sometimes the tumour is so tiny that it is difficult to detect at surgery, appearing only as a limited area of fibrosis or circumscribed thickening of the intestinal wall. In up to one-third of the patients, multiple smaller carcinoid polyps occur in the nearby intestine, most likely caused by lymphatic dissemination.[71] In a few cases additional larger carcinoid polyps have been found in proximal parts of the intestine, and these represent additional primary tumours. Among patients subjected to surgery, mesenteric metastases have been found at a high frequency. When growing close to the intestinal wall such metastases have sometimes been mistaken for primary tumours. In contrast to carcinoids located elsewhere in the gastrointestinal tract, microscopic or gross metastases have occurred in association with the smallest primary tumours.[71] Unusual large primary tumours sometimes extend directly into a conglomerate of mesenteric lymph gland metastases. The mesenteric metastases typically grow conspicuously larger than the primary tumour, and characteristically evoke a marked desmoplastic reaction with pronounced mesenteric fibrosis[71] (**Fig. 6.3**). The fibrosis might result from

Figure 6.2 • Small intestinal carcinoid, unusual entity with liver metastases but no mesenteric tumour. From Åkerström G, Hellman P, Öhrvall U. Midgut and hindgut carcinoid tumors. In: Doherty GM, Skogseid B (eds) Surgical endocrinology, 1st edn. Philadelphia: Lippincott Williams & Wilkins, 2001; pp. 448–52, with permission.

Figure 6.3 • Computed tomography image of mesenteric metastasis from a midgut carcinoid tumour, typically surrounded by fibrosis (appearing like 'hurricane centre'). From Åkerström G, Hellman P, Öhrvall U. Midgut and hindgut carcinoid tumors. In: Doherty GM, Skogseid B (eds) Surgical endocrinology, 1st edn. Philadelphia: Lippincott Williams & Wilkins, 2001; pp. 448–52, with permission.

Figure 6.4 • Intestinal venous ischaemia due to midgut carcinoid. From Åkerström G, Hellman P, Öhrvall U. Midgut and hindgut carcinoid tumors. In: Doherty GM, Skogseid B (eds) Surgical endocrinology, 1st edn. Philadelphia: Lippincott Williams & Wilkins, 2001; pp. 448–52, with permission.

local effects of serotonin, growth factors and other substances secreted from the carcinoid metastases.[70,72]

With more extensive fibrosis the distal ileal mesentery often becomes contracted and tethers the mesenteric root to the retroperitoneum, with fibrous bands attaching to the serosa of the horizontal duodenum. Occasionally fibrosis and tumour extend over parts of the transverse or the sigmoid colon.[71]

The mesenteric tumour and fibrosis can often cause partial or complete small-intestinal obstruction by kinking and fibrotic entrapment of the intestine, whereas the primary tumour only occasionally is large enough to obstruct the intestinal lumen.[71] Obstruction of the duodenum tends to occur at advanced stages. The mesenteric vessels are often encased or occluded by the growing mesenteric tumour, with resulting local venous stasis and ischaemia in the small intestine, and occasionally frank impairment of the intestinal circulation. Variable segments of the small intestine thus appear dark blue to reddish due to incipient venous gangrene (**Fig. 6.4**), or occasionally pale and cyanotic due to deficient arterial circulation.[70,71] A specific angiopathy, called vascular elastosis, occurs with advanced midgut carcinoids, and causes marked thickening of mesenteric vessel walls due to

elastic tissue proliferation in the adventitia; this contributes to the intestinal vascular impairment.[73,74] However, compression by tumour and fibrosis has in our experience been the obvious cause in patients where intestinal ischaemia was revealed at operation.[70,71]

Fibrotic attachments between intestines invariably become more pronounced after surgery and frequently create a conglomerate of distal small-intestinal loops and caecum, which becomes fixed to the posterior and anterior abdominal wall.

Distant metastases from small intestinal carcinoids occur most commonly in the liver and the patients then often present with variable features of the carcinoid syndrome. Liver metastases are often bilateral and diffusely spread; approximately 10% of the patients have fewer or dominant lesions, sometimes with conspicuous growth of individual lesions. Around 10% of patients present with liver metastases, without mesenteric lesions. Spread to extra-abdominal sites can involve the skeleton (spine and orbital framing are predilection sites), the lungs, CNS, mediastinal and peripheral lymph nodes, ovaries, breast and the skin.[70] A neck lymph gland metastasis can sometimes be the primary clinical sign of a disseminated tumour.

Clinical symptoms

The carcinoid tumours grow slowly and many patients have experienced long periods of prodromal symptoms before the disease has been clinically recognised.[70,71] Some patients have had symptoms of borborygmia or episodic abdominal pain, others have had unrecognised features of the carcinoid syndrome, with diarrhoea, discrete flush, palpitations or intolerance for specific food or alcohol.[75,76] Intestinal bleeding is generally rare with small-intestinal carcinoids due to the moderate size and submucosal location of the primary tumour. Bleeding has been mainly encountered at later stages, with larger, ulcerating primary tumours, or if mesenteric metastases have grown in the intestinal wall.[70,71] Such metastases have a special tendency to grow into the horizontal duodenum and have sometimes caused bleeding. In other cases bleeding has occurred as a result of intestinal venous stasis.

Intermittent attacks of abdominal pain may initially occur, and increase in frequency until the patient develops obvious subacute or acute intestinal obstruction requiring surgery. In 30–45% of patients the small-intestinal carcinoids are thus revealed at operation for intestinal obstruction, where the patients often have been submitted to surgery without awareness of the diagnosis.[71,77] In another 50% of patients the diagnosis becomes evident after detection of liver metastases, and some of the patients have features of the carcinoid syndrome.

CARCINOID SYNDROME

The carcinoid syndrome occurs in approximately 20% of patients with jejuno-ileal carcinoids.[3,10] Monoamine oxidase activity in the liver can generally detoxify substances released from the intestinal and mesenteric tumours, and symptoms associated with the carcinoid syndrome generally imply that the patient has liver metastases. Occasionally the syndrome may be encountered in patients with large retroperitoneal or ovarian lesions, where secretory products exceed the capacity of detoxification or can bypass the liver and drain directly into the systemic circulation. The syndrome includes flushing, diarrhoea, right-sided valvular heart disease, and bronchoconstriction. The aetiology of the carcinoid syndrome is related to release of serotonin, bradykinin, tachykinins (substance P, neuropeptide K), prostaglandins and growth factors such as platelet-derived growth factor (PDGF) and transforming growth factor β (TGF-β), as well as noradrenaline (norepinephrine).[78]

Secretory diarrhoea is the most common feature of the syndrome, but it may sometimes be mild and unspecific initially.[75,76] Diarrhoea is often most prevalent in the morning, and often meal related. The diarrhoea may, however, have many causes in carcinoid patients, especially when they have been previously operated upon, or have reached advanced disease stages.[70] Resection of the distal small intestine may cause moderate diarrhoea due to reduced bile salt absorption; other causes are a short bowel, or partial intestinal obstruction. In patients with large mesenteric tumours intestinal venous stasis or ischaemia may often contribute significantly to stool frequency. Severe watery diarrhoea and malnutrition can occasionally occur due to occlusion of main mesenteric veins, which has caused severely oedematous, fluid-leaking intestinal segments of variable length.[71,79]

Cutaneous flushing generally affects the face, neck and upper chest, and is the most typical feature of the carcinoid syndrome. Flushing may, however, be overlooked especially in females at menopause. The flush may be provoked by stress, alcohol, certain food, aged cheese, or coffee. It is often of short duration, lasting for 1–5 minutes, but may occasionally be prolonged for several hours or even days. Flushing may be severe, and when the flush has been longstanding there may be frequent telangiectases and persistent blue-cyanotic discoloration of the skin of the nose and chins.

Heart valve fibrosis, affecting tricuspid and pulmonary valves with plaquelike fibrotic endocardial thickening, is a serious and late consequence of a severe and longstanding carcinoid syndrome.[80–82] Serotonin and tachykinins may influence the heart and cause fibrosis and valvular thickening with retraction and fixation of the heart valves and subsequently regurgitation and stenosis. As many as 65% of patients with the carcinoid syndrome have tricuspid valve abnormalities, and 19% had pulmonary valve regurgitation in one series.[80,83] In less than 10%, the pulmonary degradation by monoamine oxidase activity is exceeded, and the fibrosis may involve also the left-sided heart valves, and possibly contribute to bronchoconstriction.

The carcinoid heart disease may cause progressive cardiac insufficiency with typically right-sided heart failure and severe lethargy, and used to be an important cause of death in patients with the carcinoid syndrome.[80,81,83] However, nowadays, after introduction of somatostatin analogues, patients more often die of progressive tumour disease.[9] Affected patients may require heart surgery and replacement of fibrotic heart valves with prostheses.[82] This operation may lead to substantial improvement, but can be associated with complications, especially in older persons. The heart disease can be diagnosed by echocardiography, which should always be performed prior to major abdominal surgery.

Bronchial constriction as part of the carcinoid syndrome caused by midgut carcinoids is rare.

Diagnosis

BIOCHEMISTRY

The biochemical diagnosis of small-intestinal carcinoids is often based on the demonstration of raised concentrations of the serotonin metabolite **5-hydroxyindoleacetic acid (5-HIAA)** excreted in 24-hour urine samples. The raised 5-HIAA values are specific for carcinoids, but occur only at advanced disease stages, and generally imply the presence of liver metastases.[9,70]

Determination of **plasma chromogranin A** is a more sensitive measure, which may be used for the early diagnosis of persistent or recurrent carcinoid disease. Circulating chromogranin A levels reflect the tumour load, and serial measurements have become the most important parameter for monitoring disease spread and to follow results of treatment.[9,70] The chromogranin values may also predict prognosis. However, it is a non-specific marker for any neuroendocrine tumour, and false-positive values occur with liver or kidney failure, inflammatory bowel disease, atrophic gastritis or chronic use of proton-pump inhibitors.[83]

Human choriogonadotropin (hCG-α/β) α and β subunits may be predictors of poor prognosis.[9] Exceptionally carcinoids secrete enteroglucagon and pancreatic polypeptide (PP), but PP is a non-specific marker, which may be raised in any patients with diarrhoea.[9]

Pentagastrin provocation test

Pentagastrin injection has occasionally been used to verify the presence of occult carcinoid disease by demonstrating flush and a rise in plasma peptides.[9,10]

RADIOLOGY

The primary midgut carcinoids are generally too small to be diagnosed with conventional **bowel contrast studies**.[70] At more advanced disease stages typical arcading of entrapped intestines, with segments of partial obstruction may be visualised, and occasionally signs of chronic obstruction, with thickened bowel wall. In patients with large-bowel symptoms entrapment of the sigmoid or transverse colon may be important to identify prior to surgery. Concomitant colorectal adenocarcinoma has been reported in 10–15%, and it may sometimes be necessary to exclude coexisting rectosigmoidal adenocarcinoma by endoscopy, prior to surgery or during follow-up of a small intestinal carcinoid.

Computed tomography

CT can very infrequently visualise a primary midgut carcinoid tumour, but often efficiently demonstrates mesenteric lymph node metastases, retroperitoneal extension of such masses, and liver metastases. The presence of a circumscribed mesenteric mass with radiating densities is very suspicious of a midgut carcinoid mesenteric metastasis[70] (**Fig. 6.3**).

Dynamic CT with contrast enhancement is of particular value for planning surgery, when the relation between the mesenteric metastases and the main mesenteric artery and vein is often crucially important to visualise. In cases with advanced intestinal ischaemia CT may reveal a characteristic image of universally dilated peripheral mesenteric vessels, and sometimes oedematous loops of intestine. CT is often the primary method for visualisation of liver metastases, but the sensitivity for smaller lesions in the liver is quite low. Carcinoid liver metastases are often hypervascular and CT should be performed before and after administration of i.v. contrast agent.

Magnetic resonance tomography (MR) can sometimes be more efficient than CT for demonstration of liver metastases.

Angiography

Mesenteric angiography often shows typical features in midgut carcinoids, with calibre changes, segmental occlusions, and tortuosity of mesenteric vessels, but is now seldom used in the clinical routine due to the efficiency of dynamic CT.[70] It is important to know, however, that in patients with abdominal pain, angiography cannot discriminate between intestinal obstruction and ischaemia, because the vascular impairment generally involves peripheral vessels, and laparotomy is often required to distinguish these causes.[70,71]

Ultrasound

Percutaneous ultrasound is mainly utilised to visualise liver metastases or to guide fine-needle or preferably core needle biopsy for histological diagnosis of liver metastases or the deposits in the mesentery. Ultrasound with power Doppler enhancement, and especially use of ultrasound contrast, may increase sensitivity for detection of liver metastases dramatically (unpublished results).

OctreoScan®

In nearly 90% of cases, small-intestinal carcinoids possess somatostatin receptors types 2 and 5, for which the somatostatin analogue octreotide has high affinity.[9] Somatostatin receptor scintigraphy (OctreoScan®) has detected carcinoid tumours with a sensitivity of 90%, and is being increasingly utilised to determine metastatic spread. OctreoScan® is especially efficient for detection of extra-abdominal metastases, and can visualise bone metastases better than a routine isotope bone scan, which may miss especially osteolytic metastases.[83]

Positron emission tomography (PET)

PET with the serotonin precursor 5-hydroxytryptophan, labelled with ^{11}C (5HTP-PET), is a recently introduced investigation that can identify the small-intestinal carcinoids with high sensitivity, and has been used to monitor effects of therapy.[84]

HISTOLOGY

Needle biopsy specimens from metastases are often used for diagnosis. The carcinoid tumour cells stain immunocytochemically with neuroendocrine tumour markers, mainly chromogranin A, synaptophysin and occasionally neurone-specific enolase (NSE). Reactivity with serotonin-specific antisera implies that a primary tumour should be searched for in the midgut;[8,10,70] 85% of jejuno-ileal carcinoids show reactivity for chromogranin A and serotonin.[9,10] Proliferation rate is determined with the Ki67 antibody and is invariably low in classical midgut carcinoids (<2%).[52]

Most jejuno-ileal carcinoids show a mixed insular and glandular growth pattern; occasional tumours have a pure insular and trabecular pattern and have been reported as having a slightly less favourable prognosis.[10] Rarely, tumours have an undifferentiated pattern and high proliferation rate. Since they belong to the group of neurendocrine carcinomas with poor prognosis, patients with these tumours can generally not be helped by surgery.

Surgery

Many patients with midgut carcinoids will be subjected to acute laparotomy due to intestinal obstruction without suspicion of the correct diagnosis. It is important to appreciate then that the carcinoid is common among small-bowel neoplasms, and findings at laparotomy are often typical with a tiny ileal primary tumour, and conspicuously larger mesenteric metastases with marked mesenteric desmoplastic reaction.[70,71] The primary tumour and mesenteric metastases should be removed by wedge resection of the mesentery and limited intestinal resection, and lymph node metastases should be cleared as far as possible by dissection around the mesenteric artery and its branches. This procedure is generally indicated also in the presence of liver metastases. If the surgery has been inadequately performed, because the surgeon believed he or she was facing inoperable adenocarcinoma, this will result in the primary tumour and especially the bulk of mesenteric metastases not being removed. Re-operation is then strongly recommended to remove any remaining mesenteric tumour, which can otherwise be expected to cause future abdominal complications.[70,71]

If grossly radical removal of the primary tumour and mesenteric metastases has been accomplished, midgut carcinoid patients may often remain symptom-free for long periods. However, midgut carcinoid tumours are markedly tenacious and recurrence should be watched for, as the majority of patients (>80%) will ultimately develop liver metastases if follow-up is long enough (**Fig. 6.5**).[70,85] The midgut carcinoids are unusually slow-growing tumours, and clinically overt recurrence occurs after a median of 10 years and up to 25 years.[70,85] Earlier diagnosis of such recurrence may be more sensitively based on serum chromogranin A estimates, rather than the urinary 5-HIAA measurements.

Many patients with midgut carcinoids lack acute abdominal symptoms, and instead present with liver metastases and sometimes also features of the carcinoid syndrome at the time of diagnosis. Only a few decades ago life expectancy was poor in patients with liver metastases and carcinoid syndrome, with an expected median survival of around 2 years, and abdominal surgery was not often considered.[9] Now symptoms of the carcinoid syndrome may be efficiently controlled by medical treatment with somatostatin analogues and interferon, and these and other new treatment modalities have increased life expectancy.[9,70]

Abdominal complications have become of increased concern and have appeared as a principal cause of

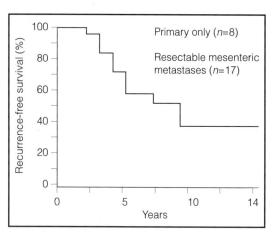

Figure 6.5 • Recurrence-free survival in midgut carcinoid patients subjected to apparently curative surgery. A majority of patients will experience recurrence during long-term follow-up. From Åkerström G, Hellman P, Öhrvall U. Midgut and hindgut carcinoid tumors. In: Doherty GM, Skogseid B (eds) Surgical endocrinology, 1st edn. Philadelphia: Lippincott Williams & Wilkins, 2001; pp. 448–52; and Makridis C, Öberg K, Juhlin C et al. Surgical treatment of midgut carcinoid tumors. World J Surg 1990; 14:377–85, with kind permission of Springer Science and Business Media.

death in patients with midgut carcinoids.[71,85] Such threatening complications have widened indications for abdominal surgery in patients undergoing medical treatment for the advanced carcinoids.

Due to continued growth and increased intestinal entrapment by mesenteric tumour or fibrosis, the patients often experience abdominal pain and will require surgery for relief of partial or complete intestinal obstruction.[71,85–87] Since incipient intestinal ischaemia may cause similar symptoms of feeding-related crampy abdominal pain, laparotomy can be urgently needed to distinguish these causes. Liberal operative intervention is indicated also because incipient venous ischaemia may contribute markedly to conditions with diarrhoea and general malaise. Occasional patients present with severe abdominal pain, weight loss, and even malnutrition and cachexia due to the intestinal ischaemia (**Fig. 6.6**).[70,71,86,87] Abdominal pain is unlikely to occur due to the carcinoid syndrome, and weight loss and malnutrition are rarely caused merely by a large tumour burden in the midgut carcinoid patients. Complications of the mesenteric tumour have been evident in a large proportion of patients with midgut carcinoids subjected to laparotomy, and are important to recognise since these patients may benefit from considerable long-term palliation following surgery.[86,87]

The natural course of the mesenterico-intestinal disease with midgut carcinoids can be variable, but surgery at an early stage is a distinct advantage, as it may provide an exceptional chance to remove the mesenteric tumour before more extensive involvement of major mesenteric vessels has occurred.[71,85–87] The authors thus advocate removal of the mesenterico-intestinal tumour as a prophylactic procedure even in asymptomatic patients considered for medical therapy. During the periods of medical treatment the patients are likely to benefit markedly from close cooperation between internists and surgeons, with liberal surgical consultations when abdominal symptoms occur.

SURGICAL TECHNIQUE

Important considerations for abdominal surgery in patients with midgut carcinoids have been outlined.[70,71,87] During surgical exploration the advanced midgut carcinoids may seem inoperable since the large mesenteric metastases with surrounding fibrosis and entrapped loops of intestine

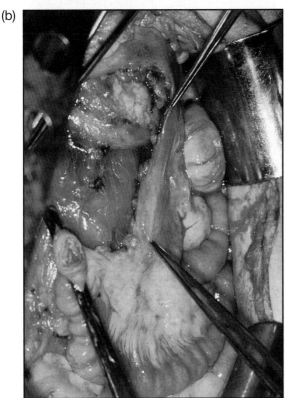

Figure 6.6 • **(a)** Computed tomography image of mesenteric tumour deemed inoperable at previous surgery, with resulting progressive intestinal vascular impairment, weight loss and cachexia. **(b)** Re-operation with mesenteric tumour removal and limited intestinal resection performed with alleviation of abdominal symptoms. Part (b) from Åkerström G, Hellman P, Öhrvall U. Midgut and hindgut carcinoid tumors. In: Doherty GM, Skogseid B (eds) Surgical endocrinology, 1st edn. Philadelphia: Lippincott Williams & Wilkins, 2001; pp. 448–52, with permission.

will frequently appear to encase the major intestinal vascular supply.[71,85,87] Incautious wedge resection in the fibrotic and contracted mesentery may easily compromise the main mesenteric artery and cause devascularisation of a major part of the small intestine and result in a short-bowel syndrome.[70,71,87] However, since the majority of these metastases originate from primary lesions in the most terminal parts of the ileum, they tend to be deposited mainly on the right side of the mesenteric artery, implying that they can often be removed without interfering with the main intestinal vascular supply. A procedure has been described where the right colon and the entire small intestinal mesenteric root is mobilised from adhesions to the retroperitoneum up to the level of the horizontal duodenum and the pancreas.[70,71,87] A large tumour deposit in the mesenteric root and fibrosis often has to be dissected from the serosa of the horizontal duodenum. With a posterior view in the elevated mesenteric root it is possible to identify the mesenteric vessels, divide the fibrotic surroundings of the mesenteric metastases, and free-dissect and debulk a major portion, or the entire tumour, from the mesenteric root (**Figs 6.6** and **6.7**). Sometimes part of the tumour may be cleaved to allow separation from the mesenteric artery and vein, since the tumour seems rarely to invade the vessel walls. The procedure can preserve the main mesenteric artery and vein, and maintain blood flow through jejunal and ileal arteries and important arcades along the intestine (**Fig. 6.6**). The larger of the mesenteric metastases (up to 10 cm in our experience) can occasionally be easier to dissect than the smaller and diffusely fibrotic ones, which may grow more diffusely around the mesenteric root. The procedure will generally permit a more limited small-intestinal resection, and thereby a reduced risk of creating a short bowel, which is likely to be very troublesome for the patient in combination with the carcinoid syndrome. Generally the right colon has to be removed together with the most terminal parts of the ileum, and occasionally fibrotic entrapment of the transverse or the sigmoid colon has to be released. In our experience, intestinal bypasses should be avoided as far as possible, because ischaemia may develop in a disengaged intestinal segment, and also because the mesenteric tumour will continue to grow and symptoms then generally progress. The bypass procedure can markedly complicate repeat surgery, which often becomes necessary in these patients.[70,71,87] Intestinal bypassing should be reserved for cases where extensive tumour growth, carcinoidosis, or fibrosis after previous operations inhibit appropriate mesenteric dissection.

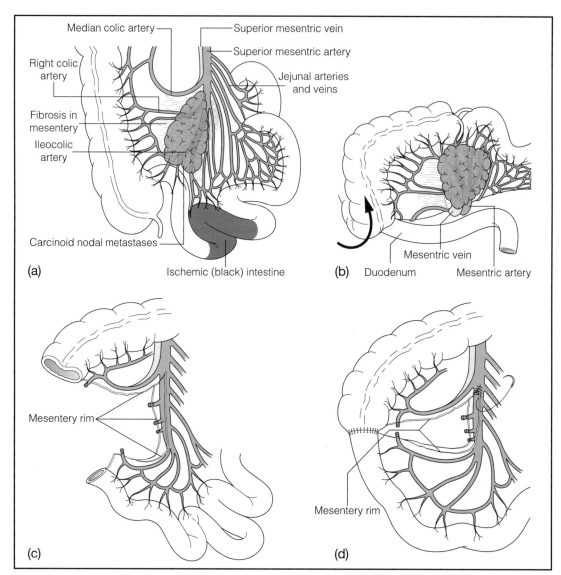

Figure 6.7 • Resection of carcinoid primary tumour and mesenteric metastasis. **(a)** Mesenteric tumour may extensively involve the mesenteric root and appear impossible to remove. **(b)** Mobilisation of caecum, terminal ileum, and mesenteric root by separation of retroperitoneal attachments, allows tumour to be lifted, approached also from posterior angle, and separated from duodenum and main mesenteric vessels, with preservation of intestinal vascular supply and intestinal length. **(c,d)** Bowel anastomosed and mesenteric defect repaired. Redrawn from Åkerström G, Hellman P, Öhrvall U. Midgut and hindgut carcinoid tumors. In: Doherty GM, Skogseid B (eds) Surgical endocrinology, 1st edn. Philadelphia: Lippincott Williams & Wilkins, 2001; pp. 448–52, with permission.

When planning dissection of mesenteric metastases it is valuable to preoperatively map the level of extension in the mesenteric root with dynamic CT investigation (**Fig. 6.8**).[70,87] For jejunal carcinoids and occasional ileal carcinoids mesenteric metastases extend high or completely surround the mesenteric root or even extend retroperitoneally above the pancreas, and these tumours have been inoperable in our experience.

Repeated surgery may sometimes be required in patients with advanced midgut carcinoids, when they suffer from chronic or intermittent abdominal

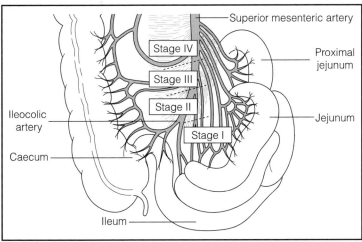

Figure 6.8 • Stages of midgut carcinoid mesenteric metastases. Stage I tumours located close to the intestine, removed by limited ileal resection. Stage II tumours involving arterial branches close to the origin in the mesenteric artery, requiring right-sided colectomy, distal ileal resection, and dissection from mesenteric vessels. Stage III tumours extending along but without encircling the mesenteric trunk, may be free-dissected. Stage IV tumours growing around the mesenteric trunk involving origins of proximal jejunal arteries, median colic artery, or extending retroperitoneally; these tumours have proved impossible to remove. Redrawn with permission from Öhrvall U, Eriksson B, Juhlin C et al. Method of dissection of mesenteric metastases in mid-gut carcinoid tumors. World J Surg 2000; 24:1402–8; and Åkerström G, Hellman P, Öhrvall U. Midgut and hindgut carcinoid tumors. In: Doherty GM, Skogseid B (eds) Surgical endocrinology, 1st edn. Philadelphia: Lippincott Williams & Wilkins, 2001; pp. 448–52.

pain due to partial or complete intestinal obstruction, or segmental intestinal ischaemia.[71] These operations may be exceedingly difficult and time consuming due to the presence of harsh fibrosis and carcinoidosis between loops of intestine, but nevertheless they are crucially important for the well-being of the patient. Re-operations, and indeed any surgery in patients with midgut carcinoid tumours, should be undertaken with great caution, since minor mistakes may easily cause intestinal fistulation, devascularisation of major parts of the small intestine, or creation of a short-bowel syndrome.[70,71,87] Duodenal fistulation can be a significant risk, which has been described in this context. Emphasising these difficulties it is recommended that the surgery for midgut carcinoids be referred to colleagues with experience in this management.

The authors have evaluated more than 200 laparotomies in patients with advanced carcinoids, including re-operations in several patients.[71,85–88] Alleviation of abdominal symptoms was often efficiently achieved by surgery, with often long duration, and was especially favourable in patients with intestinal venous stasis or ischaemia.[71]

Attempts to remove the mesenteric tumour should be undertaken as early as possible, when growth in the mesentery is less extensive.[70,71,87] If a mesenteric tumour remains our experience is that the patients will survive with medical treatment but more or less invariably reach a stage where abdominal complications represent a major threat.

Prophylactic removal of the mesenterico-intestinal tumour is strongly recommended even in the absence of abdominal symptoms, as this may prevent intestinal complications. Tardy surgical consultation may allow the disease to be increasingly difficult or impossible to manage surgically.[87]

Liver metastases

The treatment of liver metastases can use many modalities: medical treatment, surgery, radiofrequency (RF) ablation, liver embolisation, transplantation, radiolabelled octreotide therapy, and [^{131}I] metaiodobenzylguanidine (^{131}I-MIBG) therapy.[9,52,70,71] An initial period of medical treatment with somatostatin analogues and interferon can help alleviate symptoms, and slow disease progression. It also allows some time for observation and makes surgery or ablation of liver disease safer. Liver surgery is more likely to be beneficial in patients with classical midgut carcinoids with high differentiation and low proliferation rate demonstrated by the Ki67 staining.[52]

LIVER SURGERY

The majority of patients with advanced midgut carcinoids have multiple and bilaterally disseminated liver metastases, and are mainly considered for medical therapy.

In 5–10% of cases, solitary and unilateral, or grossly dominant liver metastases occur (**Fig. 6.9**). Liver surgery, consisting of formal hepatic lobectomy or parenchyma-saving liver resections should be undertaken, and this may be combined with wedge resections or simple enucleations of superficially located additional, and even bilateral lesions.[10,70,71,83,89–97] Recent developments of surgical and anaesthesiological methods now allow safe multiple wedge resections for bilobar hepatic metastases. Two-stage surgical resection may

Figure 6.9 • Computed tomography image of large midgut carcinoid metastasis within the left liver lobe. The patient had smaller metastases in contralateral liver but remained free from carcinoid syndrome 4 years after resection of the larger lesion. From Åkerström G, Hellman P, Öhrvall U. Midgut and hindgut carcinoid tumors. In: Doherty GM, Skogseid B (eds) Surgical endocrinology, 1st edn. Philadelphia: Lippincott Williams & Wilkins, 2001; pp. 448–52, with permission.

reduce the risk of liver insufficiency, with initial resection of one lobe, and removal of additional tumour after some months of liver regeneration. Preoperative portal embolisation may help induce regeneration of a hepatic lobe (without metastases) that is planned to remain after hepatic lobectomy for removal of metastatic tumour.

The debulking liver surgery may be increasingly important in patients who no longer respond to medical therapy, and larger metastases may represent cloned tumour cells that have ceased to be affected by medical therapy. Since liver surgery may considerably relieve symptoms associated with the carcinoid syndrome, it may be indicated also in the presence of concomitant or bilateral smaller metastases.

A number of reports have described series of patients who have undergone successful liver surgery with long survival and no evidence of disease,[89–97] and with significant symptom alleviation after palliative surgery.

The indications for liver surgery may be widened by the combination with other treatment modalities, especially RF ablation.[98,99]

Substantial and sustained palliation of the carcinoid syndrome and reduction of tumour markers can be expected especially after removal of large (>10 cm) dominant lesions, or if around 90% of the tumour volume can be excised or ablated (**Fig. 6.9**).[90,91] A five-year survival of 70% or more has been reported after apparently 'curative' surgery, and symptom palliation has been obtained also with non-curative resections.[89–97]

However, virtually every patient will recur with new tumour after liver resection or ablative therapy, if follow-up time is long enough. Reflecting slow progression of the carcinoid tumours, clinical symptoms (e.g. carcinoid syndrome) have reappeared 4–5 years after apparently 'curative' liver resection, but the patient may have been efficiently palliated until then.[85,91,93]

RADIOFREQUENCY ABLATION

Radiofrequency (RF) ablation has recently been introduced as an efficient and safe method for ablation of moderately large liver metastases.[98–100]

Using a needle introduced with ultrasound guidance into the tumour, the application of current with alternating radiowave-length frequency induces ionic oscillation, with production of heat around the needle leading to tissue necrosis within a range of up to 3–4 cm. RF ablation can be performed intraoperatively, laparoscopically, or repeatedly as a percutaneous ultrasound-guided procedure. Somewhat larger tumours may be coagulated by overlapping treatment, or by reduction of hepatic circulation during ablation, with hepatic artery clamping during surgery, or concomitant embolisation during percutaneous RF ablation. The efficiency of the method is good, and according to some authors equals results of surgical resection. However, tumours larger than 3 cm, and tumours close to major vessels may be inefficiently treated (due to heat loss through the perfusing vessels). Numerous reports of RF treatment are available in the literature, but so far no randomised prospective trial has yet demonstrated survival benefits or improved symptom relief after RF ablation compared with surgery.

We use RF ablation and surgery as complementary therapies, and have found that the possibility of ablation has broadened indications for surgery of bilateral tumours with the aim of cytoreduction.[100] However, the number of lesions needs to be limited, and the method is of less value in patients with numerous small metastases. Although methods for visualisation of liver metastases have improved, our experience from operations confirms that many patients have multiple small liver metastases, often not accurately visualised before surgery. A correct estimate of the spread is therefore often best achieved at laparotomy, where availability for surgical resection or RF ablation can be appropriately evaluated. Our own series has shown local recurrence after RF ablation in 10%, and a complication rate of ≈5%.[100] Since large vessels reduce the efficiency and bile ducts seem to be the most vulnerable structures we try to avoid RF treatment of tumours located in the hepatic hilum. We have utilised liver surgery and RF ablation in combination in a number of patients, although we have not yet been able to demonstrate a survival benefit for these patients. Prospective, randomised studies are needed to evaluate RF ablation and other treatment modalities for liver metastases.

LIVER EMBOLISATION

Liver tumours are generally fed mainly by arterial supply, and obstruction of the blood flow will cause tumour ischaemia. As a consequence liver metastases may be efficiently treated by selective liver artery embolisation. Embolisation with gel foam powder, sometimes performed as a repeated procedure, has provided tumour regression and symptomatic control in approximately 50% of patients during median follow-up of 7–14 months, and with resulting reduced need for somatostatin analogues and improved effects of interferon treatment.[9,10,52,101–103]

Patent portal blood flow is crucial for perfusion of the normal liver parenchyma, and angiography is performed prior to embolisation to verify a patent portal vein, and to characterise the vascular anatomy.[52,101,103] Embolisation is generally contraindicated if tumour burden relative to normal liver parenchyma exceeds 50%, and in patients with raised bilirubin and liver enzymes as signs of hepatic insufficiency. Superselective and repeated embolisations with some months interval has been performed in cases with large tumours, and in patients with recurrent tumour after previous hemihepatectomy.[101]

The procedure is associated with complications, and even mortality rates around 5%, and may cause liver insufficiency of variable degree.[102] Most common is transient elevation of liver enzymes, and two or three days of fever, nausea and abdominal pain, with disappearance of symptoms within a week.

Complications are reduced in the hands of an experienced interventional radiologist, by prophylactic octreotide infusion during the procedure, and the use of forced diuresis and haemodynamic monitoring during and after the procedure. Special caution is needed in cases where the right hepatic artery originates from the superior mesenteric artery, since mesenteric artery embolism may occur. Patients who have undergone hepatico-jejunostomy or papillotomy are more prone to develop cholangitis or hepatic abscesses afterwards.

The results of embolisation are good, although not every patient will respond as expected. Effects may be of short duration, and survival benefits still remain unclear. The success rate is lower and risks higher with extensive liver metastases. Embolisation may be used in cases of multiple unresectable metastases, but it is crucial to carefully consider if the remaining healthy liver parenchyma is sufficient to prevent liver failure in the post-embolisation period.

Chemoembolisation is arterial embolisation combined with intra-arterial infusion of chemotherapy, and may be more effective than embolisation alone with possibly more pronounced tumour reduction in some cases.[104] The treatment may have severe side effects and may be less efficient in midgut carcinoids with their typically low proliferation than in tumours with lower differentiation and higher proliferation rates.

LIVER TRANSPLANTATION

Liver transplantation may be considered for patients with liver metastases from midgut carcinoids, because of generally slow disease progression.[70,105,106] Meta-analysis of patients with endocrine tumours subjected to liver transplantation revealed a nearly 50% 1-year survival, but only 24% 5-year disease-free survival.[107] Carcinoids have been reported with more favourable survival (69% at 5 years) than endocrine pancreatic tumours.[108] Results presented so far are limited, however, and transplantation-associated immediate mortality can be high (20% or more). Low Ki67 index (<5%) in the tumour has been considered necessary to consider transplantation.[109] Few patients remain disease-free after transplantation, and the new liver may become the site for new metastases. Carcinoid tumours are unusually tenacious, and virtually all patients seem to recur with metastases after apparently radical removal of primary and regionally localised lesions.[85] Biochemical markers and imaging, even with specific methods such as OctreoScan® or 5-HTP-PET, may fail to detect spread of disease. Indications for transplantation must therefore be balanced against favourable results of medical treatment, and the proven tenacity of carcinoid tumours, which makes recurrence likely or inevitable if follow-up time is long enough.[85,93,107,108,110] It is possible that immunosuppression promotes tumour growth, and patients may live longer, with better life quality, with medical treatment. Cases considered for liver transplantation therefore have to be carefully selected, and perhaps chosen from patients

in whom liver metastases cannot be removed, are markedly space occupying or threaten to cause liver failure. However, such patients may be poor candidates for extensive surgical procedures like transplantation.[106]

Prophylaxis against carcinoid crisis

Operation and embolisation in patients with the carcinoid syndrome always entails the risk of inducing a carcinoid crisis, with hyperthermia, shock, arrhythmia, excessive flush or bronchial obstruction.

As prophylaxis to prevent crisis during surgery or intervention, patients with midgut carcinoids can be pretreated with octreotide (patient's regular dose or daily 100 µg × 3s.c.), and adrenergic drugs should generally be avoided in case of hypotension.[10,70] Patients with foregut carcinoids and atypical carcinoid syndrome are treated with octreotide, histamine blockade and cortisone, and avoidance of histamine-releasing agents (morphine and tubocurarine). In patients with carcinoid flush syndrome we routinely provide i.v. octreotide (500 µg in 500 mL saline, 50 µg/h) during surgery or embolisation procedures, and the same treatment is given if carcinoid crisis should occur.[70]

Medical treatment

Biotherapy, including somatostatin analogues and interferon, has been shown to improve clinical symptoms in 50–70% of patients with midgut carcinoids, often with significant reduction of tumour markers, and stabilisation of the disease for several years, but less often with significant tumour reduction.[9,10,52,111–115] Chemotherapy has been of little benefit in midgut carcinoids with typical low proliferation.[9,52]

Somatostatin analogues (octreotide, lanreotide) have been a breakthrough in the treatment of carcinoid tumours.[9,10,52] By binding to specific somatostatin receptors (types 2 and 5) the analogues reduce the release of bioactive peptides from tumour cells, and may also block peripheral responses of target cells. They may also inhibit tumour growth, induce apoptosis, and counteract angiogenesis.

The analogues have induced subjective and biochemical responses in up to 70% of patients with carcinoid syndrome, caused moderate tumour reduction in around 5%, and stabilisation of disease for an average of 3 years in approximately half of the patients.[111–113]

The analogues are usually given in daily doses of 50–150 μg × 3 s.c.. Higher doses (>3000 μg/day) have resulted in slightly greater tumour reduction but otherwise no greater response rate. Tachyphylaxis often occurs after 9–12 months of treatment and may often indicate a requirement for increased dosage. Long-acting formulations have become available (octreotide-LAR, lanreotide-PR, Somatuline Autogel), offering the possibility of monthly administration, and therefore are much easier to use. Side effects of all analogues include gallstone formation, pancreatic enzyme deficiency, and symptoms relating to biliary colic, sometimes necessitating cholecystectomy.[83]

Interferon α (IFN-α) reduces hormone secretion, and stimulates natural killer cells with effects on cell growth in tumours with slow progression.[9,52,114] Clinically IFN-α administration induces biochemical and subjective responses in about 50% of the patients, while antitumour effects may be seen in around 15% with doses of 15–25 × 10⁶ U/week; the duration of response is around 3 years, and stabilisation of the disease occurs in 35%.[115] Recently a pegylated form has become available (PegIntron®) for subcutaneous administration once a week, and with possible improved tolerance. Combinations of somatostatin analogue and interferon therapy may increase response rate. Interferon is associated with more adverse effects than somatostatin analogues, mainly fluelike symptoms initially, and later on chronic fatigue and sometimes depression. Autoimmune phenomena may be induced with antithyroid antibodies, causing thyroid dysfunction and occasionally other complications. Neutralising interferon antibodies may develop and interfere with the effects.[52] Some patients have to discontinue treatment, and the rather high risk of side effects has somewhat limited the use of interferon.

Radiotherapy

External radiotherapy is generally not efficient in treating carcinoid tumours but it can be used for long-term palliation of brain metastases, and especially for alleviation of pain due to bone metastases.[9,116]

Internal, or tumour-targeted radiation has been developed during recent years, using ¹³¹I-MIBG and radioactive somatostatin analogues.[117–122]

Effects of ¹³¹I-MIBG therapy have been limited, with subjective responses in 30–40% of patients and biochemical responses in less than 10%.[117] Predosing with non-labelled MIBG has resulted in prolonged biochemical and clinical responses.[118,119]

Neuroendocrine tumours, including carcinoids, express somatostatin receptor subtypes 2 and 5, which become internalised in tumour cells after binding of radiolabelled octreotide.[52,120] Remission has been seen after treating neuroendocrine tumours with [¹¹¹In]-DTPA-octreotide used for OctreoScan® examinations.[120] New compounds with beta- and gamma-emitting isotopes linked to somatostatin analogues have been developed ([⁹⁰Y-DOTA]-octreotide, [⁹⁰Y-DOTA]-lanreotide and [¹⁷⁷Lu-DOTA,Tyr³] octreotate), with affinity for different somatostatin receptors, and better tumour penetration.[121,122] Some of these compounds have shown very promising responses and mild side effects, and combinations may become of special value for this developing type of therapy.[52,121,122]

Survival

Age-adjusted overall 5-year survival for all midgut carcinoids in Sweden between 1960 and 2000 was 67%,[123] which was similar to the series from the SEER Program of the National Cancer Institute (NCI) 1973–1999.[3]

Survival has been improved during recent years, probably by active management, but remains largely dependent on the extent of disease, with the presence of liver metastases and carcinoid heart disease identified as the most significant adverse prognostic factors.[3,123,124] The importance of surgery has been documented also by survival analyses.[85,88,91,94–97] Among 314 patients treated in

Uppsala, Sweden, median survival was 12.4 years and 5-year survival rate was 91% in patients who underwent apparently grossly radical resections of mesenteric metastases, without having liver metastases.[88] The value of mesenteric resection remained, but with shorter expected survival in patients with liver metastases.[88] Patients undergoing successful surgery for mesenteric ischaemia had favourable survival prospects, with a median of 8 years.[85] The value of surgical removal of dominant or large liver metastases has also been demonstrated with extended survival and prolonged symptom palliation.[85,86,94,96,97]

Figure 6.10 • Appendiceal carcinoid, with the typical yellow colour and location in tip of the appendix. From Capella C, Solcia E, Sobin L et al. Endocrine tumours of the appendix. In: Hamilton SR, Aaltonen LA (eds) WHO Classification of tumours. Pathology and genetics of tumours of the digestive system. Lyon: IARC Press, 2000; pp. 99–101, with permission.

Patients with inoperable liver metastases in the Uppsala series had 50% 5-year survival (similar to the results in the NCI series[88,124]), and survival was 42% with inoperable liver and mesenteric lymph node metastases.[88] Survival was better for younger age groups (<50 years), and for patients who had received biotherapy.[88] Other negative factors for survival (except for liver metastases and heart disease) have been lymph gland metastases, high 5-HIAA values, old age (>75 years), tumour discovered during emergency surgery, significant weight loss, and presence of extra-abdominal metastases.[85,88,123,124]

APPENDICEAL CARCINOIDS

Appendiceal carcinoids belong to midgut carcinoids and constitute ≈10% of all gastrointestinal carcinoids, having apparently decreased in frequency.[1–3,10,125] Carcinoid is one of the most common tumours of the appendix. The majority of appendiceal carcinoids are argentaffin and originate from serotonin-producing EC cells; a few are non-argentaffin and produce other peptides.[10] The tumours appear to have a neuroectodermal origin and more benign features than other carcinoids.[125] Appendiceal carcinoids are prevalent at autopsy, and rarely attain clinical significance. Many of these carcinoids may perhaps undergo spontaneous involution, since the prevalence is reported as higher in children than in adults.[125]

Appendiceal carcinoids are often an incidental finding at surgery, and are expected to occur in 1 in 200 appendectomies,[125] but have probably frequently been overlooked. Approximately 75% of

the carcinoids are located in the tip of the appendix (**Fig. 6.10**, see also Plate 12, facing p. 212), and therefore only a few cases have had appendicitis due to an occluded appendix lumen.[125–127] Patients with appendiceal carcinoids are generally younger than those with other carcinoids, having a mean age ≈40 years, with a slight female predominance; and even children may be affected. The overall metastasis rate has been determined as 3.8%, with distant metastases in 0.7%.[1] Patients with larger tumours and metastases tend to be younger (29 years) than patients with smaller benign lesions (42 years).[10]

The majority (≈90%) of appendiceal carcinoids are <1 cm in diameter, and have minimal risk of presenting with metastases, which implies that these lesions may be treated by simple appendectomy.[10,125–128] This treatment is also apparently safe for most lesions measuring 1–2 cm, although rare cases in this group have presented with lymph node metastases.[10,125–128] Lesions >2 cm, as well as cases with residual tumour at resectional margins, or with lymph gland metastases, should be treated by right hemicolectomy. Tumours in the base of the appendix require a similar aggressive approach since they may represent colon- rather than appendix-derived tumours.

The prognosis for appendiceal carcinoids is favourable overall, with a 5-year survival rate of 91% for patients with local disease, 81% for those with regional metastases, and 28% for the few patients with distant metastases.[5,10,125]

Atypical goblet-cell carcinoid

Adenocarcinoid or goblet-cell carcinoid represents a more malignant variant, with elements of carcinoid tumours and mucinous adenocarcinomas, the most common origin being in the appendix.[125] This type has also been named 'atypical' or 'intermediate' carcinoid. The tumour is much more malignant than the classical carcinoid tumour, and more resembles classical adenocarcinoma with respect to prognosis and survival. The tumour spreads through the serosa and in the mesoappendix and intraperitoneally. Treatment for this tumour has mainly included extended ileocolic and mesenteric resection, often performed as re-operation, and additionally chemotherapy. The goblet-cell carcinoids have had unpredictable and generally less favourable survival, with a 60% 10-year survival rate.[125,129] Recently a much more aggressive therapy has been proposed, adding cytoreductive surgery and intraperitoneal heated chemotherapy.[130] The cytoreductive therapy has included omentectomy, splenectomy and peritonectomy.

COLON CARCINOIDS

Carcinoids of the colon are rare and constitute only about 5–13% of gastrointestinal carcinoid tumours.[5,10,131–133] These tumours develop preferentially in older individuals, with a mean age of 70 years, but have also occasionally been reported in children. Tumours of the proximal colon (caecum) are most common, and may infrequently (5%) be associated with the carcinoid syndrome, which does not occur in association with more distally located colonic lesions.[131,132] The tumours are generally aggressive, and have less well-differentiated histological features. They are generally large and exophytic, rather than ulcerating, apparently slow growing, and may reach conspicuous size before diagnosis. Patients then generally present with typical malignant symptoms, pain, palpable abdominal mass, and more occasionally occult rectal bleeding. Carcinoids of the colon seem to have a less pronounced tendency for regional metastases (20%) but a high incidence of liver metastases.[131–133]

Although some authors have recommended limited resection for colon carcinoids <2 cm in diameter, it is probably wise to treat all patients with hemicolectomy. Due to their slow growth rate, palliative tumour debulking may also be undertaken if possible. The 5-year survival rate for colon carcinoids has averaged 37%, slightly better than the survival for adenocarcinoma.[131,133]

RECTAL CARCINOIDS

Rectal carcinoids have previously been regarded as uncommon, but the incidence is increasing, and they constitute 1–2% of all rectal tumours. In the recent review by Modlin et al. about 13.7% of all gastrointestinal carcinoid tumours were rectal.[3] Genetic predisposition may be noted in the different annual incidence of approximately 0.35 per 100 000 in whites, and 1.2 in black people, as well as a roughly fivefold higher incidence in the Asian compared with the non-Asian North American population. The increased incidence compared with earlier reports may be due to increased awareness of the diagnosis and use of recently developed diagnostic methods, such as endosonography, as well as more accurate histopathology. The majority of rectal carcinoids are small and discovered accidentally at early stages. The overall prognosis is favourable, with up to 88.3% 5-year survival,[3] although a more thorough classification of different variants of rectal carcinoids probably is mandatory.

Presentation

The development of the tumour usually occurs in the sixth decade, about 10 years earlier than non-carcinoid rectal tumours. The majority – up to about 60% – are small, less than 1.0 cm in greatest dimension (**Fig. 6.11**, see also Plate 13, facing p. 212),[134,135] and may be discovered after presenting symptoms such as perianal pain, pruritus ani or haematochezia leading to endoscopic procedures. However, most patients are asymptomatic, and the tumours are found incidentally, which is prognostically beneficial compared with symptomatic presentation. The smaller tumours usually present as submucosal yellowish nodules, and up to 75% may be within reach of digital examination at 8 cm from the anal verge.[136] The findings at digital

Figure 6.11 • Rectal carcinoid polyp with typical yellowish colour and submucosal location. From McNevin MS, Read TE. Diagnosis and treatment of carcinoid tumors of the rectum. Chir Int 1998; 5:10–12, with permission.

palpation can be variable and described as firm, smooth or rubbery in consistency.[137] Diagnosis is made after histopathological evaluation of biopsies or after removal of the whole nodule. Patients with tumours <1 cm exhibit a low risk for metastases (<2%).[138–144]

Patients with larger tumours generally have more symptoms, and those with metastatic disease may present with generalised symptoms such as weight loss and even cachexia. The carcinoid syndrome is extremely rare among these patients, and only exceptionally present in cases with liver metastases. Occasional large tumours can be fixed to perirectal tissues, and may initially be difficult to distinguish from rectal adenocarcinoma. Previous reports, which have proposed an increased incidence of concurrent colonic adenocarcinoma,[142,145] have recently been questioned, and solid statistics have not yet been documented regarding this matter.

Tumours exceeding 1.0 cm in greatest dimension are much more prone to dissemination. Thus, patients with tumours between 1.0 and 1.9 cm have an intermediate incidence of metastatic spread (10–15%), while patients with larger tumours (>2 cm) exhibit a 60–80% incidence of distant metastases. The main sites for tumour spread are regional lymph nodes and the liver, and less commonly lung and bone.[144]

Rectal carcinoids may prognostically and in terms of management be divided up according to their size. Patients with tumours <1 cm seldom demonstrate symptoms, have a favourable outcome, are generally cured by local excision, and almost never have metastases. Patients with tumours >2 cm usually present with symptoms and the majority have metastases to regional lymph nodes, lung or liver. Thus, the smaller (<1 cm) and the larger (>2 cm) tumours have a predictable outcome, whereas the tumours measuring 1.0–1.9 cm in diameter are unpredictable.[137,146] Although the patients with smaller tumours generally may be considered as cured after tumour excision, patients with tumours measuring 1.0–1.9 cm need to be thoroughly examined for the presence of local infiltration and metastatic disease, and should also be closely surveyed. Transrectal endosonography may be used for more precise assessment of tumour extension, possible infiltration in the muscularis propria, and to reveal regional lymph node metastases. Computed tomography (CT) or magnetic resonance tomography (MRT) can clarify local tumour growth in the pelvis, and also the presence of lymph node and liver metastases. Octreotide scintigraphy (OctreoScan®) is most often negative in patients with rectal carcinoids due to lack of or few somatostatin receptors, regardless of tumour size.

Diagnosis and immunohistochemistry

The diagnosis is usually made after histopathological examination. Rectal carcinoids are derived from enterochromaffin cells of neuroendocrine origin, and display cells arranged in rosettes, ribbons or in a glandular pattern, surrounded by a dense fibrous stroma.[145–148] The cells contain acidophilic granules, and demonstrate argentaffin silver reaction (Masson staining) in 8–30%.[138,147] However, by addition of an exogenous reducing agent, a positive argyrophil reaction may occur in up to 70% of rectal carcinoids.[149,149] Cells with positive silver staining are generally also reactive with serotonin and chromogranin A antisera.[150] The most sensitive markers, however, seem to be neurone-specific enolase (NSE), being positive in 87%, and, interestingly, prostate-specific acid phosphatase (in 80–100%), which makes differentiation from prostatic carcinoma difficult.[150] A limited fraction of cells generally are positive for chromogranin A.[150,151] Two studies have concluded there is a correlation between Ki67 expression, tumour size and presence of metastases,[152,153] although the Ki67 expression generally was low. Classical tumour markers like CA19-9, CA50 and alpha-fetoprotein are poorly expressed or absent, while carcino-embryonic antigen (CEA) has been demonstated in up to 25% of cells.[153,154] The CEA expression is possibly related to the occasional rectal carcinoid tumour that exhibits histopathological signs of both adenocarcinoma and carcinoids, referred to as adenocarcinoids.[154,155] Rectal carcinoids generally show multihormonal expression, in which glucagon, somatostatin, pancreatic polypeptide, substance P, and β-endorphins may be detected.[149,156]

The immunoreactivity for the different markers is generally unevenly distributed in groups of cells exhibiting focal and patchy distribution.[149] This may indicate development of multiclonal lesions, where additional genetic derangements are prone to occur, causing more aggressive disease in fractions of tumour cells as well as in individual patients.

The tumours measuring <1 cm in diameter are only occasionally locally infiltrative, whereas tumours >2 cm almost invariably show signs of atypical histopathology, including infiltration of muscularis propria, invasion of lymphovascular and perineural structures, and a high number of mitotic figures. These tumours are frequently associated with distant metastases, local invasion and reduced survival.

It is rare that release of measurable peptides occurs in the circulation implying that s-chromogranin A or urinary 5-HIAA are less useful diagnostic or surveillance tools for rectal carcinoids. Similarly, OctreoScan® is of minor importance due to lack of or minimal expression of somatostatin receptors.

Treatment

Smaller rectal carcinoids are safely treated by local excision. No other treatment is necessary since there have been no reports of recurrence of tumours treated at this stage.[141] In patients with tumours between 1.0 and 1.9 cm in size, treatment is debated. Reports have demonstrated success with minimally invasive surgical techniques for removal of such tumours,[157–163] with similar survival as for smaller (<1.0 cm) tumours.[135]

Thus, transanal endoscopic microsurgery and even full-thickness excision have been utilised for rectal carcinoid tumours, apparently with success.[159,163] Incompletely removed polyps that are found to be carcinoids after removal, may be re-excised using such techniques.[162]

However, others strongly favour an aggressive approach with abdominoperineal or anterior resection with total mesorectal excision.[137] For tumours >2.0 cm a similar treatment debate has also taken place. Most patients with these tumours have locally infiltrative disease, and already suffer from lymph node or distant metastases to liver, lung or bone, leading some authors to suggest palliative treatment only.[140] However, recent results have documented more favourable survival rates than previously depicted.[3,138] Five-year survival for rectal carcinoids with distant metastases is about 32%, which favours an aggressive approach for this group of patients, even in the face of local invasion in the pelvis or distant lymph node, liver, lung or skeletal metastases.

Our experience of individual patients with large tumours and distant metastases supports this view. Thus we suggest surgery in these patients, in combination with chemotherapy, which can be effective in some patients. However, patients with atypical histopathological features are less likely to benefit from the aggressive surgical treatment.[146]

Although most reports demonstrate poor results of chemotherapy in rectal carcinoids, there are occasional patients who respond. To date there is no prognostic indicator selecting these patients from non-responders, which has led to wide indications for the initiation of such therapy. IFN-α and paclitaxel have in some patients resulted in reduced disease progression and also regression of metastases, and in the few patients with a positive OctreoScan®, somatostatin receptor analogues may be useful. Moreover, reports of success with such analogues in the absence of positive imaging may indicate a wider role for these agents.[164] Occasional patients with liver metastases may benefit from hepatic artery chemoembolisation. In carefully selected cases liver resection may be indicated, with the understanding, however, that these patients generally have a poor outcome and short survival.

Outcome

Prediction of outcome in rectal carcinoids should rely on several factors such as tumour size, histology (typical or atypical features), micro-invasiveness as well as presence of symptoms at presentation, but no study has yet evaluated all of these factors systematically. Nevertheless, tumour size and microinvasiveness have generally been accepted as the clinically most important factors.[141] Overall 5-year survival for patients with rectal carcinoids is about 88%, ranging between 32% for patients with distant metastases, to 91% for patients with localised disease.[3] Patients with deeply invasive tumours had a median survival of 6–7 months in one study.[165] Patients with a carcinoid tumour confined to the submucosa and smaller than 1 cm will rarely die from the disease.[141] Mean survival

after discovery of recurrence of rectal carcinoids has been reported as 4–5 months.[165]

Recommendations

Patients with tumours <1 cm in size are in most cases successfully treated by local excision, and do not require long-term follow-up. Patients with rectal carcinoid tumours measuring 1.0–1.9 cm and those >2 cm should be thoroughly investigated (MRT, CT, transrectal endosonography) for evidence of spread of disease, e.g. local or distant metastases. These patients should generally undergo surgery with the aim of achieving total tumour clearance, and the specimens should be thoroughly investigated for signs of atypical histopathology. The larger the tumour, the higher the risk for metastatic disease. There are no studies demonstrating benefit of pre-operative medical or irradiation treatment. Patients with rectal carcinoids >1 cm, including those with infiltrative or disseminated disease, need follow-up, and may require, e.g., palliation against pelvic pain. Selected individuals may be offered more aggressive medical (and surgical) treatment for distant metastases.

• **Key points**

- Carcinoids are rare tumours derived from neuroendocrine cells with wide distribution in the body. One-third occur in the lungs, bronchi and thymus, and around 70% in the gastrointestinal tract.
- Lung, thymic and occasional metastasising gastric carcinoids of sporadic type may cause an atypical carcinoid syndrome due to production of histamine.
- Carcinoids of the small intestine (midgut) with liver metastases and serotonin production are the most common cause of a classical carcinoid syndrome, with often severe and incapacitating symptoms of flush, diarrhoea and fibrotic valvular heart disease.
- Carcinoid tumours may be histologically identified with chromogranin A, synaptophysin, and for some tumours NSE stainings.
- The Ki67 antibody stain is increasingly used as a marker for tumour cell proliferation, and can help predict prognosis, and also support decisions about therapy.
- The various types of carcinoid tumour require different treatment, dependent on histological type, location and proliferation rate.
- Most carcinoid tumours are well differentiated and slow growing, and should be surgically excised when this is possible. Occasional tumours have low differentiation and a higher proliferation rate, and may respond better to chemotherapy.
- Specific tumour markers, urinary 5-HIAA excretion and especially serum chromogranin A measurements, can be used for clinical diagnosis and to monitor effects of therapy, and are also important predictors of prognosis.
- Multiple gastric carcinoids occur most commonly as a result of gastrin excess in patients with hypergastrinaemia due to chronic atrophic gastritis. These carcinoids are generally benign and can often be safely removed and controlled by endoscopy. A minority are associated with the MEN 1 Zollinger–Ellison syndrome.
- Sporadic, solitary gastric carcinoids are markedly more malignant and require more extensive surgery.
- For the midgut carcinoids surgical treatment is important, and should include efforts to remove mesenteric metastases, which may cause severe long-term abdominal complications with obstruction and ischaemia of the small bowel. Attempts can also be made to surgically remove or ablate liver metastases, since this may provide considerable palliation of the carcinoid syndrome.
- For patients with the carcinoid syndrome surgery is also combined with continous medical treatment by somatostatin analogues (in long-acting release forms) and interferon, both of which may markedly alleviate symptoms, and seem to stabilise disease and slow its progression.
- Small, non-invasive rectal carcinoids can be removed by endoscopy, whereas larger lesions are more malignant, and need wider resection, and in addition often chemotherapy.
- The diagnosis and treatment of carcinoid tumours have progressed markedly and should now include close cooperation between surgeons and internists with special interest in endocrine oncology. This collaboration is important to ensure that patients with carcinoids receive adequate surgery, and can help individualise therapy, utilising various treatment modalities. These include liver resection and radio-frequency (RF) ablation of liver metastases, and in the near future radioactively targeted somatostatin analogues.

REFERENCES

1. Godwin II JD. Carcinoid tumors, an analysis of 2837 cases. Cancer 1975; 36:560–9.

2. Modlin IM, Sandor A. An analysis of 8305 cases of carcinoid tumors. Cancer 1997; 79:813–29.

3. Modlin IM, Lye KD, Kidd M. A 5-decade analysis of 13,715 carcinoid tumors. Cancer 2003; 97:934–59.

   Excellent and valuable presentation of epidemiology and natural history in a comprehensive series of all types of carcinoid tumours.

4. Berge T, Linell F. Carcinoid tumours. Frequency in a defined population during a 12-year period. Acta Pathol Microbiol Scand [A] 1976; 84:322–30.

5. Capella C, Heitz PU, Hofler H et al. Revised classification of neuroendocrine tumors of the lung, pancreas and gut. Digestion 1994; 55(suppl. 3): 11–23.

6. Rindi G, Azzoni C, La Rosa S et al. ECL cell tumor and poorly differentiated endocrine carcinoma of the stomach: prognostic evaluation by pathological analysis. Gastroenterology 1999; 116:532–42.

7. Solcia E, Klöppel G, Sobin LA et al. Histological typing of endocrine tumors. In: WHO classification of endocrine tumors. New York: Springer-Verlag, 2000.

8. Van Eeden S, Qaedvelieg PF, Taal BG et al. Classification of low-grade neuroendocrine tumors of midgut and unknown origin. Hum Pathol 2002; 33:1126–33.

9. Öberg K. Carcinoid tumors: current concepts in diagnosis and treatment. Oncologist 1998; 3:339–45.

10. Modlin IM, Lye K, Kidd M. Carcinoid tumors. In: Schwartz AE, Persemlidis D, Gagner M (eds) Endocrine surgery. New York: Marcel Dekker, 2004; pp. 613–41.

11. Solcia E, Fiocca R, Villani L et al. Morphology and pathogenesis of endocrine hyperplasias, precarcinoid lesions, and carcinoids arising in chronic atrophic gastritis. Scand J Gastroenterol (suppl.) 1991; 180:146–59.

12. Solcia E, Bordi C, Creutzfeldt W et al. Histopathological classification of nonantral gastric endocrine growths in man. Digestion 1988; 41:185–200.

13. Solcia E, Fiocca R, Villani L et al. Hyperplastic, dysplastic, and neoplastic enterochromaffin-like-cell proliferations of the gastric mucosa. Classification and histogenesis. Am J Surg Pathol 1995; 19(suppl. 1):S1–S7.

14. Rindi G, Luinetti O, Cornaggia M et al. Three subtypes of gastric argyrophil carcinoid and the gastric neuroendocrine carcinoma: a clinicopathologic study. Gastroenterology 1993; 104:994–1006.

15. Solcia E, Capella C, Fiocca R et al. Gastric argyrophil carcinoidosis in patients with Zollinger–Ellison syndrome due to type 1 multiple endocrine neoplasia. A newly recognized association. Am J Surg Pathol 1990; 14:503–13.

16. Rindi G, Paolotti D, Fiocca R et al. Vesicular monoamine transporter 2 as a marker of gastric enterochromaffin-like cell tumors. Virchows Arch 2000; 436:217–23.

17. Kölby L, Wängberg B, Ahlman H et al. Somatostatin receptor subtypes, octreotide scintigraphy, and clinical response to octreotide treatment in patients with neuroendocrine tumors. World J Surg 1998; 22:679–83.

18. Rindi G, Bordi C, Rappel S et al. Gastric carcinoids and neuroendocrine carcinomas: pathogenesis, pathology, and behavior. World J Surg 1996; 20:168–72.

   Important article with valuable information on epidemiology and prognosis for gastric neuroendocrine tumours.

19. Cattan D, Roucayrol AM, Launay JM. Circulating gastrin, endocrine cells, histamine content, and histidine decarboxylase activity in atrophic gastritis. Gastroenterology 1989; 97:586–96.

20. Borch K, Renvall H, Liedberg G. Endocrine cell proliferation and carcinoid development: a review of new aspects of hypergastrinaemic atrophic gastritis. Digestion 1986; 35(suppl. 1):106–15.

21. Modlin IM, Kidd M, Lye KD. Biology and management of gastric carcinoid tumours: A review. Eur J Surg 2002; 168:669–83.

   Excellent review article about gastric carcinoids, in which the authors describe cellular background and important clinical features of the different gastric carcinoids.

22. Åkerström G. Management of carcinoid tumors of the stomach, duodenum, and pancreas. World J Surg 1996; 20:173–82.

23. Gough DB, Thompson GB, Crotty TB et al. Diverse clinical and pathologic features of gastric carcinoid and the relevance of hypergastrinemia. World J Surg 1994; 18:473–9.

24. Borch K. Atrophic gastritis and gastric carcinoid tumours. Ann Med 1989; 21:291–7.

25. Bordi C, Cocconi G, Togni R et al. Gastric endocrine cell proliferation. Association with Zollinger–Ellison syndrome. Arch Pathol 1974; 98:274–8.

26. Lehy T, Roucayrol AM, Miignon M. Histomorphological characteristics of gastric mucosa in patients with Zollinger–Ellison syndrome or autoimmune gastric atrophy: role of gastrin and atrophying gastritis. Microsc Res Tech 2000; 48:327–38.

27. Jensen RT. Management of the Zollinger–Ellison syndrome in patients with multiple endocrine neoplasia type 1. J Intern Med 1998; 243:477–88.

28. Chandrasekharappa SC, Guru SC, Manickam P et al. Positional cloning of the gene for multiple endocrine neoplasia-type 1. Science 1997; 276:404–7.

29. Debelenko LV, Emmert-Buck MR, Zhuang Z et al. The multiple endocrine neoplasia type I gene locus is involved in the pathogenesis of type II gastric carcinoids. Gastroenterology 1997; 113:773–81.

30. Bordi C, Falchetti A, Azzoni C et al. Aggressive forms of gastric neuroendocrine tumors in multiple endocrine neoplasia type I. Am J Surg Pathol 1997; 21:1075–82.

31. Sjöblom SM, Sipponen P, Jarvinen H. Gastroscopic follow up of pernicious anaemia patients. Gut 1993; 34:28–32.

32. Armbrecht U, Stockbrugger RW, Rode J et al. Development of gastric dysplasia in pernicious anaemia: a clinical and endoscopic follow up study of 80 patients. Gut 1990; 31:1105–9.

33. Cadiot G, Vissuzaine C, Potet F et al. Fundic argyrophil carcinoid tumor in a patient with sporadic-type Zollinger–Ellison syndrome. Dig Dis Sci 1995; 40:1275–8.

34. Granberg D, Wilander E, Stridsberg M et al. Clinical symptoms, hormone profiles, treatment, and prognosis in patients with gastric carcinoids. Gut 1998; 43:223–8.

35. Cadiot G, Cattan D, Mignon M. Diagnosis and treatment of ECL cell tumors. Yale J Biol Med 1998; 71:311–23.

36. Wilander E, El-Salhy M, Pitkänen P. Histopathology of gastric carcinoids: a survey of 42 cases. Histopathology 1984; 8:183–93.

37. Matsui K, Jin XM, Kitagawa M et al. Clinicopathologic features of neuroendocrine carcinomas of the stomach: appraisal of small cell and large cell variants. Arch Pathol Lab Med 1998; 122:1010–17.

38. Kim KM, Kim MJ, Cho BK et al. Genetic evidence for the multi-step progression of mixed glandular-neuroendocrine gastric carcinomas. Virchows Arch 2002; 440:85–93.

39. Yoshikane H, Tsukamoto Y, Niwa Y et al. Carcinoid tumors of the gastrointestinal tract: evaluation with endoscopic ultrasonography. Gastrointest Endosc 1993; 39:375–83.

40. Stridsberg M, Hellman U, Wilander E et al. Fragments of chromogranin A are present in the urine of patients with carcinoid tumours: development of a specific radioimmunoassay for chromogranin A and its fragments. J Endocrinol 1993; 139:329–37.

41. Krenning EP, Kooij PP, Pauwels S et al. Somatostatin receptor: scintigraphy and radionuclide therapy. Digestion 1996; 57(suppl. 1):57–61.

42. Borch K, Renvall H, Kullman E et al. Gastric carcinoid associated with the syndrome of hypergastrinemic atrophic gastritis. A prospective analysis of 11 cases. Am J Surg Pathol 1987; 11:435–44.

43. Stolte M. Clinical consequences of the endoscopic diagnosis of gastric polyps. Endoscopy 1995; 27:32–7.

44. Papa A, Cammarota G, Tursi A et al. Histologic types and surveillance of gastric polyps: a seven year clinico-pathological study. Hepatogastroenterology 1998; 45:579–82.

45. Hirschowitz BI, Griffith J, Pellegrin D et al. Rapid regression of enterochromaffinlike cell gastric carcinoids in pernicious anemia after antrectomy. Gastroenterology 1992; 102:1409–18.

46. Higham AD, Dimaline R, Varro A et al. Octreotide suppression test predicts beneficial outcome from antrectomy in a patient with gastric carcinoid tumor. Gastroenterology 1998; 114:817–22.

47. Wängberg B, Grimelius L, Granerus G et al. The role of gastric resection in the management of multicentric argyrophil gastric carcinoids. Surgery 1990; 108:851–7.

48. Thirlby RC. Management of patients with gastric carcinoid tumors. Gastroenterology 1995; 108:296–7.

49. Ahlman H, Kölby L, Lundell L et al. Clinical management of gastric carcinoid tumors. Digestion 1994; 55(suppl. 3):77–85.

50. Åkerström G, Hessman O, Skogseid B. Timing and extent of surgery in symptomatic and asymptomatic neuroendocrine tumors of the pancreas in MEN 1. Langenbeck's Arch Surg 2002; 386:558–69.

51. Norton JA, Fraker DL, Alexander HR et al. Surgery to cure the Zollinger–Ellison syndrome. N Engl J Med 1999; 341:635–44.

52. Öberg K, Ahlman H. Medical management of neuroendocrine gastrointestinal tumors. In: Schartz AE, Persemlidis D, Gagner M (eds) Endocrine surgery. New York: Marcel Dekker, 2004; pp. 685–96.

53. Burke AP, Sobin LH, Federspiel BH et al. Carcinoid tumors of the duodenum. A clinicopathologic study of 99 cases. Arch Pathol Lab Med 1990; 114:700–4.

54. Attanoos R, Williams GT. Epithelial and neuroendocrine tumors of the duodenum. Semin Diagn Pathol 1991; 8:149–62.

55. Thompson NW, Vinik AI, Eckhauser FE. Microgastrinomas of the duodenum: a cause of failed operations for the Zollinger–Ellison syndrome. Ann Surg 1989; 209:396–404.

56. Pipeleers-Marichal M, Somers G, Willems G et al. Gastrinomas in the duodenums of patients with multiple endocrine neoplasia type 1 and the Zollinger–Ellison syndrome. N Engl J Med 1990; 322:723–7.

57. Modlin IM, Lawton GP. Duodenal gastrinoma: the solution to the pancreatic paradox. J Clin Gastroenterol 1994; 19:184–8.

58. Sugg SL, Norton JA, Fraker DL et al. A prospective study of intraoperative methods to diagnose and resect duodenal gastrinomas. Ann Surg 1993; 218:138–44.

59. Thompson NW, Bondeson AG, Bondeson L et al. The surgical management of gastrinoma in MEN I syndrome patients. Surgery 1989; 106:1081–5.

60. Thompson NW. Surgical treatment of the endocrine pancreas and Zollinger–Ellison syndrome in the MEN 1 syndrome. Henry Ford Hosp Med J 1992; 40:195–8.

61. Pipeleers-Marichal M, Donow C, Heitz PU et al. Pathologic aspects of gastrinomas in patients with Zollinger–Ellison syndrome with and without multiple endocrine neoplasia type 1. World J Surg 1993; 17:481–8.

Important article emphasing high incidence of tiny duodenal gastrinomas as a cause of sporadic and MEN 1-related Zollinger–Ellison syndrome.

62. Griffiths DFR, Jasani B, Newman GR et al. Glandular duodenal carcinoid – a somatostatin rich tumour with neuroendocrine associations. J Clin Pathol 1984; 37:163–9.

63. Wheeler MH, Curley IR, Williams ED. The association of neurofibromatosis pheochromocytoma, and somatostatin-rich duodenal carcinoid tumor. Surgery 1986; 100:1163–9.

64. Ricci JL. Carcinoid of the ampulla of Vater: local resection or pancreaticoduodenectomy. Cancer 1993; 71:686–90.

65. Kheir SM, Helpern NB. Paraganglioma of the duodenum in association with congenital neurofibromatosis: possible relationship. Cancer 1984; 53:2491–6.

66. Burke AP, Federspiel BH, Sobin LH et al. Carcinoids of the duodenum: a histologic and immunohistochemical study of 65 tumors. Am J Surg Pathol 1989; 13:828–37.

67. Lasson Å, Alwmark A, Nobin A et al. Endocrine tumors of the duodenum: clinical characteristics and hormone content. Ann Surg 1983; 197:393–8.

68. Zyromski NJ, Kendrick ML, Nagomey DM et al. Duodenal carcinoid tumors: how aggressive should we be? J Gastrointest Surg 2001; 5:588–93.

69. Wilson RW, Gal AA, Cohen C et al. Serotonin immunoreactivity in pancreatic endocrine neo-plasms (carcinoid tumors). Mod Pathol 1991; 4:727–32.

70. Åkerström G, Hellman P, Öhrvall U. Midgut and hindgut carcinoid tumors. In: Doherty GM, Skogseid B (eds) Surgical endocrinology. Philadelphia: Lippincott Williams & Wilkins, 2001; pp. 447–59.

71. Makridis C, Öberg K, Juhlin C et al. Surgical treatment of midgut carcinoid tumors. World J Surg 1990; 14:377–85.

72. Funa K, Papanicolaou V, Juhlin C et al. Expression of platelet-derived growth factor β-receptors on stromal tissue cells in human carcinoid tumors. Cancer Res 1990; 50:748–53.

73. Anthony P, Druru RAB. Elastic vascular sclerosis of mesenteric blood vessels in argentaffin carcinoma. J Clin Pathol 1970; 23:110–18.

74. Eckhauser FE, Argenta LC, Strodel WE et al. Mesenteric angiopathy, intestinal gangrene and midgut carcinoids. Surgery 1981; 90:720–8.

75. Vinik AI, Thompson N, Eckhauser E et al. Clinical features of carcinoid syndrome and the use of somatostatin analogue in its management. Acta Oncol 1989; 28:389–402.

76. Norheim I, Öberg K, Theodorsson-Horheim E et al. Malignant carcinoid tumours. Ann Surg 1987; 206:115–25.

77. Buchanan KD, Johnston CF, O'Hare MMT et al. Neuroendocrine tumours: a European view. Am J Med 1986; 81(suppl. 6B):14–22.

78. Matuchansky C, Launay JM. Serotonin, catecholamines, and spontaneous midgut carcinoid flush: plasma studies from flushing and nonflushing sites. Gastroenterology 1995; 108:743–51.

79. Knowlessar OD, Law DH, Sleisinger MH. Malabsorption syndrome associated with metastatic carcinoid tumor. Am J Med 1959; 27:673–7.

80. Lundin L, Norheim I, Landelius J et al. Carcinoid heart disease: Relationship of circulating vasoactive substances to ultrasound-detectable abnormalities. Circulation 1988; 77:264–9.

81. Westberg G, Wängberg B, Ahlman H et al. Prediction of prognosis by echocardiography in patients with midgut carcinoid syndrome. Br J Surg 2001; 88:865–72.

82. Lundin L, Hansson HE, Landelius J et al. Surgical treatment of carcinoid heart disease. J Thoracic Cardiovasc Surg 1990; 100:552–61.

83. Ganim RB, Norton JA. Recent advances in carcinoid pathogenesis, diagnosis and management. Surg Oncol 2000; 9:173–9.

84. Öhrlefors H, Sundin A, Ahlström H et al. Positron emission tomography with 5-hydroxytryptophan in neuroendocrine tumors. J Clin Oncol 1998; 16:2534–41.

85. Makridis C, Ekbom A, Bring J et al. Survival and daily physical activity in patients treated for advanced midgut carcinoid tumors. Surgery 1997; 122:1075–82.

Survival and life-quality analyses in patients with advanced midgut carcinoids.

86. Makridis C, Rastad J, Öberg K et al. Progression of metastases and symptom improvement from laparotomy in midgut carcinoid tumors. World J Surg 1996; 20:900–7.

87. Öhrvall U, Eriksson B, Juhlin C et al. Method of dissection of mesenteric metastases in mid-gut carcinoid tumors. World J Surg 2000; 24:1402–8.

Emphasises the importance of surgery for removal of mesenteric tumours in patients with midgut carcinoids. Describes technical aspects of a surgical procedure with low rate of complications.

88. Hellman P, Lundström T, Öhrvall U et al. Effect of surgery on the outcome of midgut carcinoid disease with lymph node and liver metastases. World J Surg 2002; 26:991–7.

Demonstrates clear effect and benefit of surgery of primary tumour as well as carcinoid metastases.

89. Martin HJK Jr, Moertel CG, Adson MA et al. Surgical treatment of functioning metastatic carcinoid tumors. Arch Surg 1983; 118:537–42.

90. McEntee GP, Nagorney DM, Kvols CK et al. Cytoreductive hepatic surgery for neuroendocrine tumors. Surgery 1990; 108:1091–6.

91. Ahlman H, Wängberg B, Jansson S et al. Management of disseminated midgut carcinoid tumours. Digestion 1991; 49:78–96.

92. Norton JA. Surgical management of carcinoid tumors: role of debulking surgery for patients with advanced disease. Digestion 1994; 55(suppl. 3):98–103.

93. Ahlman H, Westberg G, Wängberg B et al. Treatment of liver metastases of carcinoid tumors. World J Surg 1996; 20:196–202.

94. Wängberg B, Westberg G, Tylén U et al. Survival of patients with disseminated midgut carcinoid tumors after aggressive tumor reduction. World J Surg 1996; 20:892–9.

Provides survival data substantiating the importance of surgical resection of liver metastases in patients with midgut carcinoids.

95. Que FG, Nagomey DM, Batts KP et al. Hepatic resection for metastatic neuroendocrine carcinomas. Am J Surg 1995; 169:36–42.

96. Söreide JA, van Heerden JA, Thompson GB et al. Gastrointestinal carcinoid tumors: long-term prognosis for surgically treated patients. World J Surg 2000; 24:1431–6.

97. Nave H, Mössinger E, Feist H et al. Surgery as primary treatment in patients with liver metastases from carcinoid tumors: a retrospective, unicentric study over 13 years. Surgery 2001; 129:170–5.

98. Buscarini L, Rossi S. Technology for radiofrequency thermal ablation of liver tumors. Sem Laparasc Surg 1997; 4:96–101.

99. Siperstein AE, Rogers SJ, Hansen PD et al. Laparoscopic thermal ablation of hepatic neuroendocrine tumor metastases. Surgery 1997; 122:1147–55.

100. Hellman P, Ladjevardi S, Skogseid B et al. Radiofrequency tissue ablation using cooled tip for liver metastases of endocrine tumors. World J Surg 2002; 26:1052–6.

Demonstrates promising results of RF for this category of tumours.

101. Allison DJ, Modlin IM, Jenkins WJ. Treatment of carcinoid liver metastases by hepatic-artery embolisation. Lancet 1977; 2:1323–5.

102. Kress O, Wagner HJ, Wied M et al. Transarterial chemoembolization of advanced liver metastases of neuroendocrine tumors – a retrospective single-center analysis. Digestion 2003; 68:94–101.

103. Jakobsen MB, Hanssen LE, Kolmanskog F et al. The effect of interferon alfa-2b treatment with or without prior hepatic artery embolization on clinical response and survival in midgut carcinoid patients. Scand J Gastroenterol 1995; 30:789–96.

104. Moertel CG, Johnson CM, McKusick MA et al. The management of patients with advanced carcinoid tumors and islet cell carcinomas. Ann Intern Med 1994; 120:302–9.

105. Gulanikar AC, Kotylak G, Bitter-Suermann H. Does immunosuppression alter the growth of metastatic liver carcinoid after orthopic liver transplantation? Transplant Proc 1991; 23:2197–2798.

106. Olausson M, Friman S, Cahlin C et al. Indications and results of liver transplantation in patients with neuroendocrine tumors. World J Surg 2002; 26:998–1004.

107. Lehnert T. Liver transplantation for metastatic neuroendocrine carcinoma: an analysis of 103 patients. Transplantation 1998; 66:1307–12.

108. Le Treut YP, Delpero JR, Dousset B et al. Results of liver transplantation in the treatment of metastatic neuroendocrine tumors. A 31-case French multicentric report. Ann Surg 1997; 225:355–64.

109. Rosenau J, Bahr MJ, von Wasielewski R et al. Ki67, E-cadherin, and p53 as prognostic indicators of long-term outcome after liver transplantation for metastatic neuroendocrine tumors. Transplantation 2002; 73:386–94.

110. Bechstein WO, Neuhaus P. Liver transplantation for hepatic metastases of neuroendocrine tumors. Ann NY Acad Sci 1994; 733:507–14.

111. Imam H, Eriksson B, Lukinius A et al. Induction of apoptosis in neuroendocrine tumors of the digestive system during treatment with somatostatin analogs. Acta Oncol 1997; 36:607–14.

112. Bousquet C, Puente E, Buscail L et al. Anti-proliferative effect of somatostatin and analogs. Chemotherapy 2001; 47(suppl. 2):30–9.

113. Öberg K. Carcinoid tumors: molecular genetics, tumor biology, and update of diagnosis and treatment. Curr Opin Oncol 2002; 14:38–45.

114. Öberg K, Funa K, Alm G. Effects of leukocyte interferon on clinical symptoms and hormone levels in patients with mid-gut carcinoid tumors and carcinoid syndrome. N Engl J Med 1983; 309:129–33.

115. Öberg K, Eriksson B, Janson ET. The clinical use of interferons in the management of neuroendocrine gastroenteropancreatic tumors. Ann NY Acad Sci 1994; 733:471–8.

116. Schupak KD, Wallner KE. The role of radiation therapy in the treatment of locally unresectable or metastatic carcinoid tumors. Int J Radiat Oncol Biol Phys 1991; 20:489–95.

117. Kölby L, Bernhardt P, Levin-Jakobsen AM et al. Uptake of meta-iodobenzylguanidine in neuro-endocrine tumours is mediated by vesicular monoamine transporter. Br J Cancer 2003; 89:1383–8.

118. Taal BG, Hoefnagel C, Boot H et al. Improved effect of ^{131}I-MIBG treatment by predosing with non-radiolabeled MIBG in carcinoid patients, and studies in xenografted mice. Ann Oncol 2000; 11:1437–43.

119. Taal BG, Zuetenhorst H, Valdes Olmos RA et al. [^{131}I]MIBG radionuclide therapy in carcinoid syndrome. Eur J Surg Oncol 2002; 28:243.

120. Valkema R, De Jong M, Bakker WG et al. Phase I study of peptide receptor radionuclide therapy with [In-DTPA]octreotide: The Rotterdam experience. Semin Nucl Med 2002; 32:110–22.

121. De Jong M, Kwekkeboom D et al. Radiolabelled peptides for tumour therapy: current status and future directions. Plenary lecture at the EANM 2002. Eur J Nucl Med Mol Imaging 2003; 30:463–9.

122. Kwekkeboom DJ, Bakker WH, Kam BL et al. Treatment of patients with gastro-entero-pancreatic (GEP) tumours with the novel radiolabelled somatostatin analogue [(177)Lu-DOTA(0),Tyr(3)] octreotate. Eur J Nucl Med Mol Imaging 2003; 30:417–22.

123. Zar N, Garmo H, Holmberg L et al. Long-term survival in small intestinal carcinoid. World J Surg 2004; 28:1163–8.

124. de Vries H, Verschueren RC, Willemse PH et al. Diagnostic, surgical and medical aspects of the midgut carcinoids. Cancer Treat Rev 2002; 28:11–25.

125. Goede AC, Caplin ME, Winslet MC. Carcinoid tumour of the appendix. Br J Surg 2003; 90:1317–22.

Succinct and comprehensive review on appendiceal carcinoids.

126. Moertel CG, Weiland LH, Nagorney DM et al. Carcinoid tumor of the appendix: treatment and prognosis. N Engl J Med 1987; 317:1699–701.

127. Capella C, Solcia E, Sobin L et al. Endocrine tumours of the appendix. In: Hamilton SR, Aaltonen LA (eds) WHO Classification of tumours. Pathology and genetics of tumours of the digestive system. Lyon: IARC Press, 2000; pp. 99–101.

128. Parkes SE, Muir KR, al-Sheyyab M et al. Carcinoid tumours of the appendix in children 1957–1986: incidence, treatment and outcome. Br J Surg 1993; 80:502–4.

129. McCusker ME, Cote TR, Clegg LX et al. Primary malignant neoplasms of the appendix: a population-based study from the surveillance, epidemiology and end-results program, 1973–1998. Cancer 2002; 94:3307–12.

130. Sugarbaker PH. Peritonectomy procedures. Surg Oncol Clin N Am 2003; 12:703–27.

131. Ballantyne GH, Savoca PE, Flannery JT et al. Incidence and mortality of carcinoids of the colon: data from the Connecticut Tumor Registry. Cancer 1992; 69:2400–5.

132. DiSario JA, Burt RW, Kendrick ML et al. Colorectal cancers of rare histologic types compared with adenocarcinomas. Dis Colon Rectum 1994; 37:1277.

133. Rosenberg JM, Welch JP. Carcinoid tumors of the colon: a study of 72 patients. Am J Surg 1985; 149:775–9.

134. Mani S, Modlin IM, Ballantyne G et al. Carcinoids of the rectum. J Am Coll Surg 1994; 179:231–48.

135. McNevin MS, Read TE. Diagnosis and treatment of carcinoid tumors of the rectum. Chir Int 1998; 5:10–12.

Comprehensive review on rectal carcinoids.

136. Jetmore A, Jetmore A, Ray J et al. Rectal carcinoids: the most frequent carcinoid tumor. Dis Colon Rectum 1992; 35:717–25.

137. Orloff M. Carcinoid tumors of the rectum. Cancer 1971; 28:175–80.

138. Soga J. Tumors of the carcinoids family: foregut endocrinomas. Acta Med Biol 1982; 29:157–201.

139. Bates HR Jr. Carcinoid tumors of the rectum. A statistical review. Dis Colon Rectum 1966; 9:90.

140. Burke M, Shepherd N, Mann CV. Carcinoid tumors of the rectum and anus. Br J Surg 1987; 74:358–61.

141. Naunheim KS, Zeitels J, Kaplan LE et al. Rectal carcinoid tumors – treatment and prognosis. Surgery 1983; 94:670–6.

142. Caldarola VT, Jackman RJ, Moertel CG et al. Carcinoid tumors of the rectum. Am J Surg 1964; 107:844–7.

143. Shirouzu K, Isomoto H, Kakegawara T et al. Treatment of rectal carcinoid tumors. Am J Surg 1990; 160:262–5.

144. Memon MA, Nelson H. Gastrointestinal carcinoid tumors: Current management strategies. Dis Colon Rectum 1997; 40:1101–18.

145. Koura AN, Giacco GG, Curley SA et al. Carcinoid tumors of the rectum: effect of size, histopathology, and surgical treatment on metastasis free survival. Cancer 1997; 79:1294–8.

146. Soga J, Tazawa K. Pathologic analysis of carcinoids: histologic re-evaluations of 62 cases. Cancer 1971; 28:990–8.

147. Taxy JB, Mendelsohn G, Gupta PK. Carcinoid tumors of the rectum, silver reactions, fluorescence and serotonin content of the cytoplasmic granules. Am J Clin Pathol 1980; 74:791–5.

148. O'Briain DS, Dayal Y, Delellis RA et al. Rectal carcinoids as tumors of the hindgut endocrine cells. A morphological and immunohistochemical analysis. Am J Surg Pathol 1982; 6:131–41.

149. Federspiel BH, Burke AP, Sobin E et al. Rectal and colonic carcinoids. A clinicopathologic study of 84 cases. Cancer 1990; 65:135–40.

150. Kimura N, Sasano N. Prostate-specific acid phosphatase in carcinoid tumors. Virchows Arch 1986; 410:247–51.

151. Onogawa S, Tanaka S, Oka S et al. Clinical significance of angiogenesis in rectal carcinoid tumors. Oncol Rep 2002; 9:489–94.

152. Shimizu T, Tanaka S, Haruma K et al. Growth characteristics of rectal carcinoid tumors. Oncology 2000; 59:229–37.

153. Hammarström S. Properties and usefulness of carcinoma associated antigens CEA, CA 19-9 and CA-50. In: Holmgren J (ed.) Tumor marker antigens. Lund: Student Literature, 1986; p. 34.

154. Ulich TR, Cheng L, Glover H et al. A colonic adenocarcinoma with argentaffin cells. An immunoperoxidase study demonstrating the presence of numerous neuroendocrine products. Cancer 1983; 51:1483–9.

155. Shousha S. Signet-ring cell adenocarcinoma of rectum: a histological and electron microscopic study. Histopathology 1982; 6:341–6.

156. Kanter M, Lechago J. Multiple malignant rectal carcinoid tumors with immunocytochemical demonstration of multiple hormonal substances. Cancer 1987; 60:1782–6.

157. Maeda K, Maruta M, Utsumi T et al. Minimally invasive surgery for carcinoid tumors in the rectum. Biomed Pharmacother 2002; 56(suppl. 1):222s–226s.

158. Akahoshi K, Fujimaru T, Nakanishi K et al. Endosonography probe-guided endoscopic resection of small flat rectal carcinoid tumor using band ligation technique. Endoscopy 2001; 33:471.

159. Msika S, Deroide G, Kianmanesh R et al. Harmonic scalpel in laparoscopic colorectal surgery. Dis Colon Rectum 2001; 44:432–6.

160. Nakagoe T, Ishikawa H, Sawai T et al. Gasless, video endoscopic transanal excision for carcinoid and laterally spreading tumors of the rectum. Surg Endosc 2003; 17:1298–304.

161. Nakagoe T, Ishikawa H, Sawai T et al. Gasless video endoscopic transanal excision of rectal tumors incompletely removed by colonoscopic snare polypectomy. J Laparoendosc Adv Surg Tech 2003; 13:99–103.

162. Ono A, Fujii T, Saito Y et al. Endoscopic submucosal resection of rectal carcinoid tumors with a ligation device. Gastrointest Endosc 2003; 57:583–7.

163. Suzuki H, Ikeda K. Endoscopic mucosal resection and full thickness resection with complete defect closure for early gastrointestinal malignancies. Endoscopy 2001; 33:437–9.

164. Hillman N, Herranz L, Alvarez C et al. Efficacy of octreotide in the regression of a metastatic carcinoid tumour despite negative imaging with In-111-pentetreotide (Octreoscan). Exp Clin Endocrinol Diabetes 1998; 106:226–30.

165. Sauven P, Ridge JA, Quan SH et al. Anorectal carcinoid tumors. Is aggressive surgery warranted? Ann Surg 1990; 211:67–71.

Seven

Clinical governance, audit and medico-legal aspects of endocrine surgery

Barnard J. Harrison and
Anthony E. Young

CLINICAL GOVERNANCE

Thou wilt learn one piece of Humility, viz. not to trust too much on thine own judgement.

Richard Wiseman
(*Severall Chirurgicall Treatises*, 1676)

We are now in the third health revolution. The first was the arrival of technology to improve care, the second the impact of financial constraints, the third, the era of accountability.[1] The measurement and regulation of clinical activity is here to stay.

The key points of Clinical Governance are to improve clinical care, avoid risk and detect adverse events rapidly. We can influence these by continued professional development, quality improvement, risk management and clinical effectiveness.

At a national level in the UK the following agencies are involved in the improvement of clinical care:

- The Department of Health (www.doh.gov.uk) sets appropriate targets and structures the service so that they can be delivered.
- NICE, the National Institute of Clinical Excellence (www.nice.org.uk), is charged with defining best practice from the welter of available evidence. NICE has not yet addressed any of the issues that specifically concern endocrine surgery.
- CHAI – previously CHI (www.chi.nhs.uk) – the Commission for Healthcare Audit and Inspection, acts to ensure that hospitals function safely and effectively. The Audit element of CHAI primarily refers to value for money audit not clinical audit.
- The NCAA, the National Clinical Assessment Authority (www.ncaa.nhs.uk), can be called on to intervene if a doctor's practice is below standard, and the General Medical Council acts when that practice falls so far from accepted standards that continued licence to practice becomes an issue.
- The Royal Colleges and professional organisations also have central roles to play in ensuring that practice is of high quality, and they have a special role in relation to education. For endocrine surgery, the British Association of Endocrine Surgeons within the UK is the relevant professional body and advises on training.
- At a local level, hospital trusts should facilitate clinical governance with audit and risk management.

More information about the practical workings of these local and national bodies can be found in *The Medical Manager*.[2]

> *Expert knowledge is often incomplete and influenced by strongly held beliefs and personal interest.*

There is ample evidence that doctors left to their own devices are not as effective as they would like to think they are, and never have been. Most surgeons would agree that unacceptable variations in standards of care and outcomes must be made to disappear yet, despite good intentions, therapeutic activity that is ineffective or unsubstantiated may take many years to disappear from clinical practice. In addition, our individual practice and the interventions that we use inevitably reflect the current fashion, albeit in the absence of any evidence base. We should not, however, lose sight of the fact that the 'evidence base' and systematic reviews may be adversely affected by subjective analysis, interpretations of variations in the results from previous studies, publication bias and missing data. Changes in clinical practice can be exciting but surgeons should be wary of advancing through errors. From an idea and hypothesis through to a technical development there should be systematic progression that ends in development and assessment of appropriate outcome measures.[3] This certainly applies to the development of minimally invasive surgery of the thyroid and parathyroid glands.[4] Are mortality and readmission rates, complications and duration of hospital stay sufficient to show that the new is an improvement on what has gone before?

Examination of new and old controversies in endocrine surgery as shown below tells us that there is currently little evidence to support a rigid approach to how we advise our patients. For example:

Thyroid disease
- Do all patients with retrosternal goitre require surgery?
- Radioiodine or surgery for patients with retrosternal goitre?
- The extent of surgery for differentiated thyroid cancer?
- The extent of lymph node surgery in differentiated and medullary thyroid cancer?
- When to complete primary surgery/re-operate in patients with medullary thyroid cancer?

Parathyroid
- The indications for surgery in patients with mild hypercalcaemia?
- What are the indications for re-operative parathyroid surgery?
- Which, if any, imaging studies are appropriate prior to first-time surgery?
- Which imaging studies are appropriate prior to re-operative surgery?
- Unilateral or bilateral neck exploration?
- Minimally invasive surgery?

Adrenal
- Transperitoneal or retroperitoneal laparoscopic surgery?
- What size of incidentaloma should be removed?
- Partial adrenalectomy in familial disease?

Pancreas
- Which preoperative localisation/regionalisation studies are required in patients with insulinoma/gastrinoma?
- When to operate on the pancreas in patients with MEN 1?

In endocrine surgery there will never be evidence based on prospective randomised controlled trials to support much of what we do, yet should we practise our craft in the manner that our peers have demonstrated to be the most effective? Critical review of our current practice will benefit our patients prior to, during and after surgery.

Guidelines should help us make decisions about what is appropriate and, in association with a review of whatever evidence there is lead to change and improvement in patient care. It should be remembered that guidelines are 'explicit' information that help us to make decisions, but the art of medicine needs as much 'tacit' as 'explicit' input.[5]

For the moment we need to stick to guidelines while remembering that they should be part of an iterative process of regular criticism and review, and that they will often need to be adapted to local circumstances. Guidelines should avoid a dogmatic approach as to what are 'appropriate' treatments.

What is good practice?

Clinical governance and quality are synonymous with achieving and maintaining good practice. As there are few if any emergencies in endocrine surgery, endocrine surgeons have ample time before any elective intervention to ask:

- Which biochemical/cytological tests and imaging studies are necessary prior to surgery, and will their results alter the management of the patient?
- Is an operation required? What is the purpose and aim of the procedure? How will this benefit the patient?
- Which operation is appropriate in this specific case?
- Does the patient understand the indications, implications and risks of surgery in order to give informed consent?

Who should perform surgery on the endocrine glands?

In the USA, thyroid operations comprise fewer than 5% of an average general surgeon's practice. This figure justifies the 1996 consensus statement on thyroid disease by the Royal College of Physicians of London and Society of Endocrinology,[6] which stated: 'each District General Hospital should have access to an experienced thyroid surgeon'. Although surgery of the endocrine glands is currently the scene of dispute between general surgeons (endocrine/upper GI/hepatobiliary, head and neck, oromaxillofacial and ENT) and urologists no individual group has an unassailable right to care for and treat the patients. The needs of the patient must come first. The introduction to the British Association of Endocrine Surgeons (BAES) guidelines states:

[the guidelines do] not define an endocrine surgeon or specify who should practice endocrine surgery... Elective endocrine surgery will not be in the portfolio of every District General Hospital, but where it is,

based on experience and caseload, it should be in the hands of a nominated surgeon with an endocrine interest. Those patients requiring more complex investigation and care as detailed in the guidelines should be referred to an appropriate centre. These rare and complex diseases will only be managed effectively by multidisciplinary teams in Units familiar with these disorders... this category includes patients with endocrine pancreatic tumours, adrenal tumours, thyroid malignancy especially medullary thyroid carcinoma, familial syndromes and those requiring reoperative thyroid and parathyroid surgery.

The advantages of subspecialisation

It is all too easy to lose sight of the important issues:

1. The experienced surgeon should be part of an experienced multidisciplinary team and should have been appropriately trained.

There is evidence from the UK to support a continued need for subspecialisation in endocrine surgery to further good practice. This is exemplified by the use of fine needle aspiration cytology (FNAC) in patients with thyroid disease and morbidity from surgery.

FNAC, in addition to clinical examination, is the most sensitive and specific test for the diagnosis of thyroid nodules and will reduce the need for surgery by at least 25% and allow the first operation for thyroid malignancy to be more appropriate. Isotope scanning and ultrasound contribute little to the diagnostic work-up of a euthyroid patient with nodular thyroid disease.

Although more than 25 years have passed since FNAC of the thyroid was introduced, a retrospective study from the South-West Thames Region found only 8% of the patients who underwent surgery had undergone preoperative needle aspiration of the thyroid;[7] 34% of 186 operations were deemed avoidable. In the same region 50 surgeons undertook a caseload of less than five thyroidectomies per year. In a retrospective study from a single district hospital only 42% of patients with thyroid cancer presenting with a thyroid nodule had preoperative FNAC.[8] The BAES audit in 1995 demonstrated that a surgeon's use of FNAC related to the number of thyroid operations performed.[9] Surgeons who performed less than 25 thyroidectomies per year used preoperative FNA in only 42% of cases overall and in 50% of the cases in which the final diagnosis was cancer. Among 107 non-specialist surgeons interviewed by postal questionnaire in the North West/ Mersey regions,[10] a median of ten thyroidectomies were performed per year; 20% of district general hospital surgeons never used FNAC. In the same study 40% of surgeons replied that they would perform nodule excision alone or subtotal lobectomy for solitary nodule, operations that are condemned as inappropriate in the management of a solitary nodule.

Complication rates of thyroid and parathyroid procedures will vary according to the experience of the surgeon, being higher in patients treated by non-specialists, as shown in Europe[11] and the USA.[12] In the UK a retrospective study from North Trent identified that over a 10-year period 32 surgeons operated on 148 patients with thyroid cancer subsequently referred to a Thyroid Cancer Clinic. Recurrent laryngeal nerve palsy and hypoparathyroidism were more common after surgery by non-specialists; more than 50% of the surgeons had treated only a single thyroid cancer patient in 10 years. A further 101 patients over the same time period were never referred to a multidisciplinary thyroid cancer clinic for consideration of adjuvant therapy.[13]

2. As the quality of the care received by the patient is paramount it should be subject to assessment by audit and benchmarking against agreed standards.

It is clear from the above studies that there is a need to collect prospective information on endocrine surgical activity in the UK, not only for issues of surgical subspecialisation, but for education and training. The BAES have initiated a long-term prospective audit that will provide much-needed information on activity and outcome. For UK

surgeons continuing membership of the Association is conditional upon providing that information, and it is likely that future GMC revalidation may require confirmation that surgeons cooperate in this sort of comparative national audit. The following standards and outcome measures are suggested as being applicable to current endocrine surgical practice.

THYROID SURGERY

Standards

- The indications for operation, risks and complications should be discussed with patients prior to surgery.
- Fine needle aspiration cytology should be performed routinely in the investigation of solitary thyroid nodules.
- The recurrent laryngeal nerve should be routinely identified in patients undergoing thyroid surgery.
- All patients scheduled for re-operative thyroid surgery should undergo preoperative examination of their vocal cords by an ENT surgeon. All patients reporting voice change after thyroid surgery should undergo examination of their vocal cords. Permanent vocal cord palsy should not occur in more than 1% of patients.
- A return to theatre to control postoperative haemorrhage should occur in less than 5% of patients.
- All patients with thyroid cancer should be reviewed by the Cancer Centre designated specialist multidisciplinary team.

Outcome measures

There should be documented evidence to support that:

- The patient was informed of the indications for surgery and its risks and complications.
- Fine needle aspiration cytology was performed in at least 90% of patients prior to operation for solitary/dominant nodule.
- The recurrent laryngeal nerve(s) were identified during a surgical procedure.
- The permanent postoperative vocal cord palsy rate is not more than 1%.

- All patients scheduled for re-operative thyroid surgery have undergone preoperative examination of their vocal cords.
- The re-operation rate for postoperative haemorrhage after thyroidectomy is less than 5%.
- Patients with thyroid malignancy have been reviewed by the specialist multidisciplinary team.

PARATHYROID SURGERY

Standards

In patients who undergo first-time operation for primary hyperparathyroidism:

- The indications for operation, risks and complications should be discussed with patients prior to surgery.
- The surgeon should identify and cure the cause of the disease in at least 95% of cases.
- All patients reporting voice change after parathyroid surgery should undergo examination of their vocal cords. Permanent vocal cord palsy should not occur in more than 1% of patients.
- All patients scheduled for re-operative parathyroid surgery should undergo preoperative examination of their vocal cords.
- Permanent hypocalcaemia should not occur in more than 5% of patients.

Outcome measures

There should be documented evidence to support that:

- The patient was informed of the indications for surgery and its risks and complications.
- After first-time parathyroid surgery, at least 90% of patients are normocalcaemic without calcium or vitamin D supplements.
- The permanent postoperative vocal cord palsy rate is not more than 1%.
- All patients scheduled for re-operative parathyroid surgery have undergone preoperative examination of their vocal cords.

ADRENAL SURGERY

Standards

There should be multidisciplinary working to agreed diagnostic and therapeutic protocols to ensure that

an appropriate strategy is developed for patients. This should include the management of the pre-operative, peroperative and postoperative metabolic syndrome.

Outcome measures

There should be documented evidence to demonstrate that all patients have been discussed with the multidisciplinary team.

Biochemical cure should be evident in at least:

- 90% of patients with phaeochromocytoma;
- 90% of patients with Conn's syndrome;
- 90% of patients with Cushing's syndrome.

PANCREATIC SURGERY

Standards

- There should be multidisciplinary working to agreed diagnostic and therapeutic protocols to ensure that an appropriate strategy is developed for patients. This should include management of the preoperative, perioperative and postoperative metabolic syndrome.
- Familial endocrine disease cases should be identified prior to surgery.
- The aims of any surgical procedure must be clearly defined prior to surgery.

Outcome measures

There should be documented evidence to demonstrate that all patients have been discussed with the multidisciplinary team.

- Insulinoma: surgery should result in biochemical cure in at least 90% of cases.
- Gastrinoma: surgery should result in biochemical cure or clinically useful response in at least 60% of cases.

Who should train the future endocrine surgeons and to what level of expertise?

Surgeons in training, when appropriately supervised and assisted by their trainers, can perform thyroidectomy safely.[14,15] Furthermore, surgeons who have completed a well-designed training programme and who have become proficient in thyroid surgery can remain proficient when they practise as general consultants.[16] In the UK the higher surgical trainee should spend at least one year in an approved unit, which should consist of:

- One or more surgeons with a declared interest in endocrine surgery.
- An annual operative workload in excess of 50 cases (verified by BAES audit).
- On site cytology and histopathology services.
- At least one consultant endocrinologist on site, holding one or more dedicated endocrinology clinics per week, with joint clinics or formal meetings held not less than once per month.
- A Department of Nuclear Medicine on site.
- On site magnetic resonance imaging (MRI) and computed tomography (CT) scanning

In practical terms flexible rotations between regions may be required for more specialised areas of endocrine practice, such as adrenal surgery.

Risk management

Risk management encapsulates the notion that all surgical activity involves some degree of risk and that the risk must be managed so as to achieve the best outcome for the patient. In the past it was sufficient merely to be properly trained, caring and conscientious; today this does not suffice.

Medical care should be given effectively and carefully; in addition it must be seen to be given effectively and carefully. However cynical one might be about the mechanics of clinical governance and however self-confident one may feel as a professional, there is now a need to take public and documented steps to ensure that risk is being managed. There is evidence that the risk management process has positive advantages in terms of delivering a high quality of care, measured as an improved process of care with better outcome. Whether or not the current bureaucratic process of clinical governance can measurably improve clinical outcome to justify its considerable expense and disruption remains to be seen.[17] We will probably never know.

STAFF ISSUES

Are the consultants properly trained and up to date with their postgraduate education in endocrine surgery? Are other consultants undertaking endocrine surgery on an occasional basis because they enjoy it rather than because they are trained in it? When appropriate, are complex patients referred to a specialist centre? The endocrine surgeon must be part of a team that includes endocrine physicians, oncologist, radiologists, cytopathologist and histopathologist, chemical pathologist and clinical/molecular geneticists.

Are trainees appropriately engaged in the process? Are surgical procedures delegated by an appropriate person in the full knowledge of the trainee's competence? Is their supervision appropriate? It is not acceptable to let a new specialist registrar undertake a thyroidectomy prior to supervised assessment of their operative competence.

COMMUNICATION ISSUES

Are patients properly informed about proposed surgery, particularly the various therapeutic options open to them in addition to the risks and implications of any choice they make (see 'Consent' below)? Are there information sheets available and in use?

PROTOCOL ISSUES

Are there written protocols in use such as the BAES Guidelines to aid clinical decision-taking, as well as local protocols for the care of patients with postoperative airway obstruction, hypocalcaemia and steroid replacement after adrenalectomy?

RECORD-KEEPING

Clear and contemporaneous evidence must be available in the notes, to show that patients were properly counselled prior to operation and warned about the risks of surgery. The operation notes should be contemporaneous, written by the operating surgeons (or at the very least countersigned by them) and should confirm that, for example, at thyroidectomy the recurrent laryngeal nerves were seen and spared and that parathyroid tissue was retained with its blood supply intact.

SUPPORT SERVICES

An increasingly common issue in litigation is delay in diagnosis or incorrect diagnosis. In this context it is imperative that the pathologists with whom you work should be competent in the specific and often difficult area of thyroid cytology and histology.

AUDIT

Remember that simply keeping audit records and having regular audit meetings is not sufficient. The audit cycle must be seen to be occurring such that what has been learned from audit is applied and the whole cycle repeated. Of course this rarely happens. A National Audit Office report has found that only one formal audit study in six had gone round the whole audit cycle and was being repeated.[18]

MEDICO-LEGAL ASPECTS OF ENDOCRINE SURGERY

Even if Trusts, teams and individual clinicians adhere conscientiously to all the requirements of good clinical governance, errors may still occur or will be thought by the patient to have occurred. In this section we cover the specific steps needed to avoid complaint and litigation in endocrine surgery, and suggest some responses should it occur, with an outline of the processes involved. In legal actions the jurisdiction that applies is that of the country in which injury occurred, and we have based our views on an interpretation of English law.

Consent

A formal process of consent in surgery is essential as it is that consent that renders surgical intervention legal. Consent requires that the patient has the **capacity** to understand the process, has the **information** about the nature and the purpose of the surgery to allow informed consent, and provides consent **voluntarily**. Failure to respect these principles means that there was effectively no consent, and the doctor is therefore open to charges of battery or to a claim of negligence. 'Battery' is the unlawful infliction of force on another person, negligence is the failure to take reasonable care. The courts have shown no enthusiasm for pursuing medical cases as battery; most cases that concern the adequacy of information given are brought under the tort of negligence.

In the hallmark UK case of Sidaway, Lord Justice Dunn said that 'the concept of informed consent forms no part of English law'.[19] There is no explicit legal meaning to the term 'informed consent' used by doctors. The case of Sidaway involved a patient who experienced spinal cord complications after an operation on a cervical vertebra as treatment for nerve root pain. She had not been informed about this particular rare complication when she gave her consent, and she claimed that she would not have had the operation if more information had been available. In this case, the patient was not warned because the neurosurgeon judged the risk to be remote, i.e. less than 1%. The problem highlights the potential gap between the 'patient standard', which is what the patient might wish to know, and the 'professional standard', which is what the doctor thinks the patient ought to or needs to know. Patients who experience a complication from an operation will, with the wisdom of hindsight, wish they had been told about a rare but damaging complication, whereas surgeons might reasonably not tell patients of all potential risks that could occur.

In the matter of consent (as in most other medico-legal issues), case law in England and Scotland tends to reflect the application of the 'Bolam test' (see below), namely that the information that the surgeon needs to give is the information that a reasonable and responsible member of the medical profession would think it proper to give in the circumstances. The amount of information that is given to validate 'informed' consent is not defined in law. The rule of thumb is that it should be any risk that is likely to occur in more than 1–2% of cases, but it is important to remember that the quality of information given for consent in medical care is an ethical not a legal requirement of a doctor and is to do with the respect for the autonomy of the patient.[20] Sidaway puts the onus on doctors to decide what information to give; the ethical requirement is merely to give what the doctors' best judgement of each patient defines as the patient's need, and to give it in terms appropriate to the patient's understanding and their education. This trend is also likely to be encouraged by the Council of Europe's Convention on Human Rights:

Biomedicine, 1997, which explicitly notes the 'need to restrain the paternalist approaches which might ignore the wishes of the patient'.[21] It is better to look at the process of 'informed' consent as part of a shared decision-making process, founded in adult debate with patients about the management of their disease. The risks and consequences of various treatment options should be discussed in sufficient detail to be understood to allow patients to make informed decisions.

In practical terms the surgeon, or somebody who is familiar with the disease and its treatment, must sign the consent form together with the patient. We recommend the use of patients' information sheets (as illustrated in the BAES Guidelines), but remember that their use does not obviate the need for detailed personal discussions between patients and surgeons (**Box 7.1**).

When things do not go smoothly

Only a tiny percentage of problems and errors mature into a complaint. It is clear that if complaints are handled effectively and promptly and if there is good and honest communication of facts, the number of complaints that mature into litigations are few. One of the virtues of proper handling of complaints is that they often show that although things did not turn out for the best, the problems that occurred were within the boundaries of those experienced in medical care and were not a sign of negligence.

Box 7.1 • Key issues in risk reduction on matters of consent

- Obtain consent well before the operation.
- Do not obtain consent after sedation has been given.
- The doctor obtaining consent should be knowledgeable about the procedure and its potential complications.
- Explain 'material risks'.
- Answer questions in an open and honest manner.
- Do not alter the consent form after the patient has signed it.
- Do not exceed the authority given by the consent form.

HANDLING COMPLAINTS

Informal complaints should be dealt with as promptly and as honestly as possible in the format of normal communication. It does no harm if there has been a degree of error to admit to that and to apologise early. We believe that if the surgeon or the person to whom the complaint has been made makes an honest and insightful assessment of the problem and considers that there has **not** been an error, there is no requirement to apologise. A verbal complaint that is dealt with orally should be recorded as a written or typed note and placed in the clinical record. Nothing should be sent out in writing without first checking the text with the Trust's complaints officer and/or your defence organisation. This is invaluable if an informal complaint subsequently turns into a formal one.

LOCAL RESOLUTION OF COMPLAINTS

Procedures that came into force in April 1996 have defined in detail how, and how speedily, hospitals must respond to complaints. These processes have some key objectives:

- Ease of access to the complaints system.
- A simple, rapid, open process.
- Fairness for complainants and staff alike.
- Lessons from complaints to be used to improve patient services.
- Investigation of complaints to be entirely separate from any subsequent disciplinary proceedings.

Complaints must be made within 6 months of the event complained about or from the moment that a patient realised that there had been a problem. The complaint can go through consecutive stages:

1. Local resolution.
2. Independent review.
3. Appeal to the health service ombudsman.

A review of the workings of the complaints system noted that it was perceived as 'biased, closed and inadequate' and that 'patients feel suspicious, frustrated and let down' and clinicians 'undervalued and beset'.[22] The same survey characterised the present processes as tending 'to investigate superficially, to analyse defensively, and to jump to conclusions about the remedy, if any action is taken at all'; little wonder therefore that complaints can turn into litigation.

COMPLAINTS THAT TURN INTO LITIGATION

As far as endocrine surgeons are concerned cases will be based in personal injury owing to an alleged breach of duty by them or their team. A complication of surgery or a delay in diagnosis will be the probable reason. There are no published figures to indicate how often endocrine surgery in the UK has led to litigation in the past and how successful that has been. The best data, although incomplete, come from the USA. In a paper presented at the annual meeting of the American Association of Endocrine Surgeons in 1993, Kern identified 62 cases of malpractice from 21 states between 1985 and 1991, for analysis. In 54% of instances the problem arose from a surgical complication, almost all during thyroid surgery; 35% arose from delayed diagnosis, equally of thyroid and adrenal disease, and 11% were from morbidity attributed to radioiodine or propylthiouracil. It is sobering to see that even 10 years ago mean payouts for successful litigation for a recurrent nerve injury approached $1 million and the maximum was $2.5 million.[23] The number of endocrine cases currently passing through the system in the USA or the UK is not known.

The first intimation of litigation will usually be a letter from the solicitor to the hospital, and this may come without patients having troubled to go through a formal complaint process first, or patients may have been through some sort of formal or informal process and not been satisfied with the outcome. Once a problem turns into a formal process of litigation it is protracted, time consuming, distressing for all concerned and, from the NHS's point of view, expensive. It is important that clinicians handle complaints in as dispassionate and efficient a way as possible, however distressed they may feel by the complaint itself and by the process of dealing with it.

The solicitor's letter

The first manifestation will normally be a solicitor's letter asking for release of copies of all the notes, X-ray films, pathology reports, etc. In NHS practice the hospital complaints or litigation officer should receive this, together with an indication that the request for release signifies or does not signify an impending action against the Trust.

At this stage you may be asked by the hospital to confirm that you are happy for copies of the notes to be released. In effect you have no choice about this, but the solicitor requesting them must give sufficient detail, setting out the expected case against the doctor, to comply with the requirements of section 33 of the Supreme Court Act, 1981. Before the release of the notes you need to make sure that they are in sensible order, that copies of all the originals are retained by the hospital and that you have reviewed any part that you or your team had in the incident that has led to the litigation. You also need to check that it is the patient who indirectly is asking for release of the files. If it is not then you will need the patient's permission to release the file. The Medical Defence Union has produced a helpful pamphlet on this subject for its members.[24]

When reviewing the notes it is in order to ensure that the filing of the notes is logical, but you must not add anything, change anything or remove anything from the notes. Do, however, refresh your memory, as it may be several years since the events occurred. If you receive a request for notes in your capacity as a private practitioner, check the notes and photocopy them, but only release them to the patient's solicitors through your medical defence organisation.

The solicitors acting for the patient will now be finding an expert and getting an initial opinion. Additionally, experience shows that they will often be applying to the Legal Aid board for a certificate to confirm that this client's costs will be covered if they are eligible. It is a sad reflection on access to justice that medical negligence litigation is not realistically affordable by any but the very rich and those receiving legal aid. There will, in any event, be a lull, the extent of which is governed only by the limitation period of three years from the time that the plaintiff could reasonably have known that he or she had a cause for action. There are, however, situations where this time may be extended, but this requires a formal plea in court to disbar a defence plea that a plaintiff's action is disbarred by lapse of time.[25]

The next communication will probably be a writ and a statement of claim from the plaintiff's solicitors, outlining in detail the allegations and often enclosing the expert's report in the details of which the claim is usually grounded. The writ formally indicates the beginning of a legal action.

Most doctors become depressed, distressed, angry or all three of these at this point, and fortunately the handling of the process from here on is not in their hands but in those of the solicitors acting for the hospital, or the medical defence organisation if the matter relates to a private patient.

If you believe that the allegation of negligence is completely unfounded, it is important at this stage to ensure that the hospital is aware of the strength of your feelings and is prepared to defend the claim rather than simply settle to reduce costs (particularly in relation to plaintiffs receiving legal aid). You may want to liaise with your medical defence organisation about this, even if it is an NHS case. Many textbooks describe the detail of the legal processes and the details of the underlying laws, principles and customs. Currently, the two most readable of these books are *Medical Negligence, a Practical Guide*[26] (written by a barrister from the point of view of the plaintiff) and *Medicine, Patients and the Law*.[27]

Essentially the case will revolve around the fact that you, the surgeon, are claimed to have been negligent. Although negligence has lay meanings as a word, it has very specific legal meanings.

MEDICAL NEGLIGENCE

Surgical cases come to court almost invariably as a result of patients suing in an action for negligence. This is a civil prosecution.

Negligence is an area considered under the civil law called tort, i.e. civil wrongs. Any formal legal action in this area only succeeds if a particular legal formula is fulfilled. The components of this formula are:

1. A relationship must exist between the parties (the surgeon and the patient), which gives rise to a **duty of care**.
2. The duty of care must have been **breached** in some way due to an unreasonable act or omission by one of the parties. This breach of the duty of care is the negligence.
3. In addition to the negligence the injured party must have experienced some '**damage**', loss or injury of a type recognised by the law.

4. The damage must have been caused **by the other party,** in this case the surgeon.
5. The action must be brought within a specified time after the injury has occurred (this is known as the **period of limitation;** see above).

Duty of care

As the NHS surgical patient will already have come under the care of a hospital, either as an outpatient or inpatient, the plaintiff will have no difficulty in establishing that the hospital Trust has a duty of care. In private practice (and this includes patients admitted to NHS pay beds) the relationship is primarily directly with the surgeon and separately with the other providers, such as the hospital, pathology laboratory, etc. The duty of care in this latter situation arises through the 'contract' that arises implicitly between the surgeon and patient.

Breaching of duty of care

A successful negligence claim requires that the patient claimant demonstrates that the defendant (Trust or surgeon) was in breach of its duty of care. In English law the breach or lack of it is determined by judging what an equivalent body of other doctors would have done in similar circumstances. This is known as the 'Bolam test'.

Bolam[28] is the legal case cited in England. In Scotland it is *Hunter* v. *Hanley*.[29] Essentially these cases have the same conclusion, which is generally favourable to the surgeon.

The more recent case of *Bolitho* v. *City and Hackney Health Authority* has slightly changed the principles behind the Bolam case. Medical evidence from eight experts was divided. The judge accepted that both bodies of evidence were respectable and concluded that he was in no position to 'prefer' one view. This was in line with Lord Scarman's view in another case that: 'a judge's preference for one body of distinguished opinion over another, also professionally distinguished, is not sufficient to establish negligence in a practitioner'.[30]

The case was appealed eventually to the House of Lords, who supported the trial judge's conclusion but added an important rider to the 'Bolam test' in that it was no longer sufficient for experts to aver that something was acceptable practice but needed to show that in 'forming their view, the experts have directed their minds to the question of comparative risks and benefits and have reached a defensible conclusion on the matter.[31] Courts in the Republic of Ireland have in general also accepted the Bolam test but have spelled out the same limitations, that the treatment supported must be logical. Experts supporting or rejecting a particular course of action must therefore ground their views in a defensible clinical assessment of the pros and cons of any particular course of action.

A recent twist to this has been the position of guidelines and protocols. Many surgeons are apprehensive that they may not, on the basis of their own experience and reading, agree with protocols that are promulgated either nationally or within their own organisation, and therefore they might feel particularly threatened if they departed from those guidelines. Guidelines and protocols hold no special status legally and they should merely be regarded as an extension of the Bolam principle, as defining the views of other reputable practitioners. A guideline should not be published unless the authors can justify their joint view with reference to normal good clinical practice and the literature. Similarly, surgeons who depart from guidelines must be able logically and clinically to defend their departure from those guidelines. It is the courts who retain the right to decide whether a particular clinical practice is acceptable or not. Expert evidence of professional habits will carry the day in most cases, but surgeons cannot rely on this with complete certainty. There seem to be only a tiny number of cases where the court has chosen not to accept the expert medical evidence.

It is hardly surprising that doctors have a duty to keep themselves informed of major developments such as might be encompassed by guidelines. That duty cannot extend to a requirement that they know everything there is to know. For example, in the case of *Crawford* v. *The Board of Governors of Charing Cross Hospital*, the plaintiff had developed a brachial palsy because of his position on the operating table. Six months prior to the event, an article had appeared in the *Lancet* warning of this danger, but the anaesthetist involved in the case had not read the article. The Court of Appeal found in favour of the anaesthetist, Lord Denning stating that:

> *It would I think be putting too high a burden on a medical man to say he has read every article appearing in the current medical press; and it would be quite wrong to suggest a medical man is negligent because he does not at once put into operation a suggestion which some contributor or other might make in a medical journal. The time may come in a particular case where a new recommendation may be so well proved, and so well known, and so well accepted that it should be adopted, this was not so in this case.[32]*

A widely promulgated guideline could, however, in Lord Denning's terms fall into a recommendation 'so well proved and so well known and so well accepted that it should be adopted'.

DAMAGE

Damage cited by plaintiffs must have been caused directly by the defendants' negligence, not, for example, simply by progression of underlying disease. Damages subsequently awarded in the UK simply aim to place defendants in the position they were in before the damage was sustained, plus an element for pain and suffering. The situation in the UK is totally different from that pertaining in the USA, where juries, not judges, decide damages, and a strong punitive element is often included.

Causation

Letters from solicitors will often use the term 'causation', a term not immediately understood by doctors (**Box 7.2**). In the legal setting 'causation' is merely the establishment of a factual and legal link between the breach of duty and the damage caused. This is often difficult to prove. Normally the 'but for' test is used. For example, 'but for the failure to take a fine needle biopsy at the first outpatient visit

Box 7.2 • Examples illustrating the legal meaning of causation

Causation	No causation
A patient comes into hospital for thyroidectomy. The cords are checked preoperatively and both move. After the operation the patient is hoarse and laryngoscopy shows one cord is not moving. The plaintiff's barrister could readily show that there was a duty of care, that there was damage and could prove causation. But it would be hard to prove negligence. Laryngeal nerve palsy ipso facto is not evidence of negligence.	A patient comes to the outpatient department with a longstanding mass in the neck. The mass is fixed to the surrounding structures. The surgeon neither biopsies the mass nor operates. Two weeks later the patient dies and the postmortem shows an anaplastic carcinoma obstructing the airway. There was a duty of care but there was no causation in that on a balance of probability failure to biopsy the mass or arrange treatment did not alter the outcome.

the patient's thyroid carcinoma would have been diagnosed 6 months earlier'. Note that in negligence cases guilt or innocence is decided on grounds of 'balance of probability' rather than 'beyond reasonable doubt', as applies in criminal cases.

EXPERT OPINIONS

Although it is for the court to decide on matters put before it – right or wrong, true or false, negligent or not negligent – it can only do so in medical cases by drawing on expert advice from clinicians and others. More importantly – and more commonly – expert advice is also used to determine whether a case needs to be put before the court or should be abandoned or settled out of court. Anyone asked to provide an expert report will usually receive with that request guidance notes advising that the expert's duty is to the court and not to the plaintiff, the defendant or the solicitor that has instructed him. Therefore:

- The report is addressed to the court.
- It contains a statement that experts understand that their duty is to the court.
- Experts may if they wish file a written request to the court for directions to assist them in carrying out their function as an expert. They do not need to give the claimant, defendant or the instructing solicitor any notice of such a request.

Reforms

The surgeon should be aware of several changes that will affect medical litigation over the next ten years:

1. Conditional/contingency fees ('no win, no fee').
2. The recommendations of the Woolf report.
3. Attempts to control the cost of legal aid.
4. The use of mediation.

NO WIN, NO FEE

The legislation to allow lawyers and their clients to come to conditional agreements about fees – the fee being conditional on the outcome of the case – came into effect in July 1995. In the UK the loser must pay the other party's costs. The option, therefore, of not having to pay your lawyer if you lose does not guarantee a risk-free exercise for the plaintiff. The 'no win, no fee' arrangement also puts greater pressure on the claimant's solicitor to check that the case is worth pursuing, and that pressure is much greater than it is in cases supported by legal aid. Overall, the system will probably reduce rather than increase the number of vexatious and speculative claims.[33] Doctors in the UK also retain the continuing privilege of the application of the 'Bolam test'.

THE WOOLF REPORT

The Woolf report[34] reviewed the whole of the civil justice system in England and Wales and recommended radical change. Medical negligence litigation did not escape Lord Woolf's attentions because he considered most cases currently to be unduly long, complex and expensive. The recommendations of the report have been summarised as follows:

1. Greater effort at prevention and early resolution of disputes. As steps towards this,

Lord Woolf recommended that medical record keeping should be better, the procedures for local resolution of problems should be clearer, and that there should be more use of mediation with jointly instructed experts where possible and a greater use of experts' meetings. Overall though, he recommended a more sparing use of experts.

2. An improved summary disposal procedure to weed out weak claims and weak defences.

3. The introduction of a system of plaintiff 'offers to settle', with sanctions where a defendant unreasonably refused to cooperate.

4. Claims of £10 000 or less to be handled by a slimmed down procedure with a limited range of legal processes conforming to tightly controlled timetables and costs.

5. Large and complex claims to be handled by a 'multitrack' process, where the management of each case legally is decided by the courts themselves rather than by lawyers.

CHANGES TO LEGAL AID LEGISLATION

The costs of legal aid are rising annually, and this is a cause of concern for the Government. Recent changes to the rules to reduce access to legal aid excluded medical negligence cases. Subsequently there have been more definite steps to limit the management of medical negligence cases to legal practices with proven expertise.

MEDIATION

Mediation is not simply a way of avoiding the expense of full-blown litigation; it is a means to resolve disputes more simply and humanely. It requires the services of trained and committed mediators. Pilot projects for mediation are underway at present and mediation is likely to form a more common way of resolving allegations of negligent care in the future. It is certain that there will be a large role for the independent, informed clinical expert to assist arbitrators.

CONCLUSIONS

The endocrine surgeon is not simply a technician; he or she must be both self-regulator and a knowledgeable member of the endocrine team.

Effective Clinical Governance will help define:

- the appropriateness and effectiveness of our interventions;
- the lack of evidence that supports some of our current practice;
- the needs for further research.

There is a clear need to improve the standards of care for patients with endocrine surgical disorders in the UK. Guidelines and audit will help surgeons pass the 'shadow line' to achieve:

...gains not only to oneself, but to the whole practice of surgery...not at the expense of overlooking how much there must always be to learn; the confidence and pride in one's own abilities that allows criticism from both within and without ... a view of medicine as a whole that can allow all its surprises and uncertainties to be one's companions throughout one's career not as spectres reflecting inadequacy, but as impartial guides who point out the way forward

R. Hayward[35]

Complaint and litigation will not go away. An increase in individualism, loss of respect for professionals, more mechanical medical processes and a good supply of well-trained, proficient lawyers is going to ensure that whatever the changes in legislation and clinical practice, litigation will continue. Risk reduction activity by surgeons should include the routine practice of documenting that an appropriate consent process has occurred and the use of patient information material. Adherence to protocols, competence-based training and career-long postgraduate education should aim to reduce the incidence of harm to the unavoidable minimum. Complaints that are not satisfactorily resolved may be better handled by processes of arbitration or mediation rather than the traditional confrontationalism of the legal process. The legal aid process is already attempting to weed out such cases.

It is the placement of that fine boundary between misadventure and negligence that is behind most medical litigation in endocrine surgery as in all other branches of medicine.

REFERENCES

1. Relman AS. Assessment and accountability. N Engl J Med 1988; 319:1220–2.

2. Young AE. The medical manager, 2nd edn. London: BMJ Books, 2003.

3. Lorenz W, Troidl H, Solomkin JS et al. Second step: testing outcome measurements. World J Surg 1999; 23:768–80.

4. Miccoli P. Minimally invasive endocrine surgery – editorial. Acta Chir Austriaca 1999; 31:195.

5. Wyatt JC. Management of explicit and tacit knowledge. J R Soc Med 2001; 94:6–9.

6. Vanderpump MP, Ahlquist JA, Franklyn JA et al. Consensus statement for good practice in the management of hypothyroidism and hyperthyroidism. The Research Unit of the Royal College of Physicians of London, the Endocrinology and Diabetes Committee of the Royal College of Physicians of London, and the Society for Endocrinology. Br Med J 1996; 313:539–44.

7. Asimakopoulos G, Loosemore T, Bowyer RC et al. A regional study of thyroidectomy: surgical pathology suggests scope to improve quality and reduce cost. Ann R Coll Surg Engl 1995; 77:425–30.

8. Vanderpump MP, Alexander L, Scarpello JH et al. An audit of the management of thyroid cancer in a district general hospital. Clin Endocrinol (Oxf) 1998; 48:419–24.

9. Chadwick DR, Harrison BJ. The role of fine-needle aspiration cytology and frozen section histology in management of differentiated thyroid cancer: the U.K. experience. Langenbeck's Arch Surg 1998; 383:164–6.

10. Peacock T, Parrott NR. Variations in the surgical practice of thyroidectomy. Br J Surg 1997; 84:1314.

11. Harness JK, van Heerden JA, Lennquist S et al. Future of thyroid surgery and training surgeons to meet the expectations of 2000 and beyond. World J Surg 2000; 24:976–82.

12. Sosa JA, Bowman HM, Tielsch JM et al. The importance of surgeon experience for clinical and economic outcomes from thyroidectomy. Ann Surg 1998; 228:320–30.

13. Miller BA, Moore S, Harrison BJ. Thyroid cancer management in North Trent. Case record review confirms the need for specialist care. Br J Surg 2000; 87:1260.

14. Runkel N, Riede E, Mann B et al. Surgical training and vocal-cord paralysis in benign thyroid disease. Langenbeck's Arch Surg 1998; 383:240–2.

15. Mishra A, Agarwal G, Agarwal A et al. Safety and efficacy of total thyroidectomy in hands of endocrine trainees. Am J Surg 1999; 178:377–80.

16. Reeve TS, Curtin A, Fingleton L et al. Can total thyroidectomy be performed as safely by general surgeons in provincial centers as by surgeons in specialised endocrine surgical units? Making the case for surgical training. Arch Surg 1994; 129:834–6.

17. Goodman NW. Accountability, clinical governance and the acceptance of imperfection. J Roy Soc Med 2000; 93:59–61.

18. National Audit Office. Clinical audit in England. London: Stationery Office, 1995.

19. *Sidaway* v. *Board of Governors of the Bethlehem Royal Hospital*. [1984] QB493 at 517, [1984] 1 All ER 1018 at 1030, CA.

20. Davies M. Textbook on medical law. London: Blackstone Press, 1996; pp. 166–74.

21. Medical Law Monitor 1997; 4(10):6.

22. Hill AP, Baeza J. Dealing with things that go wrong. Lancet 1999; 354:2099–100.

23. Kern KA. Medicolegal analysis of errors in diagnosis and treatment of surgical endocrine disease. Surgery 1993; 114:1167–74.

24. Hoyte P. Can I see the records? London: Medical Defence Union, 1996.

25. Finch J. Speller's law relating to hospitals, 7th edn, section 5.2. London: Chapman & Hall Medical, 1993.

26. Lewis C. Medical negligence, a practical guide, 4th edn. London: Butterworths, 1998.

27. Brazier M. Medicine, patients and the law. London: Penguin, 1992.

28. *Bolam* v. *Friern Hospital Management Committee* [1957]; 2 All ER 118, [1957] 1 WLR 582.

29. *Hunter* v. *Hanley*. 1955 SC 200.

30. *Maynard* v. *West Midlands Regional Health Authority* [1984] 1 WLR 634 at 639.

31. *Bolitho* [1997] 4 All ER 771.

32. Cited by Mason JK, McCall Smith RA. Law and medical ethics. London: Butterworths, 1994; p. 202.

33. Barton A. Conditional fees: access to justice for all. Clin Risk 1997; 3:130–1.

34. Lord Woolf. Access to justice. London: Stationery Office, 1996.

35. Hayward R. The shadow-line in surgery. Lancet 1987; 1:375–6.

Plate 1 • Computed tomography (CT)-enhanced SPECT scan. This image shows a mediastinal parathyroid adenoma identified precisely by SPECT enhancement and CT. The top two rows of images mark the parathyroid adenoma on CT scan (crosshair). The bottom row of images mark the parathyroid adenoma on SPECT scan.

Plate 2 • Parathyroid adenoma. This photomicrograph demonstrates the characteristic hypercellularity, loss of fat, loss of lobulation, and oxyphilic change of adenomatous degeneration (×40).

Plate 3 • Parathyroid hyperplasia. This photomicrograph demonstrates the characteristic hypercellularity, loss of fat and retained lobulation of parathyroid hyperplasia (×40).

Plate 4 • Parathyroid carcinoma. This photomicrograph demonstrates the characteristic thickened fibrous septa, nuclear atypia and capsular invasion of parathyroid carcinoma (×40).

Plate 5 • Conventional open parathyroidectomy: left superior parathyroid adenoma and normal inferior parathyroid gland.

Plate 6 • Multiglandular disease: four-gland hyperplasia.

Plate 7 • Endoscopic parathyroidectomy by lateral approach – trocar position.

Plate 8 • Endoscopic parathyroidectomy by left lateral approach: recurrent laryngeal nerve and superior parathyroid adenoma.

Plate 9 • Secondary hyperparathyroidism: four-gland hyperplasia.

Plate 10 • Large retrosternal goitre causing respiratory distress. Specimen resected without the need of a sternotomy.

Plate 11 • Total thyroidectomy for papillary thyroid cancer with right-sided modified neck dissection to remove involved cervical nodes.

Plate 12 • Appendiceal carcinoid, with the typical yellow colour and location in tip of the appendix. From Capella C, Solcia E, Sobin L et al. Endocrine tumours of the appendix.

Plate 13 • Rectal carcinoid polyp with typical yellowish colour and submucosal location.

Plate 14 • Fine-needle aspiration cytology of a pleomorphic adenoma showing epithelial and mucinous components.

Plate 15 • Pathological specimen showing the cut surface of a pleomorphic adenoma of the parotid gland.

Eight

The salivary glands

Zenon Rayter

THE PAROTID GLAND

Diseases of the parotid are relatively uncommon, but this salivary gland has one of the greatest diversities of pathology. Most lesions are of an inflammatory nature although some arise from a post-traumatic, systemic or uncertain pathogenesis. There is also a wide spectrum of neoplastic conditions, some of which are unique to the parotid gland. The differential diagnosis of a parotid mass remains an important aspect of a surgeon's training.

Embryology

The mouth is developed partly from the stomodaeum and partly from the cephalic portion of the foregut. By the growth of the head end of the embryo and formation of the head fold, the pericardial area and the oral or buccopharyngeal membrane come to lie on the ventral surface of the embryo. With the further expansion of the brain and the bulging of the pericardium, the oral membrane comes to lie at the bottom of the depression bounded by these two prominences.[1] This depression constitutes the stomodaeum, or primitive mouth (**Fig. 8.1**). The parotid gland can be recognised in human embryos as 8 mm long and arising from the epithelial lining of the mouth, appearing as an elongated furrow running dorsally from the angle of the mouth between the mandibular arch and maxillary process. The

groove, which is converted into a tube, loses its connection with the epithelium of the mouth[1] (except at its anterior end) and grows dorsally into the substance of the cheek. This tube persists as the parotid duct, and its blind end proliferates to form the gland. Subsequently, the size of the oral fissure is reduced, and the parotid duct opens on the inside of the cheek at some distance from the angle of the mouth. The epithelial buds enlarge, elongate and branch, initially forming solid structures, but they eventually cannalise, creating lumina. The lining epithelial cells of the ducts, tubules and acini then differentiate both morphologically and functionally, and the contractile myoepithelial cells become placed around the acini.[2] The interaction between the parenchymal and stromal elements with the autonomic system is necessary for normal salivary gland development and function; sympathetic nerve stimulation leads to acinar differentiation whereas parasympathetic nerve stimulation is required for overall glandular growth.[2]

Prior to the complete development of the parotid gland, the lymphatic system begins to emerge in the mesoderm. Because of this, in the adult there are unique intraglandular lymph nodes and lymphatic channels. In addition, salivary epithelial cells can be included within these lymph nodes. This unusual situation is believed to have a role in the development of Warthin's tumours and possibly lymphoepithelial cysts.[3] As parotid epithelial buds grow

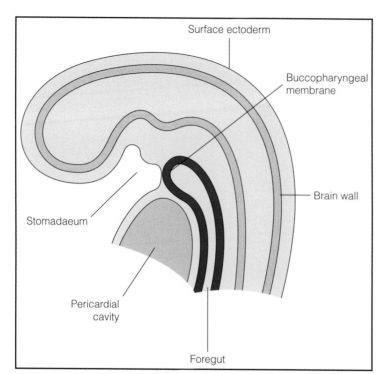

Figure 8.1 • Sagittal section of the cephalic end of a 25-day embryo illustrating the development of the mouth prior to the appearance of the parotid gland.

and branch, they extend between and around the division of the facial nerve, incorporating the distal portion of this nerve within the gland.[2]

Anatomy

The parotid gland occupies the irregular space bounded behind by the external auditory meatus, the mastoid process and the sternomastoid muscle, in front by the mandible and its attached muscles, and medially by the styloid process and its attached muscles. It extends upwards as far as the zygomatic arch and forwards, both deep and superficial to the ramus of the mandible. The gland is separated from the skin by the general investing layer of the deep fascia of the neck, which above the angle of the mandible passes over the gland and fuses with the masseter muscle on the outer aspect of the ramus of the mandible. The fascia is attached to the zygomatic arch and becomes continuous with the temporal fascia. There is no true capsule to the parotid gland, and the lobules of gland substance fill the available space and conform to the shape of the surrounding structures. The duct of the gland (Stensen's duct) follows the masseter muscle to its anterior edge,

where it turns medially through buccinator to open on to the mucous membrane of the cheek opposite the crown of the upper second molar tooth. As Stensen's duct passes over the masseter, it may receive the duct of an accessory parotid gland, which is found overlying the masseter muscle in approximately 20% of people, usually related cranial to Stensen's duct.

The facial nerve emerges from the mastoid at the stylomastoid foramen lateral to the styloid process and almost immediately enters the parotid. Before entering the parotid gland, the facial nerve gives off branches to the stylohyoid, the posterior belly of the diagastric muscle and the occipitalis muscles. The main trunk of the nerve (the pes anserinus, or goose's foot) then usually divides into its upper and lower divisions two-thirds of the way to the mandible. The two divisions are the temporo-zygomatic and the cervicofacial branches, which pass through the parotid gland superficial to the retromandibular vein.[4] The two divisions divide into peripheral branches. The nerves to the fore-head muscles and the upper and lower eyelids arise from the temporozygomatic branch, and the buccal branch and nerves to the upper and lower lips arise

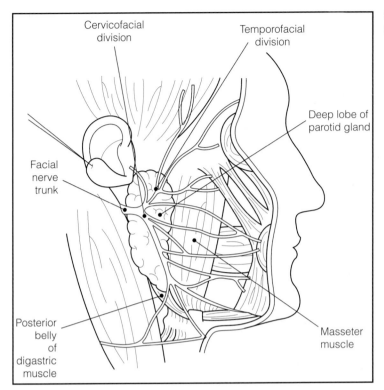

Figure 8.2 • Surgical anatomy of the parotid salivary gland.

from the cervicofacial branch (**Fig. 8.2**). Variations to this pattern are common. This division of the parotid gland by the facial nerve into superficial and deep lobes is important when operating on parotid lesions.

The external carotid artery enters the deep surface of the parotid and divides at about the level of the neck of the mandible into the superficial temporal artery, which emerges from the upper edge of the gland, and the maxillary artery, which passes medially out of the gland. In the substance of the gland are numerous lymph nodes. The anterior surface of the gland is in contact with the mandible and the masseter and medial pterygoid muscles. The posterior surface is in contact below with the mastoid process and the sternomastoid and digastric muscles and above with the external auditory meatus. Medially, the gland is separated by the digastric muscle from the internal jugular vein and the styloid process, and by the stylohyoid muscle from the internal carotid artery. Above, the gland is in contact with the capsule of the mandibular joint. The postganglionic nerve supply of the gland runs in the auriculotemporal nerve from the otic

ganglion. The preganglionic fibres arise in the inferior salivary nucleus in the medulla oblongata, run in the glossopharyngeal nerve and its tympanic branch to the lesser petrosal nerve and so enter the otic ganglion. The parotid and periparotid lymph glands drain primarily into the internal jugular chain nodes, with some drainage going to the upper spinal accessory chain of nodes.

Physiology

The physiological control of parotid gland secretion is almost entirely by the autonomic nervous system. If the parasympathetic innervation is interrupted, glandular atrophy occurs. If sympathetic innervation is interrupted, there is little effect.[5] Normal saliva is 99.5% water but contains salts and mucins, amylase and maltase. The total volume of saliva produced may be up to 1500 mL/day, 45% of which is produced by the parotid glands. Saliva moistens food, allowing it to be swallowed easily. Other functions of the salivary glands are to moisten mucous membranes and to inhibit bacterial invasion, which is mediated by the secretion of secretory immunoglobulin A. Finally, the salivary glands assist in the excretion of heavy metals and inorganic and organic materials and in the maintenance of water balance.

Developmental abnormalities

Developmental abnormalities of the parotid glands are rare. When they do occur, other facial abnormalities may be present and are associated with xerostomia, sialadenitis and dental caries. Parotid gland agenesis has been reported with hemifacial microstomia, mandibulofacial dysostosis, cleft palate and anophthalmia.[6] Recently, agenesis of one parotid gland has been reported with sialosis of the contralateral parotid.[7] Hypoplasia of the parotid gland has been reported in the Melkersson–Rosenthal syndrome, and congenital fistula formation of the ductal system has been associated with branchial cleft abnormalities, accessory parotid ducts and diverticula.[8]

Ectopic location of salivary gland tissue can occur in many sites, including the external auditory canal and middle ear cleft, the anterior mandible, the inner-posterior mandible (Stafne cyst), the pituitary gland and even the cerebellopontine angle.[8]

Investigation of the parotid gland

CLINICAL EVALUATION

Most lesions of the parotid gland are either due to tumour, inflammatory conditions or obstruction of Stensen's duct. The commonest presentations of parotid pathology are therefore swelling of the whole gland (in inflammatory conditions and obstructions of the duct) or a solitary mass in the parotid region. It should be possible for the clinician to make this distinction,[9] which is important as a mass nearly always implies a neoplasm. In the assessment of a parotid mass, particular attention should be paid to the presence or absence of facial palsy, as its presence strongly suggests malignancy.[10] Other important aspects of the clinical examination are fixity and site of the lesion within the parotid. Thus, a recent study concluded that 96% of tumours in the tail of the gland (that region lying inferiorly) were benign if there was no facial palsy, pain,

trismus or fixation.[10] This may be useful in the assessment of frail elderly patients in whom fine-needle aspiration is not performed.

In assessing any parotid mass, the patient should be asked to clench teeth to contract the masseter muscles; this allows the examiner to assess if the swelling is due to hypertrophy of the masseter or whether the mass is in the substance of the muscle (haemangioma or myxoma). Complete examination of all the other salivary glands should be performed to ascertain whether multiple masses are present (as in Warthin's tumour) or whether other glands are involved in a systemic disease (as in Sjögren's syndrome). All glands should be examined bimanually and each duct orifice inspected and palpated. No examination is complete without examination of the pharynx to ascertain the presence of a parapharyngeal tumour, which may be shaped like a dumb-bell and present as a parotid mass. The diagnosis of a parotid mass is not usually difficult, but clinicians should bear in mind the rarer causes of an apparent parotid mass (Box 8.1).

RADIOLOGY

The choice of imaging modalities has increased dramatically recently and the emphasis is now on

Box 8.1 • Differential diagnosis of a parotid mass not caused by a parotid tumour

- Sebaceous cyst
- Enlarged preauricular lymph node
- Branchial cyst
- Dental cyst
- Lipoma
- Lymphangioma
- Mandibular tumours
- Myxoma of the masseter
- Neuroma of the facial nerve
- Facial vein thrombosis
- Temporal artery aneurysm
- Mastoiditis
- Hypertrophic masseter
- Winged mandible

ultrasonography, computed tomography (CT) and magnetic resonance imaging (MRI). As a general rule, inflammatory lesions are probably best imaged using CT, whereas tumours are best imaged by MRI. Ultrasonography is also useful for the evaluation of both parotid lesions in children and tumours.[11]

Plain X-ray films

These are rarely used now as most parotid calculi are radiotranslucent and are better visualised by ultrasonography or CT. Plain films may be useful in differentiating some of the extrasalivary causes of sialomegaly.

Sialography

This remains the most detailed method of visualising the duct system but is now rarely used except in the assessment of suspected sialectasis. In congenital saccular sialectasis, the characteristic snowstorm appearance is seen, and strictures and clubbing of the duct system may be demonstrated. In advanced cystic sialectasis, large collections of contrast may be seen. It can occasionally be useful for identifying a stenosis of the duct, which can be dilated with an inflatable balloon. Sialography is contraindicated in the presence of active infection or allergy to the contrast medium.

Computed tomography

If the patient's history is suggestive of inflammatory disease, CT will identify the actual disease and may also identify the calculi responsible.[12] Usually, little extra information is obtained with the use of contrast.[11]

Magnetic resonance imaging

This is probably the preferred method of imaging a mass suspected of being a tumour (**Figs 8.3** and **8.4**). This is sometimes combined with contrast and is useful in assessing perineural tumour spread in parotid malignancies.[13] MRI studies are usually performed as 3-mm-thick slices with a 1-mm inter-slice gap. Non-contrast T1- and T2-weighted sequences and then T1-weighted, postcontrast, fat-suppressed images are obtained. Axial views are obtained for all sequences and sagittal and coronal views obtained as required.[11,14] Normally, the facial nerve is not imaged. The recent use of high-

Figure 8.3 • MRI scan of a pleomorphic adenoma of the parotid gland.

Figure 8.4 • MRI scan of maltoma of the parotid gland.

resolution three-dimensional Fourier-transformed MRI has allowed the facial nerve to be consistently visualised on contiguous scans.[15] MRI is also particularly useful in lesions situated within the deep lobe of the parotid.

Recent advances in MRI are MR sialography and digital subtraction sialography. The latter technique in particular has shown very good results in the investigation of suspected ductal salivary gland disease as it is able to depict not only the main duct system and first- and second-order branches, but also third-order branches. In a recent study, digital subtraction sialography had a sensitivity and specificity of 96% and 100% respectively in the diagnosis of chronic sialadenitis, and a sensitivity and specificity of 90% and 98% in the diagnosis of sialolithiasis.[16]

Ultrasonography

This was traditionally used to differentiate between solid and cystic masses in the parotid gland and to identify salivary calculi. It can also be used to identify the more advanced stages of autoimmune disease (Sjögren's syndrome) and to differentiate between lymphomatous and non-lymphomatous nodes,[17] although not with sufficient accuracy to avoid biopsy. Ultrasonography is particularly useful in children, in whom exposure to radiation is to be avoided. For lesions that have spread beyond the capsule, it does not provide the detailed anatomical information obtained with CT and MRI.[18–20]

Other radiological techniques

Radionuclide salivary gland scans are based on the fact that salivary glands normally concentrate technetium pertechnetate (^{99m}Tc) and some masses excessively accumulate the radionuclide, especially Warthin's tumours and oncocytomas.[21,22] Radionuclide scans are rarely used now that CT and MRI are freely available. Angiography was useful in the investigation of tumours situated in the parapharyngeal space to differentiate salivary gland tumours from chemodectoma of the carotid or from a nerve sheath tumour. Its use has also been superseded by CT and MRI. MRI spectroscopy is still a relatively new procedure and is based on the fact that salivary tumours express increased quantities of phosphates compared with normal. This is detectable by means of phosphorus-31 spectroscopy,[23] but this is primarily an investigative and research tool.

FINE-NEEDLE ASPIRATION CYTOLOGY

Fine-needle aspiration cytology (FNAC) of a discrete parotid mass remains controversial.[24] Its proponents argue that it has a high diagnostic accuracy, may influence the decision to operate, may allow planning of the most appropriate operative procedure and allows better-informed preoperative

counselling.[25–28] Its detractors argue that it is not sufficiently accurate at diagnosing low-grade malignant lesions, and that the decision to operate is clinically based and the extent of the surgery is not influenced by the cytology, since in the parotid gland more radical surgery for a malignant lesion does not influence outcome.[24] However, all authorities are agreed that FNAC does not cause tumour seeding and that it is free of any major morbidity. A recent survey of 34 institutions with a major interest in salivary gland tumours concluded that approximately one-third of surgical oncologists did not employ FNAC, one-third always employed it and one-third employed it selectively.[24]

Numerous series now attest to the accuracy of FNAC (**Table 8.1**).[25,29–36]. FNAC is particularly accurate in the diagnosis of pleomorphic adenoma,[25] and a study highlighting the features of infarction and squamoid metaplasia achieved an accuracy of up to 88% for adenolymphoma.[27]

Even proponents of the technique have emphasised the pitfalls in diagnosis and have concluded that atypical pleomorphic adenoma is difficult to distinguish from monomorphic adenoma, mucoepidermoid carcinoma and adenoid cystic carcinoma.[37]

Laser scanning slide-based cytometry may improve the positive predictive value for malignancy by analysng the DNA index of cells, as the majority of malignant tumours are aneuploid whilst virtually all benign tumours are diploid.[29] FNAC is useful if lymphadenopathy is suspected due to sarcoid, tuberculosis[26] and lymphoma. It may assist in distinguishing a parotid lesion from other local structures such as a branchial cyst, lymph node or even submandibular gland. It can often confirm a benign neoplasm in an elderly, unfit patient for whom surgery would carry significant risk. It is essential to discriminate between a parotid lesion and a secondary deposit from a melanoma or squamous cell lesion. A typical example of a cytological smear obtained by fine-needle aspiration of a pleomorphic adenoma is shown (**Fig. 8.5**, see also Plate 14, facing p. 212).

In the current climate of informed consent, the most useful role of FNAC may be in preoperative counselling of the patient.

Table 8.1 • Accuracy of fine-needle aspiration cytology (only series with more than 100 patients)

Authors	No. of Patients	No. with histology	Sensitivity (%)	Specificity (%)	Accuracy (%)
Eneroth et al.[30]	1000	690	64	95	89
Layfield et al.[31]	171	171	91	98	92
Lindberg and Akerman[32]	860	461	67	85	81
O'Dwyer et al.[33]	341	341	73	94	93
Persson and Zettergren[34]	362	216	86	99	70
Qizilbash et al.[35]	160	101	88	99	95
Shaha et al.[25]	160	NS	95	98	97
Filopoulos et al.[37]	129	121	95	97.6	96.7

NS = not stated.

Figure 8.5 • Fine-needle aspiration cytology of a pleomorphic adenoma showing epithelial and mucinous components.

SIALOMETRY

Salivary gland output can be determined from individual major salivary glands or from the aggregate fluid in the oral cavity (termed whole saliva). Secretions can be collected in a resting (unstimulated) state or after gustatory or mechanical stimulation. Whole saliva collection is a useful screening technique to determine overall gland function in patients suspected of xerostomia (dry mouth) and may be particularly useful in the diagnosis of Sjögren's syndrome (see below). However, it is infrequently used as it is quite a cumbersome technique. A simpler method for the determination of salivary gland hypofunction is the recently described candy weight loss test. A standard weight of hard sugar candy is incubated for 3 minutes between the dorsum of the tongue and hard palate. The decrease in candy weight correlates well with salivary flow and with subjective reports of dry mouth.[38]

SIALOENDOSCOPY

Advances in technology have enabled the development of miniendoscopes to directly view the distal portions of the ducts of the major salivary glands. There are three types of miniendoscope: flexible, rigid and semirigid. The rigid endoscope provides a better image than the flexible endoscope, but its main disadvantage is the inability to negotiate sharp corners. The semirigid endoscope combines properties of both rigid and flexible endoscopes and also has the advantage of allowing the passage of miniaturised surgical tools. The semirigid endoscope is only 1 mm in diameter and can be used with two types of outer sleeve: an exploration unit (1.3 mm in diameter) and a treatment unit (2.3 mm in diameter). The latter has three channels: one for the endoscope; one that will accept a surgical device up to 1 mm in diameter; and a third that is an irrigation port.

Indications for sialoendoscopy are:

• Calculi in the proximal portion of the major salivary gland duct.

- Screening the ductal system for residual calculi.
- To confirm evidence of ductal dilatation or stenosis seen on sialography or ultrasound scanning.
- To investigate recurrent episodes of major salivary gland swelling without obvious cause.

The sialoendoscope can be used in conjunction with an intracorporeal lithotripter for stone fragmentation. It is important to leave a 2-mm diameter polyethylene tube in the duct after endoscopy, ideally for up to 2 weeks, to prevent obstruction and to allow any residual calculi to be washed out of the system. It also reduces duct stenosis. In their series of 236 salivary gland endoscopies, Nahleili and Baruchin failed to perform the technique in only 4% of cases.[39] Intraoperative failure to remove or eliminate obstruction occurred in only 10% of 170 patients, and late failures due to recurrent obstruction occurred in only 7% of 170 cases. Complications following sialoendoscopy include swelling of the salivary gland, which subsides spontaneously after a few hours, and infection in 3% of cases.[39,40]

Infections of the parotid gland

BACTERIAL INFECTIONS

Bacteria usually reach the gland by retrograde infection from the mouth, although rarely infection may be blood borne. The commonest causative organisms are *Staphylococcus aureus*, *Streptococcus viridans*, *Streptococcus pyogenes*, *Haemophilus influenzae*, *Escherichia coli* and *Streptococcus pneumoniae*.[41] Infection is usually unilateral and may involve intraparotid and periparotid lymph nodes. The aetiology of acute parotitis is usually due to debility and dehydration after major surgery or due to serious medical disease, but may be idiopathic, secondary to obstruction of Stensen's duct (usually due to calculi) or a complication of septicaemia.

The clinical features are of a painful swelling of the side of the face and fever. Pus or purulent fluid may be expressed from Stensen's duct. Untreated, the condition may progress to a parotid abscess, which may subsequently extend to the upper neck or to the parapharyngeal space. The treatment of acute bacterial parotitis consists of oral hygiene,

correction of dehydration and appropriate antibiotics. Signs of improvement are usually evident within 48 hours. If no improvement after this time has occurred, a parotid abscess should be suspected. CT[42] not only confirms the diagnosis but allows planning of the most appropriately sited incision to drain the abscess to spare the branches of the facial nerve. If no abscess is present and fulminating parotitis is suspected, decompression of the parotid gland should be considered.[43] Recurrent subacute and chronic parotitis is more common than an acute infection and is usually due to parotid calculi (see below).

VIRAL INFECTIONS

The commonest infection of the parotid glands is mumps.[44] It can also occur in the submandibular and sublingual glands. Mumps is most reliably diagnosed during epidemics or by measuring serum antibody titres. It usually affects children between the ages of 4 and 12 years. Common manifestations of active disease include bilateral or occasionally unilateral parotid swelling, fever, chills, joint pain and myalgia. Uncommon manifestations include epididymitis, orchitis, pancreatitis, thyroiditis, meningoencephalitis and unilateral sensorineural hearing loss. The treatment relies on isolation of the patient, adequate hydration and nutrition, and measures to relieve symptoms.

Other viruses that can cause acute viral parotitis include Coxsackie viruses, parainfluenza viruses (types 1 and 3), influenza virus type A, herpesvirus, echovirus and choriomeningitis virus.[41,45] Although Epstein–Barr virus and cytomegalovirus can be found in saliva, they do not seem to directly infect the major salivary glands. The same seems to pertain to the human immunodeficiency virus.[46]

However, two large studies of HIV-positive women have concluded that xerostomia is more common in these patients, and their salivary glands may be enlarged (in 4.3%) and tender (in 6.9%). These clinical findings are positively associated with viral load.[47,48]

GRANULOMATOUS AND OTHER DISEASES

These diseases may affect the intraparotid and extraparotid lymph nodes, and the parenchyma of the parotid gland can also be affected. The chief granulomatous diseases affecting the major salivary glands include sarcoidosis, tuberculosis, atypical mycobacterial infection, syphilis, cat-scratch fever, toxoplasmosis and actinomycosis.[49,50] In practice, not all of these diseases produce histologically recognisable granulomata.

Sarcoidosis

This is a systemic disease characterised by non-caseating granulomas involving many organs. Its presumed aetiology is infectious. The parotid glands are affected in 10–30% of patients and occasionally may be the only manifestation of the disease. It usually presents as a non-tender, painless, chronic enlargement of the gland, which may mimic malignancy. CT and MRI reveals multiple, benign, non-cavitating masses. The major differential diagnosis is lymphoma, although if the lesion is solitary it may be difficult to distinguish between other benign lesions.

 If FNAC excludes a neoplasm, incisional biopsy may be performed and will confirm the diagnosis.[50]

Most cases resolve with treatment of the generalised condition.

Tuberculosis

Primary involvement of the salivary glands is rare. Usually, the salivary gland disease arises from a focus in the tonsils and spreads to the salivary gland via the regional lymph nodes. FNAC is often a helpful diagnostic procedure. Treatment is with appropriate antituberculous chemotherapy, and surgery is rarely necessary.

Cat-scratch fever

This diagnosis is suggested by a history of cat scratch followed by fever, malaise and enlargement of the salivary glands and lymph nodes. Identification of the causative organism is often difficult. Treatment consists of incision and drainage of any abscess and antibiotic chemotherapy of secondary infection.

Toxoplasmosis

Infection by *Toxoplasma gondii* causes asymptomatic lymphadenopathy and in the parotid gland may be indistinguishable from the above granulomatous diseases. Active and previous infection can be confirmed on serological testing.

Actinomycosis

Infection by *Actinomyces israelii* is usually caused by spread of the organism from dental, periodontal or intestinal disease. Parenchymal disease is characterised by granulomatous inflammation with abscess and fistula. 'Sulphur granules' may also be found. The treatment of choice is with long-term penicillin.

Autoimmune disease

Autoimmune disease affecting the salivary glands is best considered as Sjögren's syndrome. This is a systemic disorder of the exocrine glands that occurs either alone (primary Sjögren's syndrome) or with any other connective tissue disease (secondary Sjögren's syndrome). The diagnosis is suspected when two or more of the following clinical features are present: keratoconjunctivitis sicca, xerostomia and a connective tissue disease, which is usually rheumatoid arthritis.[51] Usually the lacrimal and salivary glands are affected but other exocrine glands can also be involved.[52]

The incidence of Sjögren's syndrome is difficult to establish, but among the autoimmune diseases it is probably second in frequency only to rheumatoid arthritis.[52] The adult form of the disease is ten times more common than the childhood form, and children are less likely to develop the advanced features.[53] It is important to establish the diagnosis early in children because many cases may spontaneously resolve by puberty, and this knowledge may avoid unnecessary surgery.

The adult form of the disease is most common between the ages of 40 and 60 years, with a male to female ratio of 1:9. It tends to be progressive. The incidence of parotid enlargement varies from 25 to 55% of cases, and either parotid or submandibular gland enlargement occurs in 80% of all cases of Sjögren's syndrome. The risk of developing non-Hodgkin's lymphoma is estimated to be 44 times greater than in normal controls.[8] Local radiotherapy or immunosuppression may further increase this risk.

Two types of pathological appearance are evident in the salivary glands: the benign lymphoepithelial lesion, occurring primarily in the parotid glands, and focal lymphocytic sialadenitis, occurring in the other major and minor salivary glands.[54] Studies with monoclonal antibodies have shown that lymphocytes in labial salivary glands contain more than three times as many T-helper cells (CD4+) as T-suppressor cells (CD8+).[55]

The diagnosis is most reliably made by labial salivary gland biopsy, and usually biopsy of the parotid gland is not required unless this is the only gland affected.[50,54] The suspicion of malignant lymphoma should be borne in mind in this subset of patients. Sialography is the most useful radiological adjunct to diagnosis, showing a normal central duct system and numerous peripheral punctate collections of contrast material uniformly scattered throughout the gland. Eventually, larger globular collections of contrast material may also be seen scattered uniformly throughout the gland, and MRI findings of these globular changes are diagnostic.[42]

The management of patients with Sjögren's syndrome involves reducing the patient's symptoms and preventing irreversible damage to the teeth and eyes. Thus, attention should be paid to treating and preventing dental caries, treating oral candidiasis, stimulating the remaining salivary glands to produce more saliva and selectively using saliva substitutes.[54] Stimulation of the salivary glands may be accomplished by local gustatory stimuli, such as mints or chewing gum, or by systemic sialagogues. Immunosuppressive therapy with ciclosporin A has shown some promise.[56] The combination of prednisolone and chlorambucil has also been shown to decrease disease progression.[57] Finally, corticosteroid irrigation of the parotid duct has been shown to significantly increase salivary flow rate compared with saline irrigation in a controlled study, and this benefit seemed to be sustained for a mean of 8.4 months.[58]

Obstructive parotid gland disease

STRICTURE OF STENSEN'S DUCT

This may be caused by repeated infection, iatrogenic injury, congenital abnormality, trauma or through compression by a tumour. The clinical features are of pain and swelling of the parotid gland associated with eating. The diagnosis is established by sialography, which may also establish whether calculi are present. Distal duct or orifice stricture can now be treated by repeated duct dilatation, and surgery is seldom indicated. In patients who fail to respond, a formal stenotomy or marsupialisation of the duct orifice may be required. Duct reimplantation or excision of the gland are rarely required. Proximal duct stricture is more difficult to deal with, and alternative forms of treatment may be duct ligation (usually leading to atrophy of the gland) or, rarely, radiotherapy.

SIALOLITHIASIS

Stone formation in the parotid gland is less common than in the submandibular gland. It may be primary or secondary. Stasis or slow clearance of salivary gland secretions occurs with one or more predisposing factors, including anatomical alterations in the duct, damaged duct epithelium from infection or trauma, stricture, alteration of the physicochemical composition of salivary secretions and systemic metabolic disease (particularly hyperparathyroidism and hyperuricaemia). A history of recurrent progressive glandular swelling, initially associated with meals, is common. The stone may occasionally be palpated along the course of Stensen's duct. Diagnosis is best made by sialography. Treatment depends on the location of the stone. If located superficially in the cheek, the stone may be removed via the oral cavity. If located in the proximal duct or in the hilum of the gland, the stone may be removed by parotidectomy. Multiple small stones may be dealt with by irrigation, stenting and ductoplasty.

Advances in technology have enabled the development of extracorporeal shockwave lithotripsy for the treatment of salivary gland stones. The stones have to be detectable by an ultrasound imaging system. The development of a machine with a smaller shockwave focus (2.4 mm wide by 25 mm long) has removed the need for analgesia. The technique is best reserved for stones that are not hidden by bone. Complete disintegration of parotid calculi can be achieved in 22–37% of patients, and residual small fragments pass spontaneously or can be removed by irrigation. The majority of patients (63–97%) are rendered asymptomatic. Complications of the procedure include petechiae at the point of entry of the shock wave (36%), slight pain in the treated gland (22.5%) and ductal haemorrhage (64%) which resolves spontaneously. Patients with chronically infected glands are also at risk of an acute infection after the procedure.[59,60]

SIALECTASIS

This is a disease of unknown aetiology in which progressive destruction of the alveoli and paren-chyma of the gland is accompanied by duct stenosis and cyst formation as the alveoli coalesce. Most patients are thought to have congenital sialectasis and in children it may mimic mumps, although mumps seldom recurs. Approximately 50% of children have no symptoms by the time they reach adulthood, and only a small proportion require treatment.[61] The typical presentation is painful enlargement of one salivary gland after eating. The attack regresses after a few hours but is made worse by eating again. Attacks vary in frequency and are due to the main ducts being blocked by stones or epithelial debris. The diagnosis may be confirmed by sialography. Surgery to remove stones may be necessary, and occasionally the gland may require excision.

CYSTS IN THE PAROTID GLAND

Cystic lesions account for up to 5% of parotid masses, but if neoplasms are excluded then the number of true cysts is greatly diminished.[3] Cystic lesions may be solitary or multiple. Solitary cysts may be due to obstruction of the ductal system from any cause[8] or may be a lymphoepithelial cyst probably formed owing to intranodal inclusions.[3] Rarer causes of solitary cystic lesions of the parotid are dermoid cyst, necrotic metastatic lymph node or cystic degeneration in low-grade mucoepidermoid carcinoma, papillocystic variant of acinic cell carcinoma or oncocytic cystadenoma. Lympho-epithelial cysts have occasionally been reported in association with Castleman's disease or angio-follicular lymph node hyperplasia.[62] Multiple cysts most often occur in Warthin's tumour and in HIV infection when they are associated with multiple cervical lymphadenopathy.[42]

POST-IRRADIATION SIALADENITIS

This is due to irradiation of the gland as part of the planned treatment for head and neck malignancy. After 4000 cGy, the gland atrophies and xerostomia

results. Characteristic findings on CT and MRI have been described.[42] External beam irradiation is a tumour promoter, and an increased incidence of malignancy of the parotid gland occurs after 10 to 25 years.[52]

Tumours of the parotid gland

CLASSIFICATION AND STAGING

There have been a variety of classifications of salivary gland tumours but the most widely used is the World Health Organization's (WHO) classifi-cation based on the classic work by Thackray and Sobin (**Table 8.2**).[63] The TNM staging of parotid tumours is illustrated in **Box 8.2** and is based on that described by Hermanek and Sobin.[64]

AETIOLOGY

Radiation

The strongest evidence implicating high-dose ionising radiation in the development of salivary gland tumours has been provided by studies of the survivors of the atomic bombs in Hiroshima and Nagasaki in 1945. The most recent study, which had a follow-up of 37 years, confirmed an increased incidence of benign and malignant neoplasms of the salivary glands. This was especially so for Warthin's tumour and mucoepidermoid carcinoma.[65]

Low-dose radiation, ultraviolet radiation and iodine-131 therapy have also been implicated.[66,67]

Viruses

Only for the Epstein–Barr virus is there any convincing evidence for a viral role in salivary gland tumorigenesis. Several studies have now demonstrated a close association between Epstein–Barr virus and undifferentiated carcinoma in tumours with lymphoid stroma.[68,69]

The detection of the virus in a clonal form and the expression of its viral oncoprotein in neoplastic epithelial cells from the above mentioned carcinomas adds further evidence to support this association.[70]

Smoking

Only adenolymphoma (Warthin's tumour) seems to be commoner in smokers (see 'Adenolymphoma' below).

Table 8.2 • WHO classification of salivary gland tumours[63]

Tumour type	Approximate proportion of all salivary tumours (%)
Benign epithelial tumours:	
Pleomorphic adenoma	48
Adenolymphoma (Warthin's)	18
Monomorphic adenoma	<1
Malignant epithelial tumours	
Mucoepidermoid tumour	4
Acinic cell tumour	2
Carcinomas:	16
Adenoid cycstic	
Carcinoma ex-pleomorphic adenoma	
Adenocarcinoma	
Epidermal carcinoma	
Undifferentiated carcinoma	
Non-epithelial tumours	4
Haemangioma	
Lipoma	
Neurofibroma	
Unclassified tumours	8
Tumours from neighbouring organs or metastases	
Lymphomas	
Allied conditions	<1
Benign lymphoepithelial lesions	

Box 8.2 • TNM classification of parotid tumours[64]

T	Primary tumour
TX	Not assessable
T0	No evidence of primary tumour
T1	Tumour <2 cm without extraparenchymal extension
T2	Tumour >2–4 cm without extraparenchymal extension
T3	Tumour >4–6 cm or tumour with extraparenchymal extension without seventh nerve involvement
T4	Tumour >6 cm or tumour invading skull base or seventh nerve

N	Regional lymph nodes
NX	Not assessable
N0	Regional nodes not involved
N1	Metastasis in a single ipsilateral node, <3 cm
N2	Metastasis in a single ipsilateral node >3–6 cm Metastasis in multiple ipsilateral nodes, none >6 cm Metastasis in bilateral or contralateral nodes, none >6 cm
N3	Metastasis in a lymph node >6 cm

M	Distant metastases
MX	Not assessable
M0	No distant metastases
M1	Distant metastases present

Stage			
1	T1/2	N0	M0
2	T3	N0	M0
3	T1/2	N1	M0
4	T4	N0	M0
	T3/4	N1	M0
	Any T	N2/3	M0
	Any T	Any N	M1

Miscellaneous

Exposure to silica dust and kerosene are associated with the development of salivary gland neoplasms. Dietary factors implicated are high cholesterol intake and low intake of vitamins and dark-yellow vegetables.

MOLECULAR BIOLOGY OF SALIVARY GLAND TUMOURS

A variety of chromosomal and molecular changes have been described in benign and malignant tumours. In future, they may become useful in diagnosis, prognosis and even treatment. However, there are still no data on the genetic mechanisms responsible for the development of salivary gland tumours. Some of the more consistent findings are summarised.

Chromosomal rearrangements

Translocations of genetic material have been noted on chromosome 8 in pleomorphic adenomas, chromosome 11 in mucoepidermoid carcinomas, and chromosome 6 in adenoid cystic carcinomas. In pleomorphic adenomas, the best characterised translocation is frequently t(3,8)(p21;q12) and involves band 8q12 in 40% of cases. This involves a developmentally regulated zinc finger gene (*PLAG1*), while the expression of β-catenin is reduced.[71,72] In mucoepidermoid carcinomas of the minor salivary glands, a t(11,19)(q21;p3.1) translocation has been described,[73] whilst in adenoid cystic carcinoma there is an increased frequency of the t(6,9)(q23;p21) translocation.[74] Interleukin-6, an autocrine growth regulator, may play a part in salivary tumour cell growth and may have prognostic significance.[75,76]

Monosomy and polysomy

Alterations in the number of chromosomes have been described in benign and malignant tumours. Loss of the Y chromosome occurs in malignant adenocarcinomas, as well as polysomy of chromosomes 3 and 17. Of interest is the description of monosomy of chromosome 17, as the *p53* tumour suppressor gene is located on this chromosome.[77]

Allelic loss and microsatellite instability

Allelic loss has been demonstrated on chromosomal regions 12p and 19q in pleomorphic adenomas and adenoid cystic carcinomas, and >50% loss at 2q, 5p, 12p and 16q in mucoepidermoid carcinomas.[78] Most pleomorphic adenomas also exhibit allelic loss on chromosome 8, whilst loss of heterozygosity (LOH) is found in 53% of malignant and 41% of benign tumours.[73] Of clinical interest is that malignant tumours exhibiting LOH also exhibit aggressive tumour characterisitcs. In a recent study, LOH on the long arm of chromosome 6 was frequently observed and this was associated with a significant decrease of thrombospondin 2, a potent inhibitor of tumour growth and angiogenesis. This decreased expression was significantly associated with increased microvessel counts, indicating an association with angiogenesis, especially in adenoid cystic and mucoepidermoid carcinomas.[79]

Proto-oncogenes and tumour suppressor genes

The *p53* tumour suppressor gene, located on chromosome 17 (p13) is altered in some benign and many malignant tumours. The mutated *p53* gene product accumulates in the nucleus of neoplastic cells and can be detected in 11% of benign tumours and up to 67% of malignant tumours. Its expression is statistically associated with regional and distant metastases and a decreased disease-free and actuarial survival compared with those patients whose tumours express only low levels of the mutation or wild-type p53.[77,80–83]

Amplification of the c-*erbB2* (*HER2/neu*) oncogene and overexpression of its protein have been demonstrated in almost 35% of salivary gland carcinomas, with a clear correlation with tumour aggressiveness in some studies.[84,85] This has potential therapeutic implications, as an antibody to the HER2/Neu protein is available and is currently used in breast cancer patients whose tumours strongly express HER2/Neu. However, a more recent study has detected this overexpression in only 16% of adenoid cystic carcinomas and only 3% expressed strong (3+) immunohistochemical staining.[86] This is the only group of tumours against which the antibody is likely to have any therapeutic benefit.

Other proto-oncogene abnormalities described are alterations in c-*fos*,[87] c-*kit*[88] and epidermal growth factor receptor.[89] Also of interest is the observation of an increased expression of cyclooxygenase-2 in benign and malignant tumours.[90]

BENIGN EPITHELIAL PAROTID NEOPLASMS

Pleomorphic adenoma

This is the most common salivary gland tumour, accounting for 50% of all salivary gland tumours and approximately 80% of parotid tumours, and so called because of its mixed epithelial and mesenchymal elements. A study has suggested that epithelial-mesenchymal transition occurs within this tumour.[91]

The annual incidence of parotid pleomorphic adenoma in the UK is approximately 1.4 per 100 000 people.[92,93] The peak age of incidence is in the fifth decade, and women are more commonly affected than men. The commonest site within the parotid gland is in the tail,[10,92] with most tumours lying superficial to the facial nerve.

The history is usually that of a slowly growing painless mass in the parotid, and pain and facial palsy are rare. The latter should prompt consideration of a malignant lesion. Fortunately, malignant transformation of a previously benign pleomorphic adenoma is rare.[92]

The diagnosis is primarily clinical, and it has been argued that radiological and cytological investigations are unnecessary,[24,92] although FNAC is useful in distinguishing between benign and malignant neoplasms and in determining pleomorphic adenoma from Warthin's tumour.[27] Radiological confirmation of a truly single lesion may be accomplished using ultrasonography or MRI and may show the depth of the neoplasm. The value of this is in preoperative counselling of the patient in the likelihood of a neuropraxia. Treatment is usually by some form of superficial or total conservative parotidectomy, with identification of the facial nerve during surgery (see 'Surgery of the parotid gland' below). An example of an excised parotid tumour is shown in **Fig. 8.6** (see also Plate 15, facing p. 212).

Pleomorphic adenoma recurs, and the reasons for this have been hotly debated. When the surgical management in the early 20th century was local excision (for fear of damaging the facial nerve), local recurrence was in the order of 20–45%.[92] By the 1940s, superficial parotidectomy with dissection of the facial nerve was being advocated, and this reduced local recurrence. In 1957, Patey and Thackray demonstrated that small tumour buds protrude from the tumour surface into the surrounding tumour capsule.[94] This came to be accepted as the cause for local recurrence, but was disproved by Nicholson and Gleave who practised the technique of 'extracapsular dissection' for 45 years with results that were equally as good as those for superficial parotidectomy.[95] It is therefore clear that the main factor regarding recurrence was incomplete surgical excision, and the same group confirmed a recurrence rate of only 1.6% after a median follow-up of 12.5 years. This low rate of local recurrence has also been achieved by other groups.[96] This also explains the paradox that preserving the facial nerve did not increase the risk of tumour recurrence despite the observation that in 50% of patients, a branch of the nerve was in direct contact with the tumour capsule.[92] Other factors said to contribute to local recurrence are young age at presentation[97] and inadequate surgical margins.[98,99] Rupture of the capsule as a cause of local recurrence has recently been disputed.[64] Radiotherapy in such patients is regarded as unhelpful.[98] Most pleomorphic adenomas are probably best treated by superficial parotidectomy with identification and preservation of the facial nerve.

Local recurrence of pleomorphic adenomas may be uninodular or multinodular,[97] and this distinction is important. When uninodular disease is treated by surgery alone there is a failure rate of 15% at 15 years; with multinodular disease the failure rate is 43% but is reduced to 4% by the addition of postoperative radiotherapy.[97]

However, no randomised studies exist to examine which patients may benefit from this treatment. The type of surgery, not surprisingly, is not standardised for such an uncommon procedure and depends on the type, site and extent of the local recurrence. It is not surprising that the incidence of temporary and permanent facial nerve damage is greatly increased in this situation.

Adenolymphoma (Warthin's tumour)

Warthin described only two patients with this tumour over a 35-year period, and initially called it papillary cystadenoma lymphomatosum.[100] It is apparent that its incidence has been increasing since its description, and it may now constitute 18% of all salivary gland neoplasms (**Table 8.2**) and up to 33% of all parotid neoplasms.[101,102]

Figure 8.6 • Pathological specimen showing the cut surface of a pleomorphic adenoma of the parotid gland.

The highest incidence of tumours confined almost entirely to the parotid gland occurs in the sixth and seventh decades, with a male:female ratio of 1.6:1.[102] Smoking has been noted to be a strong aetiological factor and may explain the increasing incidence of this tumour and the change in its sex distribution over the past 70 years.[102,103]

Clinically, this tumour presents as an ovoid, smooth lump containing cystic spaces filled with fluid and lined by papillary epithelium set in a lymphoid stroma. The epithelium develops from parotid duct cells as a result of metaplasia, forming two layers. Lining the cysts, the inner layer of epithelium is formed largely by tall columnar cells called oncocytes, whereas the basal layer of epithelium is formed by small, elongated irregular cells containing oval vesicular nuclei.[102] The most satisfactory explanation for the inclusion of lymphoid stroma lies in the embryological development of the parotid gland (see 'Embryology' above) and that the tumour is due to a cellular response to the epithelium by the included residual lymphatic tissue. It has been proposed that adenolymphoma is not a benign neoplasm but a manifestation of a delayed hypersensitivity reaction, and that the trigger for the reaction is metaplasia of the ductal epithelium secondary to a metabolic or nutritional defect,[104] such as one caused by smoking.[102] In up to 10% of patients, the lesions are multiple and occasionally bilateral, either synchronously or asynchronously.

Preoperative diagnosis has recently been improved by attention to specific cytological features of squamoid metaplasia and infarction.[27] Ultrasonography allows the detection of previously unsuspected multiple lesions within the same gland and occasionally identifies occult contralateral lesions. A correct preoperative diagnosis allows the correct surgical procedure to be planned. Because these tumours are benign and do not recur locally, a conservative surgical approach to their excision has been advocated in the form of 'controlled enucleation'.[102,105] This allowed a reduction in temporary facial neuropraxia from 43% for superficial parotidectomy to 8% for controlled enucleation.[102] This procedure is unsuitable for multiple lesions and identification of the facial nerve is then required, especially for lesions in the deep portion of the gland.

Monomorphic adenoma

This is a rare benign tumour characterised by a proliferation of epithelial elements in the absence of cells of mesenchymal origin. In practice, preoperative diagnosis is difficult and distinguishing it from a low-grade acinic cell carcinoma may be impossible. Treatment should ensure an adequate margin of excision, and most are therefore treated by superficial parotidectomy.

Oncocytoma

This rare benign tumour usually affects elderly people and may originate in the salivary glands. It presents as a slow-growing painless lump that is well circumscribed and soft. Histologically, this tumour is characterised by tetrahedral cells with eosinophilic cytoplasm, and treatment is by surgical excision.

MALIGNANT EPITHELIAL PAROTID NEOPLASMS

Tumours of variable malignancy

Mucoepidermoid tumours Since their description in 1945, there has been some debate as to the true biological nature of these tumours. One view has been that their biological nature is related to grade. Thus, low-grade tumours behave more like pleomorphic adenomas whereas high-grade tumours behave more aggressively and metastasise. A more recent view is that their behaviour is not related to histological appearance and that even apparently low-grade tumours may metastasise, and even initially aggressive tumours may be cured with appropriate treatment.

Mucoepidermoid tumours can arise in any salivary gland, but 90% occur within the parotid (**Table 8.2**). The age of presentation is wide, and these tumours may even occur in childhood, although the peak incidence lies in the fourth decade. The sex distribution is equal. These tumours may in addition be subdivided according to grade, which has a bearing on survival.[106-108] Thus, if all grades of tumour are included, mortality may be as low as 8.7%.[106] Spiro has shown that the overall survival of 434 patients with mucoepidermoid tumours was of the order of 70%.[107] For intermediate- and high-grade tumours, survival may fall to as little as 22.5%.[108]

Acinic cell tumour This accounts for approximately 2% of all parotid tumours and, like Warthin's tumour, it may be bilateral in 3% of patients. It is uncommon outside the parotid gland. It occurs in childhood, but its peak age of incidence is in the fifth decade. It may also occur in intraparotid lymph nodes. Although its biological behaviour is variable, in general it has a better prognosis than muco-epidermoid tumours, and survival over 20 years has been reported to be between 75 and 84%.[106,107] Approximately 10% metastasise.

Carcinomas of the parotid gland

Adenoid cystic carcinoma This histological type of cancer accounts for only 10% of salivary neoplasms. Only about 20% arise within the parotid, and they form only 2% of all parotid tumours.[109] The median age of presentation for patients with tumours arising in the parotid gland is 43 years, 10 years younger than for patients whose tumours arise in other salivary glands.[109] Histologically, these tumours contain round or oval cells forming strands or clusters in a myxomatous connective tissue matrix. The islands or strands of tumour cells interconnect to enclose characteristic cystic spaces, presenting a cribriform, cylindromatous pattern of growth. Classification into three grades is feasible but has not been found to be clinically useful.[110,111]

This tumour has a predilection for neural spread, and this may account for the high proportion of patients (18%) who present with some degree of facial weakness. The incidence of lymph node spread is relatively low (6–10%),[109,110] and the incidence of distant metastases is high (40%).[111]

Survival from adenoid cystic carcinoma tends to be better for parotid sites compared with other salivary gland sites, with 5-year and 10-year survival in the order of 42% and 25%, respectively. Local recurrence seems to be improved with the addition of postoperative radiotherapy but overall survival is apparently unaffected.[109]

The most important factor influencing survival seems to be stage at presentation,[109,111] and the previously reported finding that grade of tumour is an important determinant of survival of adenoid cystic carcinoma[112] has not been confirmed by later studies.[109,111]

Carcinoma ex-pleomorphic adenoma This is sometimes described as a malignant mixed parotid tumour,[110] because the histological features show some characteristics of a benign mixed tumour (pleomorphic adenoma) with other areas containing carcinoma cells. These tumours comprise 18% of parotid cancers[110] and may arise as either malignant transformation in a longstanding pleomorphic adenoma (occurring in 10% after 15 years) or as a carcinoma arising in a mixed cell tumour. Lymph node metastases occur in approximately 20% of patients, and survival at 5 and 10 years has been reported to be 63% and 39%, respectively.[110]

Adenocarcinoma This comprises 10% of malignant tumours of the parotid and approximately 3% of all salivary gland tumours. The sex incidence is equal, and this tumour occasionally occurs in children. The histological pattern varies from trabecular to tubular, solid, papillary or mucus-secreting varieties without epidermoid differentiation. They may be low, intermediate or high grade and this, along with stage at presentation, influences survival, which may be as low as 19% at 10 years with high-grade lesions.[107,110]

Epidermoid carcinoma This is rare, occurring in only 3% of malignant parotid tumours, and is characterised by exhibiting epidermoid or squamous differentiation. It may be difficult to differentiate from squamous cell carcinoma arising in other sites.[110] It is an aggressive tumour, presenting clinically with pain, skin fixation, ulceration, facial nerve palsy and metastatic spread to lymph nodes in 50% of patients.[110] Survival is poor and depends on grade of tumour and stage at presentation.

Undifferentiated (anaplastic) carcinoma This is a rare tumour, invariably of high grade and with a poor prognosis.

BENIGN NON-EPITHELIAL PAROTID NEOPLASMS

Within the parotid gland, these tumours are rare. **Haemangiomas** of the parotid may be primary or secondary, involving the parotid from a primary site nearby such as the skin overlying the gland or the infratemporal fossa.[3] Some tumours may spontaneously regress, and treatment by embolisation is preferable to surgery.[113] **Lipomas** usually lie lateral to the parotid gland and are unilateral. They need to be distinguished from fatty infiltration of the parotid, which is usually bilateral. There are three types of **lymphangiomas**: simple lymphangioma, cavernous lymphangioma and cystic hygroma. Cavernous lymphangiomas are prone to recur after excision because they are almost impossible to remove completely. Cystic hygromas almost always involve the parotid gland and submandibular space and may require several excisions for complete removal.[113]

LYMPHOMAS OF THE PAROTID

Malignant lymphoma of the parotid is a rare condition, accounting for only 2% of lymphomas of the head and neck.[78] They are usually described as mucosa-associated lymphoid tissue (MALT) lymphomas, which histologically exhibit centrocyte-like cell proliferation surrounding B-cell reactive follicles. They may be surgically excised, but successful treatment with radiotherapy alone has been described, with a good prognosis.[114]

Management of patients with a parotid neoplasm

Since most benign tumours occur in the superficial lobe of the parotid, the standard operation since the 1950s has been superficial parotidectomy with dissection and preservation of the facial nerve. This is also true for low-grade parotid carcinomas such as the mucoepidermoid tumours and acinic cell tumours, which uncommonly present with lymph node metastases.[92] Total conservative parotidectomy (with facial nerve preservation) may be indicated for these tumours depending on the size of the tumour and its position within the parotid gland, especially if located in the deep lobe. The aim of the surgery is to achieve a clear margin of excision around the tumour to minimise the risk of local recurrence. A variation on this procedure is subtotal parotidectomy, which has been described as a conservative resection of the superficial lobe with less than a full facial nerve dissection.[115] The merits of this procedure are that for benign and low-grade malignant lesions, surgical clearance is adequate with the advantage of a reduction in the postoperative complication rate, especially that of facial nerve paresis.

Postoperative radiotherapy may be given after excision of a low-grade carcinoma if the surgical margin is involved by tumour,[92] but its use after surgery for pleomorphic adenoma is controversial.[116] Postoperative radiotherapy may have a place in the management of patients with recurrent pleomorphic adenoma, especially in patients in whom recurrences are multinodular. In this situation, the addition of postoperative radiotherapy is associated with a significantly improved rate of local control.[97]

The treatment of Warthin's tumour has hitherto also been by superficial parotidectomy, but increasingly some authorities have advocated an even more conservative approach and have recommended enucleation.[103,105] The rationale for this approach has been the zero recurrence rate after complete excision and the greatly reduced incidence of facial nerve paresis compared with superficial parotidectomy (8% vs. 43% respectively).[102]

The management of patients with overtly malignant tumours is primarily surgical, the extent of surgery depending on the stage at presentation. Facial nerve paresis and clinically detectable lymphadenopathy both occur in approximately 20% of patients,[107,109,110] and careful clinical staging is essential. An accurate preoperative diagnosis is also highly desirable using either FNAC or even a Tru-cut biopsy.[117] Imaging of the head and neck, as well as the chest, with CT scanning has been advocated,[117] although MRI is probably better for evaluating tumours.[42] This allows better visualisation of the primary tumour – notably any deep-lobe extension – and may identify fixity to surrounding structures. It is also useful in identifying clinically occult lymph node metastases. Finally, MRI allows for better preoperative counselling of the patient, especially if the extent of the surgery is likely to sacrifice the facial nerve or if immediate reconstructive surgery is contemplated. Prophylactic radical cervical lymphadenectomy has been advocated in the past and is much more controversial.[118–120] It is unnecessary in all patients in whom lymph node metastases are only suspected, and studies suggest that local recurrence is unlikely if a jugulodigastric lymph node examined by frozen section at operation is free from tumour.[121] Postoperative radiotherapy may be required, and an oncologist should be involved early in the management of these patients.

SURGERY OF THE PAROTID GLAND

Superficial conservative parotidectomy

Superficial conservative parotidectomy is indicated for benign tumours and low-grade malignant tumours confined to the superficial lobe of the parotid.

The patient is positioned in the supine position with the neck slightly extended and the head turned away from the surgeon. The table is inclined in a slightly head-up position to reduce venous congestion, and a small 'peanut' swab is placed in the external auditory canal to protect the tympanic membrane. The towels are arranged so that the ipsilateral eye and corner of the mouth can be viewed when necessary during stimulation of the facial nerve. During general anaesthesia, muscle relaxants should be avoided.

The incision begins near the top of the pinna in the preauricular crease, runs inferiorly until the point at which the ear lobe joins the face and then sweeps posteriorly and upwards beneath and behind the ear lobe. The incision is then extended inferiorly along the anterior border of the sternomastoid for 2 cm. The incision is then deepened through the superficial fascia and platysma, and the anterior skin flap is mobilised superficial to the parotid gland as far as its anterior border. The skin flap and the ear lobe may then be retracted out of the operative field with sutures. The great auricular nerve is identified lying on the deep cervical fascia investing the sternomastoid muscle. The sternomastoid muscle is separated from the posterior border of the parotid gland, and the great auricular nerve is divided at the point where it crosses on to the parotid gland. The posterior border of the parotid gland is then separated from the mastoid process and the cartilaginous external meatus, opening up a sulcus between the parotid gland and these structures, which is extended inferiorly between the gland and the sternomastoid muscle. This sulcus is further deepened to expose the posterior belly of the digastric muscle, which is then followed upwards to a point where it dips beneath the mastoid process. Great care must be taken to avoid damage to the facial nerve at this point.

The sulcus between the posterior border of the parotid and the external meatus and mastoid process is deepened by carefully dividing the fibrous septa bridging it, and the main trunk (pes anserinus)

of the facial nerve is identified. Identification of the facial nerve is facilitated by the use of a nerve stimulator, but even so, great caution must be maintained during this and the subsequent dissection. The nerve has a characteristic appearance and usually has a tiny blood vessel on its surface. The parotid gland is then retracted forwards, and the plane between the nerve and the superficial lobe is dissected forwards until the bifurcation of the nerve is identified. A haemostat is now slid over the upper division of the nerve and the blades opened. Glandular tissue overlying the posterior blade is divided with a knife or scissors to divide the posterior border of the gland. Keeping the superficial lobe retracted, the plane between the nerve and the superficial lobe is gently dissected so as to eventually identify all the branches of the nerve, keeping the scissors used for dividing the septa of the gland in a forward direction. It is important to remember that the smaller branches of the facial nerve become more superficial as the dissection proceeds distally, and great care is needed to ensure that none of the peripheral branches of the nerve are damaged as the superficial lobe is dissected away from the nerve. The superficial lobe can then be mobilised sufficiently to allow it to be pedicled anteriorly.

The buccal branch or branches are then traced downwards and the superficial lobe eventually severed. Small bleeding vessels may be tied off with a fine absorbable suture. It is usual to see the retromandibular vein lying vertically deep to the branches of the facial nerve and emerging from the tail of the remaining gland just posterior to the mandibular branch.

The platysma may be sutured as a separate layer but is often deficient in the superior part of the wound. A small suction drain is used to drain the cavity, and the skin is sutured with a subcuticular absorbable suture. The drain may be removed on the first postoperative day and the patient discharged.

Variations to this procedure are the partial superficial parotidectomy[122] and the conservative parotidectomy by the peripheral approach, in which the branches of the facial nerve (usually the cervical branch) are identified first, with subsequent proximal dissection to the main trunk of the nerve.[123]

Total conservative parotidectomy

Total conservative parotidectomy is indicated for benign neoplasms arising in the deep lobe of the gland, chronic parotitis secondary to longstanding duct obstruction, and tuberculous parotitis. It may also be indicated for recurrent pleomorphic adenoma, low-grade malignant tumours and, occasionally, high-grade tumours in which the facial nerve is not involved. It is contraindicated for tumours in which the nerve is involved.

The operation involves removal of the superficial and deep lobes of the gland, with preservation of the facial nerve. A superficial parotidectomy is first performed. The branches and main trunk of the facial nerve are dissected off the underlying deep lobe using small scissors to divide the fascial attachments of the nerve to the underlying gland. This manoeuvre is facilitated by lifting the branches with a nerve hook. The deep lobe is separated with scissors from the posterior border of the ascending ramus of the mandible and from the temporo-mandibular joint. The deep aspect of the gland is gently separated from its underlying bed with small scissors, which are introduced above and below the main trunk of the nerve. Any attachments of the gland to the styloid process are divided. The upper and lower ends of the retromandibular vein and any anterior branches are divided between ligatures. The more deeply placed external carotid artery may not have to be interrupted if it does not actually penetrate the gland but lies deep to it. However, it often perforates the deep lobe, and that portion may have to be excised with the specimen. If so, the artery is divided at the lower border of the gland above the posterior belly of digastric and stylohyoid muscles and superiorly where it becomes the superficial temporal artery. The internal maxillary and transverse facial branches of the external carotid artery are then also divided, enabling the deep lobe to be dissected off its bed in a downward direction. The wound is closed as described for superficial parotidectomy.

Radical parotidectomy

High-grade carcinoma of the parotid gland is the primary indication for radical parotidectomy. It is only occasionally indicated for recurrent pleomorphic adenoma when, for technical reasons, there is little chance of preserving the facial nerve.

Histological confirmation of malignancy is desirable prior to surgery and this may be performed pre-operatively with a Tru-cut biopsy.[117]

The patient is positioned as described for superficial parotidectomy. In some patients, radical parotidectomy may be accompanied by a radical or functional neck dissection to remove regional lymph nodes also involved by tumour. An incision similar to that described for superficial parotidectomy is performed. This may need to be extended inferiorly to accommodate a radical neck dissection. The following description applies to the parotid gland and does not take into account radical neck dissection in continuity. The posterior limits of the dissection are defined in the same way as for superficial parotidectomy, thus dissecting the posterior border free from the sternomastoid muscle to expose the posterior belly of the digastric muscle. The gland is freed superiorly from the mastoid process and external auditory meatus. The retromandibular vein is then ligated and divided at the tail of the parotid. The parotid gland is then elevated to reveal the posterior belly of the digastric and the stylohyoid muscles, and the external carotid artery is ligated and divided just before it enters the deep aspect of the gland above the stylohyoid muscle. The soft tissues at the tail of the parotid gland are further incised in a forward direction until the angle of the mandible is reached. Starting at the lower border of the mandible and dissecting upwards along a vertical line anterior to the parotid gland, the soft tissues overlying the ascending ramus are divided down to bone all the way up to the zygomatic arch. The structures divided during this dissection include subcutaneous fat, branches of the facial nerve, the transverse facial artery and veins, the parotid duct and the masseter muscle. The cut peripheral branches of the facial nerve may be tagged with a suture for ease of identification if a nerve graft is contemplated.

A periosteal elevator is used to push the soft tissues of the specimen backwards to the posterior border of the ascending ramus of the mandible. The soft tissues overlying the zygomatic arch are incised down to the bone as far back as the pinna. Branches of the upper division of the facial nerve are divided during this step and may also be tagged with a suture. The superficial temporal artery and vein are divided at the point where they cross the arch. The incision is now carried inferiorly between the parotid gland and the cartilage of the external auditory meatus to join the earlier line of separation of the posterior border of the parotid gland.

By retracting the tail of the specimen superiorly, the gland is dissected away from its bed with scissors, starting from below and working upwards. It is separated from the posterior border of the mandible, from the styloid process, which lies deep to it, and from the anterior aspect of the bony external meatus, below which the facial nerve is divided as it emerges from the stylomastoid foramen. The specimen can now be retracted downwards and laterally sufficiently to expose the maxillary artery and veins so that they can be divided between ligatures or clamps. A nerve graft consisting of branches of the cervical plexus derived from a common stem can now be inserted between the divided trunk and branches of the facial nerve and sutured in place. The wound is closed as described for superficial parotidectomy.

Locally advanced tumours may require resection of adjacent tissues such as muscle, bone or overlying skin (extended radical parotidectomy), and this may necessitate soft tissue reconstruction such as a cervical cutaneous flap or pectoralis major, latissimus dorsi and trapezius flaps. A free flap such as the radial forearm flap provides a good cosmetic result.

POSTOPERATIVE COMPLICATIONS

Facial nerve injury

After superficial parotidectomy, permanent nerve injury occurs in only 1% of patients.[95] Transient nerve paresis occurs much more commonly, in 30–43%.[95,102] After total conservative parotidectomy, permanent and transient nerve paresis increase to 6% and 60% respectively,[97] and 90% of transient injuries recover within 12 months.[92] Clearly, more limited resection of the parotid gland is associated with a marked reduction of transient facial paresis to approximately 8%.[102]

Several techniques have been described to repair a divided facial nerve and consist of faciohypoglossal transposition, end-to-end anastomosis and cable graft anastomosis. The comparison of the results of such surgery has been facilitated by the development of facial function scoring systems such as the House–Brackmann scale.[124] Results of these techniques indicate an improvement in facial function in two-thirds of patients.[125]

Frey's syndrome

This consists of discomfort, sweating and occasionally redness of the skin overlying the parotid area, which occurs during and after eating. It is due to the severed ends of the parasympathetic secretomotor fibres growing into the skin; the fibres are then stimulated by eating, causing vasodilatation and sweating. It may occur in up to 60% of patients postoperatively, but only 20% of patients actually complain about it.[113] The frequency with which it occurs varies with the extent of resection of the parotid gland.[95,96] The condition usually resolves spontaneously but if persistent it may be treated by tympanic neurectomy, which divides the parasympathetic pathway. A variety of topical agents have been tried to alleviate these symptoms and a clinical trial using 1% glycopyrrolate roll-on lotion or cream has been found to be effective in controlling gustatory sweating for up to 3 days.[126] It is claimed that the incidence of clinical Frey's syndrome can be reduced to 3% with the use of a synthetic implant (expanded polytetrafluoroethylene) placed in the cavity after superficial parotidectomy.[127]

Salivary fistula

This is uncommon and due to the excessive production of saliva from the remaining deep lobe after superficial parotidectomy. In most patients it resolves spontaneously after a few weeks, but if it does persist, the deep lobe of the gland may be removed; an alternative to this is to irradiate the remaining parotid gland. The use of a fascial flap has been advocated to prevent this complication.[128]

Hypoaesthesia of the ear lobe

It is common for patients to experience some hypoaesthesia of the preauricular region and the lower half of the pinna due to division of the posterior branch of the great auricular nerve. This usually improves with time and does not require any specific treatment.

Neuroma

Occasionally a neuroma may arise from the cut end of the posterior branch of the great auricular nerve. This complication should be borne in mind before concluding that the swelling is a recurrence of a parotid tumour.

RADIOTHERAPY

A major proportion of parotid tumours are radiosensitive.[129] Postoperative radiotherapy has been recommended for all patients with malignant salivary tumours[106] but local recurrence is rare after complete excision of low-grade tumours, and radiotherapy is probably best reserved for those patients with high-grade tumours.[130] More recent studies indicate that not only does radiotherapy improve local control of malignant salivary gland tumours, it also improves -year survival.[131–135]

A review of the evidence for the use of postoperative radiotherapy has recently been published.[135]

Radiotherapy alone may achieve temporary local control in approximately 30% of patients and may produce a sufficient reduction in tumour bulk to facilitate subsequent excision.[136,137]

THE SUBMANDIBULAR GLAND

Diseases of the submandibular gland are less common than those of the parotid. Furthermore, the pattern of disease is slightly different, with stones in the gland or its duct being more common than tumours, which are also less diverse in their histological features. The submandibular gland may be affected by the same infections and autoimmune diseases as the parotid, and these will not be described again.

Embryology

The submandibular gland develops as an epithelial outgrowth from the floor of the alveololingual groove. It increases rapidly in size by giving off numerous branching processes, which later acquire lumina. At first, the connection of the submandibular outgrowth with the floor of the mouth lies at the side of the tongue, but the edges of the groove in which it opens come together from behind forwards and form the tubular part of the submandibular duct. As a result, the orifice of the duct is shifted forwards until it comes to lie below the tip of the tongue, close to the median plane. The submandibular gland becomes encapsulated before the emergence of the lymphatic system in the mesoderm, and this explains why the spectrum of benign tumours differs from that of the parotid.[2]

Anatomy

The submandibular gland is the second largest salivary gland, being about half the weight of the parotid. It occupies most of the submandibular triangle of the neck and is folded around the dorsal free edge of the mylohyoid muscle. Although there are no separate lobes to the gland, by convention it is often described as having a superficial and deep lobe. The larger superficial lobe lies in the submandibular triangle, superficial and caudal to the mylohyoid. It lies deep to the skin and platysma and is crossed superficially by the cervical branch of the facial nerve. This is extremely important to know as the nerve may be damaged by an incision placed too high in the neck when excision of the gland is to be performed. The smaller, deep lobe lies between the mylohyoid and hyoglossus muscles. The duct (Wharton's duct) arises from this deep portion and passes forwards adjacent to the sublingual gland to the papilla in the floor of the mouth to the side of the frenulum of the tongue. Posteriorly, the gland is grooved by the facial artery. The lingual nerve lies on the hyoglossus above the gland but crosses the duct first on its outer (mandibular) aspect and then recrosses it on its deeper (lingual) aspect. The hypoglossal nerve lies between the gland and the hyoglossus and then runs forwards, inferior to the duct. In front of the hyoglossus, the nerve passes deep to the duct to reach the muscles of the tongue. The digastric and stylohyoid muscles lie inferior to the more superficial part of the gland.

The arteries supplying the submandibular gland are branches of the facial and lingual arteries, and the venous drainage follows that of the arteries. The nerves are derived from the submandibular ganglion, through which the gland receives parasympathetic fibres from the chorda tympani branch of the facial nerve, the lingual branch of the mandibular nerve and sympathetic fibres. Lymphatic drainage is to the submandibular and upper deep cervical lymph nodes.

The submandibular gland is a mixed serous and mucous gland, with about 10% of the acini being mucinous. By contrast with the parotid, adipose tissue is not a prominent component of the glandular parenchyma.

Physiology

The submandibular glands contribute approximately 45% of the total volume of saliva. As with the parotid gland, control of secretion is by the autonomic nervous system.[138]

Developmental abnormalities

Atresia of one or more major salivary gland ducts – usually the submandibular or sublingual glands – is rare and is associated with xerostomia and possibly the development of a retention cyst.[6,8]

Investigation of the submandibular gland

CLINICAL EVALUATION

Most lesions of the submandibular gland are due to obstructive stone disease and only occasionally due to tumour. The gland should be palpated bimanually and any degree of fixity noted. Stones may be palpated in the gland itself or in Wharton's duct on the floor of the mouth, and the duct orifice should be inspected. Cervical lymphadenopathy should be noted and all other salivary glands should be inspected to determine whether the submandibular enlargement is part of a generalised disease.

The diagnosis of a submandibular mass is usually obvious but may easily be mistaken for an enlarged submandibular lymph node mass.

RADIOLOGY

The indications for radiological investigation of the submandibular gland are similar to those of the parotid.[42] Submandibular stones are nearly always radio-opaque and therefore plain films are much more useful. Sialography (**Fig. 8.7**) is also more informative and is especially helpful in locating the position of a stone within the duct system. This enables a decision to be made as to whether a stone

Figure 8.7 • Sialogram of the submandibular gland showing calculus obstruction.

can be removed from a duct via the floor of the mouth or whether submandibular gland excision is more appropriate. The indications for ultrasonography, CT and MRI are similar to those for the parotid gland.[42]

FNAC

The major problem in evaluating the submandibular region has been in distinguishing between chronic sialadenitis and squamous cell carcinoma.[25] FNAC is valuable, however, in distinguishing metastatic carcinoma from squamous carcinoma of the oral cavity. Primary salivary gland tumours in the submandibular region pose similar diagnostic problems to those in the parotid region, and these have been described above. Lymphoma and tuberculosis are quite common in the submandibular lymph nodes, and FNAC is useful in making a diagnosis. The diagnosis of other benign conditions such as lipoma or neurofibroma are difficult on FNAC. Diagnostic accuracy of submandibular masses is similar to that of parotid masses.[25]

SIALOMETRY

Wharton's duct can be cannulated to assess submandibular gland output and composition, and this may be helpful in confirming a hyposecretory state.

SIALOENDOSCOPY

This is identical to that described for the parotid gland.[39,40]

INFECTIONS

Bacterial and viral infections are much less common than in the parotid gland. Even primary tuberculosis of a salivary gland seems to occur less frequently in the submandibular gland compared with the parotid (27% vs. 70%).[49] The principles of diagnosis and treatment are the same as those outlined for the parotid gland.

AUTOIMMUNE DISEASES

The submandibular glands are commonly involved in Sjögren's syndrome, and the principles in diagnosis and treatment are the same as for parotid gland involvement.

OBSTRUCTIVE SUBMANDIBULAR GLAND DISEASE

Stricture of Wharton's duct

This may occur due to repeated infection, trauma due to stones or iatrogenic injury, congenital abnormalities or compression by a tumour. Treatment options are similar to those for Stensen's duct.

Sialolithiasis

The most common sites for a salivary gland calculus are within the submandibular gland or its duct. Calculi are almost 50 times more common in the submandibular gland than in the parotid[43] because the saliva is more mucinous. Other predisposing causes are the same as for the parotid gland.

The clinical features are of recurrent painful swelling of the gland before or during meals. To reproduce the swelling at the time of examination, the patient can be given some fruit juice to sip. The orifices of Wharton's duct are then examined and compared. Saliva will be seen issuing from the unaffected side but not from the side of the swollen gland. If the stone is in Wharton's duct, it can often be palpated in the floor of the mouth. The diagnosis may be confirmed by sialography.

If the stone lies in the duct, it can be removed from the floor of the mouth. If the stone is in the hilum of the gland or is associated with other stones in the gland itself, excision of the gland is curative. Recent technological advances have allowed the introduction of sialoendoscopy and intracorporeal shockwave lithotripsy and extracorporeal shockwave lithotripsy as described for the parotid gland.[59,60]

TUMOURS OF THE SUBMANDIBULAR GLAND

Classification and staging

Submandibular gland tumours are classified as illustrated in **Table 8.2**, and according to the TNM classification as used for parotid tumours (**Box 8.2**). It should be emphasised that tumours of the submandibular gland are extremely uncommon. They comprise 4–8% of all salivary tumours; also, 57–66% of all submandibular neoplasms are benign.[93,106,107] The commonest tumour is a pleomorphic adenoma. Diagnosis is confirmed by FNAC. Imaging of the gland with ultrasonography and MRI may be useful if malignancy is suspected due to local fixity, especially to the mandible.

Treatment

Benign tumours are adequately treated by complete excision of the gland. Malignant tumours should be staged appropriately. Surgery may involve simple excision of the gland if this is sufficient to obtain clear margins. However, fixity to surrounding structures or involved lymph nodes requires a radical excision, radical neck dissection and reconstruction. Early involvement with a reconstructive surgeon and oncologist is mandatory. Radiotherapy is recommended postoperatively in most patients with malignant disease and in those undergoing surgery for recurrent pleomorphic adenoma.[106] It seems that survival is related to the histological type of the cancer and the stage at presentation and is similar to that quoted for parotid cancers.

Surgery of the submandibular gland

REMOVAL OF DUCT CALCULUS

This may be performed under general or local anaesthesia if the stone is near the duct orifice. The tissues immediately behind the stone are grasped with tissue forceps, which steadies the stone, elevates it and prevents inadvertent dislocation proximally down the duct. An incision in the floor of the mouth is made on to the stone in the long axis of the duct and the stone retrieved. Haemostasis is achieved if necessary and the wound left unsutured.

EXCISION OF THE SUBMANDIBULAR GLAND

The most common indication for excision of the submandibular gland is recurrent swelling and pain due to stones in the gland or in the proximal portion of Wharton's duct. Other indications are after acute phlegmonous sialadenitis and recurrent sialectasis. Neoplasia is an absolute indication for excision and may need to be combined with a radical neck dissection for malignant disease.

The patient is positioned in the supine position, with a small sandbag under the shoulders and the head turned in the opposite direction. A horizontal skin incision is made well below the mandible, preferably in a skin crease just above the hyoid bone to avoid the lowest branch of the facial nerve. The incision should overlap the sternomastoid posteriorly and extend to just beyond the limit of the gland anteriorly. The incision is deepened through the fat and platysma to the level of the deep cervical fascia, which is then incised along the anterior border of the sternomastoid and horizontally above the hyoid bone to expose the fascial condensation around the gland. This is incised horizontally at the lower border of the gland.

The upper flap, consisting of skin, subcutaneous fat, platysma, deep cervical fascia and the fascial capsule superficial to the gland, is now elevated by sharp dissection. The dissection proceeds from below upwards and the tissues are retracted. The common facial or anterior facial vein is divided between ligatures, and the lower border of the gland is grasped by suitable traction forceps and lifted up. This reveals the common tendon of the digastric muscle and the hyoglossus muscle. The gland is separated from the muscular floor of the submandibular triangle using sharp dissection, and the hypoglossal nerve with its venae comitantes is identified on the hyoglossus muscle. The anterior segment of the gland is released from the mylohyoid muscle. Traction on the gland is applied forwards and upwards, and the stylohyoid and posterior belly of the digastric is retracted downwards and backwards. The facial artery is identified as it emerges from its position deep between these muscles and divided proximal to the gland between strong ligatures, freeing the gland posteriorly.

The gland is retracted downwards and its superior fascial attachments to the mandible divided. This exposes the facial artery and anterior facial vein, which are divided between ligatures as close to the gland as possible to avoid the mandibular branch of the facial nerve. A blunt retractor is inserted deep to the posterior free border of the mylohyoid, exposing the deep part of the gland. Traction on the gland drags down the lingual nerve, which should be separated from the gland. Traction in a downward and lateral direction exposes the duct, which is ligated and divided. Haemostasis is secured and the wound closed by suturing the platysma and skin. A suction drain may be employed if desired but is often unnecessary.

POSTOPERATIVE COMPLICATIONS

Paralysis of the depressor anguli oris due to damage of the mandibular branch of the facial nerve is the commonest complication. Hypoglossal nerve palsy leads to deviation of the tongue to the affected side and eventually fasciculation and wasting. It is uncommon and requires no action in a unilateral palsy. Lingual nerve damage is very uncommon and results in paraesthesiae or loss of taste in the homolateral half of the tongue. Should this be troublesome, division of the lingual nerve relieves the symptoms but results in loss of taste.

• **Key points**

- A wide range of investigational techniques is now available for the evaluation of the salivary glands. The biggest recent technological advance has been the development of the sialoendoscope.
- The vast majority of patients with infective and inflammatory conditions do not require surgery.
- Recent advances have been made in our understanding of the molecular mechanisms related to the development of malignant neoplasms. Of special importance is the finding that a (small) proportion of malignant tumours express the HER2/Neu protein. This may have important therapeutic implications as it already has in the treatment of patients with breast cancer whose tumours also express this protein.

REFERENCES

1. Langman J. Medical embryology. Baltimore: Williams and Wilkins, 1963; pp. 195–211.

2. Sperber GH. Craniofacial embryology, 4th edn. London: Wright, 1989; pp. 188–91.

3. Batsakis JG. Tumours of the head and neck: clinical and pathological considerations, 2nd edn. Baltimore: Williams and Wilkins, 1979.

4. Davis RA, Anson BJ, Budinger JM et al. Surgical anatomy of the facial nerve and parotid gland based upon a study of 350 cervico-facial halves. Surg Gynecol Obstet 1956; 102:385–412.

   Large postmortem study.

5. Snyderman NL, Suen JY. Neoplasms. In: Cummings CW, Schuller DE (eds) Otolaryngology – head and neck surgery, vol. 2. St Louis: Mosby Year Book, 1986; pp. 1027–69.

6. Johns ME. The salivary glands: anatomy and embryology. Otolaryngol Clin North Am 1977; 10:261–71.

7. Kelly BA, Black MJM, Soames JV. Unilateral enlargement of the parotid gland in a patient with sialosis and contralateral parotid aplasia. Br J Oral Maxillofac Surg 1990; 28:409–12.

8. Mason DK, Chisholm DM. Salivary glands in health and disease. London: WB Saunders, 1975; pp. 37–69.

9. Hobsley M. Salivary tumours. Br J Hosp Med 1973; 10:555–62.

10. Phillps DE, Jones AS. Reliability of clinical examination in the diagnosis of parotid tumours. J R Coll Surg Edinb 1994; 39:100–2.

11. Yousem DM. Head and neck imaging. Radiol Clin North Am 1998; 36:941–66.

12. Bryan RN, Miller RH, Ferreyro RI et al. Computed tomography of the salivary glands. Am J Roentgenol 1982; 139:547–54.

13. Parker GD, Harnsberger HR. Clinical-radiologic issues in perineural tumour spread of malignant diseases of the extra-cranial head and neck. Radiographics 1991; 11:383–99.

14. Chaudhuri R, Bingham JB, Crossman JE et al. Magnetic resonance imaging of the parotid gland using the STIR sequence. Clin Otolaryngol 1992; 17:211–17.

15. McGhee RB Jr, Chakeres DW, Schmalkbrock P et al. The extra-cranial facial nerve: high resolution three-dimensional Fourier transform MR imaging. Am J Neuroradiol 1992; 14:465–72.

16. Kalinowski M, Heverhagen JT, Rehberg K et al. Comparative study of MR sialography and digital subtraction sialography for benign salivary gland disorders. Am J Neuroradiol 2002; 23:1485–92.

17. Ahuja A, Ying M, Yang WT et al. The use of sonography in differentiating cervical lymphomatous lymph nodes from cervical metastatic lymph nodes. Clin Radiol 1996; 51:186–90.

18. Diederich S, Roos N, Bick U et al. Diagnostic imaging of the salivary glands in children and adolescents. Radiologie 1991; 31:550–7.

19. Kawamura H, Taniguchi N, Itoh K et al. Salivary gland echography in patients with Sjögren's syndrome. Arthritis Rheum 1990; 33:505–10.

20. Mann W, Wachter W. Ultrasonic diagnosis of the salivary glands. Laryngorhinootologie 1988; 67:355–61.

21. Brandwein MS, Huvos AG. Oncocytic tumours of major salivary glands: a study of 68 cases with follow-up of 44 patients. Am J Surg Pathol 1991; 15:514–28.

22. Cogan MI, Gill PS. Value of sialography and scintigraphy in diagnosis of salivary gland disorders. Int J Oral Surg 1981; 10:216–22.

23. Vogl TJ, Dadashi A, Jassoy A et al. The 31-phosphorus spectroscopy of space occupying lesion of the salivary glands. The clinical results and differential diagnosis. Rofo Fortschr Geb Rontgenstr Neuen Bildgeb Verfahr 1993; 158:31–8.

24. McGurk M, Hussain K. Role of fine needle aspiration cytology in the management of the discrete parotid lump. Ann R Coll Surg Engl 1997; 79:198–202.

25. Shaha A, Webber C, DiMaio T et al. Needle aspiration biopsy in salivary gland lesions. Am J Surg 1990; 160:373–6.

26. Rodriguez HP, Silver CE, Moisa II et al. Fine needle aspiration of parotid tumours. Am J Surg 1989; 158:342–3.

27. Lewis DR, Webb AJ, Lott MF et al. Improving cytological diagnosis and surgical management of parotid adenolymphoma. Br J Surg 1999; 86:1275–9.

28. Pitts DB, Hilsinger RL, Karandy E et al. Fine needle aspiration in the diagnosis of salivary gland disorders in the community hospital setting. Arch Otolaryngol Head Neck Surg 1992; 118:479–82.

29. Gerstner A, Mueller AK, Machlitt J et al. Slide based cytometry for predicting malignancy in solid salivary gland tumours by fine needle aspirate biopsies. Cytometry 2003; 53B:20–5.

30. Eneroth CM, Franzen S, Zajicek J. Cytologic diagnosis on aspirate from 1000 salivary gland tumours. Acta Otolaryngol 1967; 1:168–71.

31. Layfield LJ, Tan P, Glasgow BJ. Fine-needle aspiration of salivary gland lesions. Comparison with frozen sections and histologic findings. Arch Pathol Lab Med 1987; 111:346–53.

32. Lindberg LG, Akerman M. Aspiration cytology of salivary gland tumours: diagnostic experience from six years of routine laboratory work. Laryngoscope 1976; 86:584–94.

33. O'Dwyer P, Farrar WB, James AG et al. Needle aspiration biopsy of major salivary gland tumours. Its value. Cancer 1986; 57:554–7.

34. Persson PS, Zettergren L. Cytological diagnosis of salivary gland tumours by aspiration biopsy. Acta Cytol 1973; 17:351–4.

35. Qizilbash AH, Sianos J, Young JE et al. Fine needle aspiration biopsy cytology of major salivary glands. Acta Cytol 1985; 29:503–12.

Refs 30–35 include large numbers of patients with histopathological correlation.

36. Filopoulos E, Angeli S, Daskalopoulou D et al. Preoperative evaluation of parotid tumours by fine needle biopsy. Eur J Surg Oncol 1998; 24:180–3.

37. Orell SR, Nettle WJS. Fine needle aspiration biopsy of salivary gland tumours. Problems and pitfalls. Pathology 1988; 20:332–7.

38. Wolff A, Herscovici D, Rosenberg M. A simple technique for the determination of salivary gland hypofunction. Oral Surg Oral Med Oral Pathol Oral Radiol Endod 2002; 94:175–8.

39. Nahleili O, Baruchin AM. Long term experience with endoscopic diagnosis and treatment of salivary gland inflammatory diseases. Laryngoscope 2000; 110:988–93.

40. Arzoz E, Nahleili O. Salivary gland endoscopy. In: McGurk M, Renehan A (eds) Controversies in the management of salivary gland disease. Oxford: Oxford University Press, 2001; pp. 271–83.

41. Miglets AW. Infections, Part III. Clinical entities. In: Cummings CW, Fredrickson JM, Harker LA (eds) Otolaryngology – head and neck surgery, vol. 2. St Louis: Mosby Year Book, 1986; pp. 999–1006.

42. Yousem DM. The radiologic clinics of North America; head and neck imaging, vol. 36. Philadelphia: WB Saunders, 1998; pp. 949–50.

43. Harding Rains AJ, Ritchie HD (eds). Bailey and Love's short practice of surgery, 16th edn. London: HK Lewis, 1975; pp. 537–8.

44. Moss-Salentijn L, Moss L. Development and functional anatomy. In: Rankow RM, Polayes IM (eds) Diseases of the salivary glands. Philadelphia: WB Saunders, 1976; pp. 17–31.

45. Al-Deeb SM. Herpes simplex encephalitis mimicking mumps. Clin Neurol Neurosurg 1993; 95:49–53.

46. Chapnick JS, Noyek AM, Berris B et al. Parotid gland enlargement in HIV infection: clinical/imaging findings. J Otolaryngol 1990; 19:189–94.

47. Navazesh M, Mulligan R, Barron Y et al. A 4-year longitudinal evaluation of xerostomia and salivary gland hypofunction in the Women's Interagency HIV Study participants. Oral Surg Oral Med Oral Pathol Oral Radiol Endod 2003; 95:1079–2104.

48. Mulligan R, Navazesh M, Komaroff E et al. Salivary gland disease in human immunodeficiency virus-positive women from the WIHS study. Oral Surg Oral Med Oral Pathol Oral Radiol Endod 2000; 89:702–9.

49. Rabinov K, Weber AL. Radiology of the salivary glands. Boston: G Hall, 1985; pp. 153–66.

50. Marx RE, Hartman KS, Rethman KV. A prospective study comparing incisional labial to incisional parotid biopsies in the detection and confirmation of sarcoidosis, Sjogren's disease, sialosis and lymphoma. J Rheumatol 1988; 15:621–9.

Although not a randomised study, it does confirm this technique in the diagnosis of Sjögren's disease.

51. Work WP, Hecht DW. Inflammatory diseases of the major salivary glands. In: Paparella MM, Shumrick DA (eds) Otolaryngology, vol. 3. Philadelphia: WB Saunders, 1973; pp. 258–65.

52. Hudson NP. Manifestations of systemic disease. In: Cummings CW, Fredrickson JM, Harker LA et al. (eds) Head and neck surgery, vol. 2. St Louis: Mosby Year Book, 1986; pp. 1007–13.

53. Bloch KJ. Sjogren's syndrome. In: Stein JH (ed.) Internal medicine. Boston: Little Brown, 1983; pp. 1034–6.

54. Daniels TE, Fox PC. Salivary and oral components of Sjogren's syndrome. In: Fox RI (ed.) Rheumatic disease clinics of North America, vol. 18. Philadelphia: WB Saunders, 1992; pp. 571–89.

55. Fox RI, Carstens SA, Fong S et al. Use of monoclonal antibodies to analyse peripheral blood and salivary gland lymphocyte subsets in Sjögren's syndrome. Arthritis Rheum 1982; 25:419–26.

56. Drosos AA, Skopouli FN, Costopoulos JS et al. Cyclosporin A (CyA) in primary Sjögren's syndrome: a double blind study. Ann Rheum Dis 1986; 45:732–5.

57. Vasil'ev VI, Simonova MV, Safonova TN et al. [Comparative evaluation of the treatment of Sjögren's syndrome with anti-rheumatic preparations.] Ter Arkh 1988; 60:67–72.

58. Izumi M, Eguchi K, Nakamura H et al. Corticosteroid irrigation of parotid gland for treatment of xerostomia in patients with Sjögren's syndrome. Ann Rheum Dis 1998; 57:464–9.

59. Reimers M, Vavrina J, Schlegel C. Results after shock wave lithotripsy for salivary gland stones. Schweiz Med Wochenschr 2000; (suppl.) 125:122S–126S.

60. Escudier M, Katz P, Capaccio P. Extracorporeal lithotripsy for salivary calculi: results and future roles. In: McGurk M, Renehan A (eds) Controversies in the management of salivary gland disease. Oxford: Oxford University Press, 2001; pp. 257–69.

Good example of the prospective evaluation and audit of a new surgical technique.

61. Thackray AC. Sialectasis. Arch Middlesex Hosp 1955; 5:151.

62. Santonja C, Garcia-Aroca J, Colomar PJ. Castleman's disease and lymphoepithelial cysts of the parotid in childhood. Histopathol 1997; 30:369–72.

63. Thackray AC, Sobin LH. In: Thackray AC, Sobin LH (eds) Histological typing of salivary tumours. Geneva: World Health Organisation, 1972; pp. 16–25.

64. Hermanek P, Sobin LH. TNM classification of malignant tumours. Berlin: Springer-Verlag, 1987; pp. 30–2.

65. Saku T, Hayashi Y, Takahara O et al. Salivary gland tumours among atomic bomb survivors, 1950–1987. Cancer 1997; 79:1465–75.

66. Katz AD, Preston Martin S. Salivary gland tumours and previous radiotherapy to the head or neck. Am J Surg 1984; 147:345–8.

67. Hoffman DA, McConahey WM, Fraumeni JF Jr et al. Cancer incidence following treatment of hyperthyroidism. Int J Epidemiol 1982; 11:218–24.

68. Atula T, Grenman R, Klemi P et al. Human papilloma virus, Epstein–Barr virus, human herpesvirus 8 and human cytomegalovirus involvement in salivary gland tumours. Oral Oncol 1998; 34:391–5.

69. Sheen TS, Tsai CC, Ko JY et al. Undifferentiated carcinoma of the major salivary glands. Cancer 1997; 80:357–63.

70. Kuo T, Hsueh C. Lymphoepithelioma-like salivary gland carcinoma in Taiwan: a clinicopathological study of nine cases demonstrating a strong association with Epstein–Barr virus. Histopathology 1997; 31:75–82.

71. Voz ML, Astrom AK, Kas K et al. The recurrent translocation t(5;8) (p13;q12) in pleomorphic adenomas results in upregulation of PLAG 1 gene expression under control of the LIFR promoter. Oncogene 1998; 16:1409–16.

72. Kas K, Voz ML, Roijer E et al. Promoter swapping between the genes for a novel zinc finger protein and beta-catenin in pleomorphic adenomas with t(3;8) (p21;q12) translocation. Nat Genet 1997; 15:170–4.

73. El Naggar AK, Hurr K, Kagan J et al. Genotypic alterations in benign and malignant salivary gland tumours: histogenetic and clinical implications. Am J Surg Pathol 1997; 21:691–7.

74. Nordkvist A, Gustaffson H, Juberg Ode M et al. Recurrent rearrangements of 11q 14-22 in mucoepidermoid carcinoma. Cancer Genet Cytogenet 1994; 74:77–83.

75. Gallo O, Bani D, Toccafondi G et al. Characterization of a novel cell line from pleomorphic adenoma of the parotid gland with myoepithelial phenotype and producing interleukin-6 as an autocrine growth factor. Cancer 1992; 70:559–68.

76. Gandour Edwards R, Kapadia SB, Gunnerlock PH et al. Immunolocalization of interleukin-6 in salivary gland tumours. Hum Pathol 1995; 26:501–3.

77. Li X, Tsuji T, Wen S et al. A fluorescence in situ hybridization (FISH) analysis with centromere-specific DNA probes of chromosomes 3 and 17 in pleomorphic adenomas and adenoid cystic carcinomas. J Oral Pathol Med 1995; 24:398–401.

78. Johns MM 3rd, Westra WH, Califano JA et al. Allelotype of salivary gland tumours. Cancer Res 1996; 56:1151–4.

79. Kishi M, Nakamura M, Nishimine M et al. Loss of heterozygosity on chromosome 6q correlates with decreased thrombospondin-2 expression in human salivary gland carcinomas. Cancer Sci 2003; 94:530–5.

80. Gallo O, Bianchi S, Giovannucci Uzzielli ML et al. p53 oncoprotein overexpression correlates with mutagen-induced chromosome fragility in head and neck cancer patients with multiple malignancies. Br J Cancer 1995; 71:1008–12.

81. Gallo O, Franchi A, Bianchi S et al. p53 oncoprotein expression in parotid gland carcinomas is associated with clinical outcome. Cancer 1995; 75:2037–44.

82. Kamio N. Coexpression of p53 and c-erbB2 proteins is associated with histological type, tumour stage and cell proliferation in malignant salivary gland tumours. Virchow's Arch 1996; 428:75–83.

83. Pignataro L, Capaccio P, Carboni N et al. P53 and cyclin X D1 protein expression in carcinomas of the parotid gland. Anticancer Res 1998; 18:1287–90.

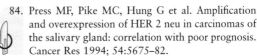

84. Press MF, Pike MC, Hung G et al. Amplification and overexpression of HER 2 neu in carcinomas of the salivary gland: correlation with poor prognosis. Cancer Res 1994; 54:5675–82.

This observation may prove to be therapeutically important.

85. Sugano S, Mukai K, Tsuda H et al. Immuno-histochemical study of c-erbB2 oncoprotein over-expression in human major salivary gland carcinoma: an indicator of aggressiveness. Laryngoscope 1992; 102:923–7.

This may be prognostically important.

86. Dori S, Vered M, David R et al. HER2/neu expression in adenoid cystic carcinoma of salivary gland origin: an immunohistochemical study. J Oral Pathol 2002; 31:463–7.

87. Birek C, Lui E, Dardick I. C-fos oncogene under-expression in salivary gland tumours as measured

by in situ hybridization. Am J Pathol 1993; 142:917–23.

88. Jeng YM, Lim CY, Hsu HC. Expression of the c-kit protein is associated with certain subtypes of salivary gland carcinoma. Cancer Lett 2000; 154:107–11.

89. Vered M, Braunstein E, Buchner A. Immuno-histochemical study of epidermal growth factor receptor in adenoid cystic carcinoma of salivary gland origin. Head Neck 2002; 24:632–6.

90. Sakurai K, Urade M, Noguchi K et al. Increased expression of cyclooxygenase-2 in human salivary gland tumours. Pathol Int 2001; 51:762–9.

91. Aigner T, Neureiter D, Völker U et al. Epithelial-mesenchymal transdifferentiation and extracellular matrix gene expression in pleomorphic adenomas of the parotid salivary gland. J Pathol 1998; 186:178–85.

92. McGurk M. Parotid pleomorphic adenoma. Br J Surg 1997; 84:1491–2.

93. Renehan A, Gleave FN, Hancock BD et al. Long-term follow-up of over 1000 patients with salivary gland tumours treated in a single centre. Br J Surg 1996; 83:1750–4.

Includes a large series of patients.

94. Patey DH, Thackray AC. The treatment of parotid tumours in the light of pathological study of parotid-ectomy material. Br J Surg 1957; 45:477–87.

95. McGurk M, Renehan A, Gleave EN et al. Clinical significance of the tumour capsule in the treatment of parotid pleomorphic adenomas. Br J Surg 1996; 83:1747–9.

96. Leverstein H, van der Wal JE, Tiwari RM et al. Surgical management of 246 previously untreated pleomorphic adenomas of the parotid gland. Br J Surg 1997; 84:399–403.

97. Renehan A, Gleave EN, McGurk M. An analysis of the treatment of 114 patients with recurrent pleomorphic adenomas of the parotid gland. Am J Surg 1996; 172:710–14.

A large series of a relatively uncommon event.

98. Stevens KL, Hobsley M. The treatment of pleo-morphic adenomas by formal parotidectomy. Br J Surg 1982; 69:1–3.

99. Buchanan C, Stringer SP, Mendenhall WM et al. Pleomorphic adenoma: effect of tumour spill and inadequate resection on tumour recurrence. Laryngoscope 1994; 104:1231–4.

100. Warthin AS. Papillary cystadenoma lymphomatosum. A rare teratoid of the parotid region. J Cancer Res 1929; 13:116–25.

101. Kennedy TL. Warthin's tumour: a review indicating no male predominance. Laryngoscope 1983; 93:889–91.

102. Ebbs SR, Webb AJ. Adenolymphoma of the parotid: aetiology, diagnosis and treatment. Br J Surg 1986; 73:627–30.

A good study confirming previous suspicions of an association of smoking with adenolymphoma of the parotid gland.

103. Cadier M, Watkin G, Hobsley M. Smoking pre-disposes to parotid adenolymphoma. Br J Surg 1992; 79:929–30.

104. Allegra SR. Warthin's tumour: a hypersensitivity disease? Hum Pathol 1971; 2:403–20.

105. Heller KS, Attie JN. Treatment of Warthin's tumour by enucleation. Am J Surg 1988; 156:294–6.

106. Gleave EN, Whittaker JS, Nicholson A. Salivary tumours – experience over thirty years. Clin Otolaryngol 1979; 4:247–57.

107. Spiro RH. Salivary neoplasms: overview of a 35-year experience with 2807 patients. Head Neck Surg 1986; 8:177–84.

108. Guzzo M, Andreola S, Sirizzotti G et al. Mucoepidermoid carcinoma of the salivary glands: clinicopathological review of 108 patients treated at the National Cancer Institute of Milan. Ann Surg Oncol 2002; 9:688–95.

109. Spiro RH, Huvos AG, Strong EW. Adenoid cystic carcinoma: factors influencing survival. Am J Surg 1979; 138: 579–83.

110. Spiro RH, Huvos AG, Strong EW. Cancer of the parotid gland. Clinicopathological study of 288 primary cases. Am J Surg 1975; 130:452–9.

Refs 106–110 include large numbers of patients with long follow-up.

111. Spiro RH, Huvos AG. Stage means more than grade in adenoid cystic carcinoma. Am J Surg 1992; 164:623–8.

112. Perzin KH, Gullane PJ, Clairmont AA. Adenoid cystic carcinoma arising in salivary glands: a cor-relation of histological features and clinical course. Cancer 1978; 42:265–82.

Another large study that usefully stimulated debate.

113. Maran AGD. The salivary glands. In: Cuschieri A, Giles GR, Moosa AR (eds) Essential surgical practice, 3rd edn. Oxford: Butterworth-Heinemann, 1995; pp. 5991–6000.

114. Balm AJM, Delaere P, Hilgers FJM et al. Primary lymphoma of mucosa associated lymphoid tissue (MALT) in the parotid gland. Clin Otolaryngol 1993; 18:528–32.

115. Helmus C. Subtotal parotidectomy: a 10-year review (1985–1994). Laryngoscope 1997; 107:1024–7.

116. Watkin GT, Hobsley M. Influence of local surgery and radiotherapy on the natural history of pleo-morphic adenomas. Br J Surg 1986; 73:74–6.

Although a useful study with some evidence, it lacks the power of a randomised controlled trial.

117. Ball ABS, Thomas JM. Salivary glands. In: Allen-Mersh TG (ed.) Surgical oncology. London: Chapman & Hall Medical, 1996; pp. 93–9.

118. Rosenfeld S, Sessions DG, McSwain B et al. Malignant tumours of salivary gland origin: a review of 184 cases. Ann Surg 1966; 163:726–35.

119. Stennert E, Kisner D, Jungehuelsing M et al. High incidence of lymph node metastases in salivary gland cancer. Arch Otolaryngol Head Neck Surg 2003; 129:720–3.

120. Korkmaz H, Yoo GH, Du W et al. Predictors of nodal metastases in salivary gland cancer. J Surg Oncol 2002; 80:186–9.

Useful study that highlights factors to be considered when planning treatment.

121. Ball ABS, Rajagopal G, Thomas JM. Malignant epithelial parotid tumours. Ann R Coll Surg Engl 1990; 72:247–9.

122. Yamashita T, Tomoda K, Kumazawa T. The usefulness of partial parotidectomy for benign parotid gland tumours. Acta Otolaryngol 1993; (suppl.) 500: 113–16.

This study confirms the utility of a more conservative surgical approach to the management of benign tumours.

123. Chan S, Gunn A. Conservative parotidectomy by the peripheral approach. Br J Surg 1981; 68:405–7.

124. House JW. Facial nerve grading systems. Laryngoscope 1983; 93:1056–9.

125. Saeed SR, Ramsden RT. Rehabilitation of the paralysed face: results of facial nerve surgery. J Laryngol Otol 1996; 110:922–5.

126. Hays LL, Novack AJ, Worsham JC. The Frey syndrome: a simple effective treatment. Otolaryngol Head Neck Surg 1982; 90:419–25.

127. Dulguerov P, Quinodoz D, Cosendai G et al. Prevention of Frey syndrome during parotidectomy. Arch Otolaryngol Head Neck Surg 1999; 125:833–9.

128. Jianjun Y, Tong T, Wenzhu S et al. The use of a parotid fascia flap to prevent postoperative fistula. Oral Surg Oral Med Oral Pathol Oral Radiol Endod 1999; 87:673–5.

129. Borthne A, Kjellevold K, Kaalhus O et al. Salivary gland malignant neoplasms: treatment and prognosis. Int J Radiat Oncol Biol Phys 1986; 12:747–84.

130. Guillamondegui OM, Byers RM, Luna MA et al. Aggressive surgery in treatment for parotid cancer: the role of adjunctive postoperative radiotherapy. J Roentgenol Radium Ther Nucl Med 1975; 123:49–54.

131. North CA, Lee DJ, Piantadosi S et al. Carcinoma of the salivary glands treated by surgery or surgery plus postoperative radiotherapy. Int J Radiat Oncol Biol Phys 1990; 18:1319–26.

132. Armstrong JG, Harrison LB, Spiro RH et al. Malignant tumours of major salivary gland origin. A matched pair analysis of the role of combined surgery and postoperative radiotherapy. Arch Otolaryngol Head Neck Surg 1990; 116:290–3.

Refs 131 and 132 have highlighted the role of combined treatment modalities in achieving local control of malignant salivary gland tumours.

133. Douglas JG, Koh WJ, Austin-Seymour M et al. Treatment of salivary gland neoplasms with fast neutron radiotherapy. Arch Otolaryngol Head Neck Surg 2003; 129:944–8.

134. Simpson JR, Thawley SE, Matsuba HM. Adenoid cystic salivary gland carcinoma: treatment with irradiation and surgery. Radiology 1984; 151:509–12.

135. Slevin N, Frankenthaler R. The role of radiotherapy in the management of salivary gland cancer. In: McGurk M, Renehan A. Controversies in the management of salivary gland disease. Oxford: Oxford University Press, 2001; pp. 163–72.

136. Corcoran MO, Cook HP, Hobsley M. Radical surgery following radiotherapy for advanced parotid carcinomas. Br J Surg 1983; 70:261–3.

137. Gallegos NC, Watkin G, Cook HP et al. Further evaluation of radical surgery following radiotherapy for advanced parotid carcinoma. Br J Surg 1991; 78:97–100.

138. Wotson S, Mandel ID. The salivary secretions in health and disease. In: Rankow RM, Polayes IM (eds) Diseases of the salivary glands. Philadelphia: WB Saunders, 1976; pp. 32–53.

Index